Recent Advances in Hematology-?

Recent Advances in Hematology-3

Editors

Renu Saxena MD FIMSA
Professor and Head
Department of Hematology
All India Institute of Medical Sciences (AIIMS)
Ansari Nagar, New Delhi-110029, India

President
Indian Society of Hematology and Transfusion Medicine (2009-2010)
Delhi Society of Hematology (2005-2007)
Fellow International Medical Sciences Academy
Coordinator, ISHTM-AIIMS EQAP Program
Ex-Editor, Delhi Society of Hematology, Newsletter

HP Pati MD
Professor
Department of Hematology
All India Institute of Medical Sciences (AIIMS)
Ansari Nagar, New Delhi-110029, India
General Secretary, Indian Society of Hematology and Transfusion Medicine
Senior Specialist, Armed Forces Hospital, Kuwait

Manoranjan Mahapatra MD (Med) FICP FIACM
Associate Professor
Department of Hematology
All India Institute of Medical Sciences (AIIMS)
Ansari Nagar, New Delhi-110029, India
Fellow of Indian College of Physicians
Fellow of Indian Academy of Clinical Medicine
Fellow of Indian Society of Hematology and Transfusion Medicine

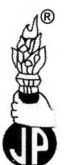

JAYPEE BROTHERS MEDICAL PUBLISHERS (P) LTD
New Delhi • St Louis (USA) • Panama City (Panama) • London (UK) • Ahmedabad
Bengaluru • Chennai • Hyderabad • Kochi • Kolkata • Lucknow • Mumbai • Nagpur

Published by
Jitendar P Vij

Jaypee Brothers Medical Publishers (P) Ltd

Corporate Office
4838/24 Ansari Road, Daryaganj, **New Delhi** - 110002, India,
Phone: +91-11-43574357, Fax: +91-11-43574314

Registered Office
B-3 EMCA House, 23/23B Ansari Road, Daryaganj, **New Delhi** - 110 002, India
Phones: +91-11-23272143, +91-11-23272703, +91-11-23282021
+91-11-23245672, Rel: +91-11-32558559, Fax: +91-11-23276490, +91-11-23245683
e-mail: jaypee@jaypeebrothers.com, Website: www.jaypeebrothers.com

Offices in India
- **Ahmedabad,** Phone: Rel: +91-79-32988717, e-mail: ahmedabad@jaypeebrothers.com
- **Bengaluru,** Phone: Rel: +91-80-32714073, e-mail: bangalore@jaypeebrothers.com
- **Chennai,** Phone: Rel: +91-44-32972089, e-mail: chennai@jaypeebrothers.com
- **Hyderabad,** Phone: Rel:+91-40-32940929, e-mail: hyderabad@jaypeebrothers.com
- **Kochi,** Phone: +91-484-2395740, e-mail: kochi@jaypeebrothers.com
- **Kolkata,** Phone: +91-33-22276415, e-mail: kolkata@jaypeebrothers.com
- **Lucknow,** Phone: +91-522-3040554, e-mail: lucknow@jaypeebrothers.com
- **Mumbai,** Phone: Rel: +91-22-32926896, e-mail: mumbai@jaypeebrothers.com
- **Nagpur,** Phone: Rel: +91-712-3245220, e-mail: nagpur@jaypeebrothers.com

Overseas Offices
- **North America Office, USA,** Ph: 001-636-6279734
  e-mail: jaypee@jaypeebrothers.com, anjulav@jaypeebrothers.com
- **Central America Office, Panama City, Panama,** Ph: 001-507-317-0160
  e-mail: cservice@jphmedical.com   Website: www.jphmedical.com
- **Europe Office, UK,** Ph: +44 (0) 2031708910, e-mail: info@jpmedpub.com

Recent Advances in Hematology-3

© 2011, Jaypee Brothers Medical Publishers (P) Ltd

All rights reserved. No part of this publication should be reproduced, stored in a retrieval system, or transmitted in any form or by any means: electronic, mechanical, photocopying, recording, or otherwise, without the prior written permission of the editors and the publisher.

> This book has been published in good faith that the material provided by contributors is original. Every effort is made to ensure accuracy of material, but the publisher, printer and editors will not be held responsible for any inadvertent error(s). In case of any dispute, all legal matters are to be settled under Delhi jurisdiction only.

First Edition: **2011**
ISBN 978-81-8448-888-3
Typeset at JPBMP typesetting unit
Printed at Sanat Printers, Kundli.

Contributors

Ajay Gogia MD
Department of Medical Oncology
All India Institute of Medical Sciences
Ansari Nagar, New Delhi-110029
India

Amit Upadhyay MD
Consultant
Sunflag Pahuja Center for Blood Disorders
Sunflag Hospital Sector 16A
Faridabad-121002
India

Arijit Biswas PhD
Institute of Hematology and Transfusion Medicine
Room No. 2.308
Sigmund Freud Street-25
Bonn, 53127
Germany

Ashok Kumar MD
Director and Head
Department of Rheumatology
Fortis Flt Lt Rajan Dhall Hospital
Vasant Kunj, New Delhi-110070
India

Deepak Dabkara MD
Department of Medical Oncology
All India Institute of Medical Sciences
Ansari Nagar, New Delhi-110029
India

Deepanjan Panda MD
Department of Medical Oncology
All India Institute of Medical Sciences
Ansari Nagar, New Delhi-110029
India

Gundu HR Rao PhD
Professor
Laboratory Medicine and Pathology
Lillehei Heart Institute, MMC 609
University of Minnesota
Minneapolis, MN 55455
USA

Hemant Gopal MD
Clinical Associate
Department of Rheumatology
Fortis Flt Lt Rajan Dhall Hospital
Vasant Kunj, New Delhi-110070
India

HP Pati MD
Professor
Department of Hematology
All India Institute of Medical Sciences (AIIMS)
Ansari Nagar, New Delhi-110029
India

Kanjaksha Ghosh MD MRCP MRCPI FRCPath FACP (USA) FICP FAMS FNASc
Director
National Institute of Immunohematology (ICMR)
13th Floor, NMS Bldg
KEM Hospital Campus
Parel, Mumbai-12
India

Kevin W Song MD FRCPC
Division of Hematology
Department of Medicine
Vancouver General Hospital
Hematology, 10th Floor, 2775 Laurel St Vancouver, British Columbia
Canada

Lalit Kumar MD
Department of Medical Oncology
All India Institute of Medical Sciences
Institute Rotary Cancer Hospital
Room 245, Ansari Nagar
New Delhi-110029
India

Manoranjan Mahapatra MD (Med) FICP FIACM
Associate Professor
Department of Hematology
All India Institute of Medical Sciences
Ansari Nagar, New Delhi-110029
India

Matthew D Seftel MBChB MPH MRCP FRCPC
Section of Hematology/Oncology
Department of Internal Medicine
University of Manitoba
Winnipeg, Manitoba
Canada

MB Agarwal MD
Department of Hematology
Bombay Hospital Institute of
Medical Sciences
Mumbai
India

Neelam Varma MD
Professor and Head
Departments of Internal Medicine and Hematology
Postgraduate Institute of Medical Education and Research (PGIMER)
Chandigarh
India

Neelam Marwaha MD FAMS FISHTM
Department of Transfusion Medicine
Postgraduate Institute of Medical Education and Research
Chandigarh
India

Niranjan Rathod MD
Seninor Resident (Academic)
Department of Hematology
All India Institute of Medical Sciences
Ansari Nagar, New Delhi-110029
India

Prashant Sharma MD DM
Senior Resident and DM Student
Hematology Department
All India Institute of Medical Sciences
Ansari Nagar, New Delhi-110029
India

Rajat Kumar MD (Med) DNB (Med) FRCP (London) FRCP (Edin) FRCPC
Professor
University of Manitoba
CancerCare Manitoba
675 McDermot Avenue, Winnipge
MB R3E 0V9
Canada

Ravi Ranjan PhD
Department of Hematology
All India Institute of Medical Sciences
Ansari Nagar, New Delhi-110029
India

Renu Saxena MD FIMSA
Professor and Head
Department of Hematology
All India Institute of Medical Sciences (AIIMS)
Ansari Nagar, New Delhi-110029
India

S Varma MD
Departments of Internal Medicine and Hematology
Postgraduate Institute of Medical Education and Research (PGIMER)
Chandigarh
India

Sanjeev Kumar Gupta MD DM
Department of Hematology
All India Institute of Medical Sciences
Ansari Nagar, New Delhi-110029
India

Seema Tyagi MD
Associate Professor
Department of Hematology
All India Institute of Medical Sciences
Ansari Nagar, New Delhi-110029
India

Shyam Rathi MD DM
Senior Resident (Academic)
Department of Hematology
All India Institute of Medical Sciences
Ansari Nagar, New Delhi-110029
India

Contributors

Suhail Akhter MSc
All India Institute of Medical Sciences
Room No 154, Department of
Hematology, 1st Floor, IRCH Building
AIIMS, Ansari Nagar
New Delhi-110029
India

Tulika Seth MD
Assistant Professor Hematology
All India Institute of Medical Sciences
Ansari Nagar, New Delhi-110029
India

Tuphan Kanti Dolai MD DM
Assistant Professor
Department of Hematology
NRS Medical College, Kolkata-14
India

VP Choudhry MD
Director
Sunflat Pahuja Center for
Blood Disorders
Sunflag Hospital Sector 16A
Faridabad-121002

Director
Hematology Department
Paras Hospital, Gurgaon
India

Preface

The *Recent Advances in Hematology-3* offers the state-of-the-art chapters by distinguished experts in the field. The contributors have critically examined and analyzed into perspective some of the contemporary advances and developments and rising torrent of valuable literature of various aspects of hematology. These are unique in providing the depth and breadth of knowledge as also a stimulus for further discussion and future research.

We are indeed grateful to our distinguished contributors for readily responding to our requests and reposing confidence in our editorship.

Thanks are also due to our Advisory Editorial Board for helping us in the editorial matters and attending promptly to our requests and queries.

Finally, we express our indebtedness to M/s Jaypee Brothers Medical Publishers (P) Ltd, New Delhi, India and their staff for the skillful production qualities of the volume.

Renu Saxena
HP Pati
Manoranjan Mahapatra

Contents

1. The Rare Coagulation Disorders 1
   Ravi Ranjan

2. Autologous Stem Cell Transplantation for Multiple Myeloma ... 19
   Kevin W Song

3. Role of Autologous Stem Cell Transplantation in
   Hematological Malignancies 29
   Lalit Kumar, Deepak Dabkara, Ajay Gogia, Deepanjan Panda

4. Evidence-based Management of Fever in the
   Neutropenic Patient 49
   Matthew D Seftel

5. Thrombin-activable Fibrinolysis Inhibitor (TAFI):
   An Important Contributor in the Fibrinolytic System 60
   Arijit Biswas, Suhail Akhter, Renu Saxena

6. Pathobiology, Prognostication and Management of
   Low-risk Myelodysplastic Syndrome 67
   HP Pati, Shyam Rathi

7. Antiphospholipid Syndrome—Recent Insights 77
   Ashok Kumar, Hemant Gopal

8. Fanconi Anemia 94
   Tulika Seth

9. Chronic Lymphoproliferative Disorders (CLPDs) 99
   S Varma, Neelam Varma

10. Aspirin Resistance: Expectations and Limitations 110
    Gundu HR Rao

11. Hemovigilance 129
    Neelam Marwaha

12. Allogeneic Hematopoietic Stem Cell Transplantation
    in Hematologic Disorders 141
    Rajat Kumar

13. The Battle of Cancer is to be Won by Targeted Therapy 159
    MB Agarwal

14. **Thalassemia Screening and Control Program** 167
    VP Choudhry, Amit Upadhyay

15. **Pathophysiology of Bleeding in Dengue Virus Infection: A Holistic View** 178
    Kanjaksha Ghosh

16. **Approach to Polycythemia** 187
    Manoranjan Mahapatra, Shyam Rathi

17. **Aplastic Anemia: Issues in Management** 194
    Manoranjan Mahapatra, Tuphan Kanti Dolai, Niranjan Rathod

18. **Secondary Leukemia** 211
    Seema Tyagi, Prashant Sharma

19. **Current Pathogenesis and Therapy in Essential Thrombocythemia** 226
    VP Choudhry

20. **Current Management of Idiopathic Thrombocytopenic Purpura** 238
    Tulika Seth

21. **Minimal Residual Disease (MRD) Detection in Acute Leukemia** 246
    Seema Tyagi, Sanjeev Kumar Gupta

Index 261

Plate 1

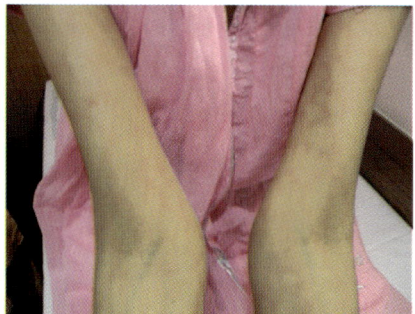

Fig. 7.1: Livedo reticularis over the forearms in a patient with APS

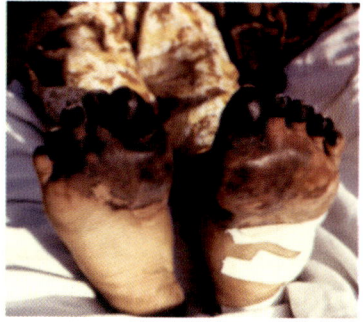

Fig. 7.2: Digital gangrene in another patient with APS secondary to SLE

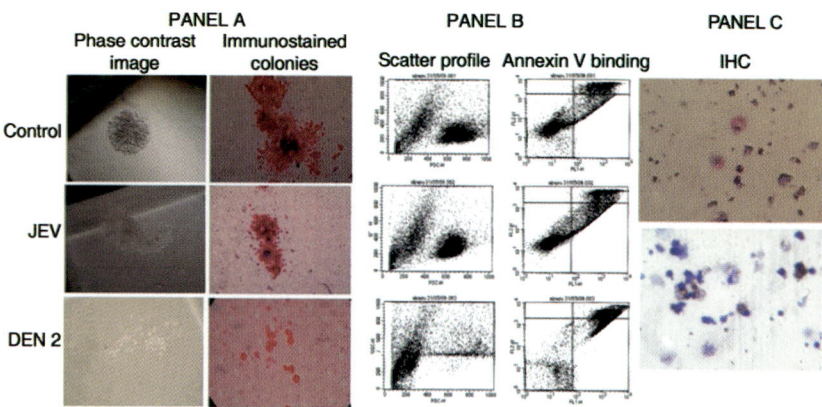

Fig. 15.1: Panel A: Total suppression of CFU-Meg by dengue virus infection *in vitro*. Panel B showing increased apoptosis and increased annexin binding in megakaryocyte precursors in culture on exposure to DEN-2 virus. Panel C showing immunohistochemistry of dengue virus positive Meg precursors. Upper figure is without infection

Chapter 1

The Rare Coagulation Disorders

Ravi Ranjan

SUMMARY

Deficiencies of rare coagulation factors are heritable abnormalities of hemostasis that may present significant difficulties in diagnosis and management. This chapter summarizes the various rare coagulation disorders such as disorders of fibrinogen (FI), and deficiencies of prothrombin (FII), factor V, combined deficiency of FV and FVIII, FVII, FX, the combined vitamin K-dependent factors, FXI and FXIII. Based on both collective clinical experience and the literature, guidelines for management of bleeding complications are suggested with specific advice for surgery, spontaneous bleeding, management of pregnancy and the neonate. The chapter describes the various clinical phenotypes, prevalence, diagnosis and molecular basis of these rare coagulation disorders and gives a brief idea about the molecular biology of these factors.

KEYWORDS

Fibrinogen, Prothrombin, Factor V, Factor VII, Factor X, Factor XIII, Mutation

INTRODUCTION

The rare coagulation disorders are heritable abnormalities of hemostasis that may present significant difficulties in diagnosis and management to clinicians. The common feature shared by these disorders is that their overall population frequency is low (with the exception of factor XI deficiency). Consequently, diagnosis and monitoring of affected individuals may require specialist phenotypic and molecular investigations that are not widely available. There may be considerable interindividual variation in bleeding phenotype amongst affected individuals resulting at least in part from the molecular heterogeneity of the rare coagulation disorders. The bleeding risks in affected individuals may therefore be difficult to assess. Since, there are few long-term prospective studies of large cohorts of patients, reliable information about clinical management is often scarce. Coagulation factor support may require the prescription of unlicensed treatment products that are not readily available.

Although the rare coagulation disorders are uncommon, most hospitals will have a handful of individuals with one or more disorders. Some may have significant number of affected individuals because of the prevalence of these disorders in populations in which consanguineous marriage is common. Particular emphasis is placed on prophylaxis and the management of surgical patients, pregnant mothers and affected neonates.

INHERITED ABNORMALITIES OF FIBRINOGEN (FACTOR I DEFICIENCY)

Background

Fibrinogen is a 340 kDa protein that is synthesized in the liver. It has a plasma concentration of approximately 1.5-3.5 g L^{-1} and a half-life of around 4 days. The FI molecule is a homodimer, each half consisting of three nonidentical polypeptide chains termed Aα, Bβ and γ.

Fibrin is produced by proteolytic cleavage of FI by thrombin with the release of fibrinopeptides A and B and generation of insoluble fibrin monomer followed by polymerization. FI is also important in primary hemostasis for normal platelet aggregation.

Definitions

1. Afibrinogenemia refers to the total absence of FI measured by an antigenic assay.
2. Hypofibrinogenemia is a decreased level of normal FI.
3. Dysfibrinogenemia is characterized by structural abnormality of the FI molecule resulting in altered functional properties.

Afibrinogenemia/hypofibrinogenemia has an estimated prevalence 1:1 000 000.[1]

Clinical Phenotypes

Afibrinogenemia is associated with umbilical, mucosal, musculoskeletal, central nervous system (CNS) and intra-abdominal bleeding tendency of variable severity including life-threatening, spontaneous events,[2,5] recurrent miscarriage with both antepartum and postpartum hemorrhage.[3,4] In hypofibrinogenemia the bleeding pattern is similar but appears to follow a milder course and bleeding may follow invasive procedures.

Dysfibrinogenemia patients may have bleeding postpartum or with surgery and dental extraction with delayed wound healing and dehiscence. Umbilical stump, CNS and soft tissues bleeding are associated with lower levels. Thrombosis is also associated with these patients. Pregnant women are at risk of bleeding following vaginal delivery, cesarean section and with regional analgesia.

Diagnosis

Afibrinogenemia

There is a marked prolongation of the PT, APTT and thrombin time (TT). The bleeding time is often prolonged. FI levels are undetectable by both functional (Clauss) and antigenic assays.

Hypofibrinogenemia

Coagulation tests are prolonged in proportion to the FI deficiency. TT is the most sensitive test. The total clottable and immunogenic FIs are both reduced to a similar level as the functional FI.

Dysfibrinogenemia

TT is usually prolonged but in rare cases may be normal or shortened. It is important to exclude the effect of heparin and interference with fibrin polymerization. The reptilase time is usually prolonged but may be shortened or sometimes normal. The PT and APTT may be prolonged but are less sensitive than the TT. The functional FI by Clauss method will be low. A definitive diagnosis requires the demonstration of a molecular defect.

Molecular Basis for Inherited Abnormality of Fibrinogen

The three FI subunits (Aα, Bβ and γ) are encoded by three different genes clustered in a region of 50 kb on chromosome 4 (q28-30), FGA, FGB and FGG. The FGA is 5.4 kb in length and consists of six exons. It encodes two different transcripts by alternative splicing at the 3'-end. The major isoform (α), which represents 99% of mRNA, is coded by exons 1-5. The extended αE variant is produced by the addition of 236 amino acids encoded by exon 6. The FGB consists of eight exons and is 8.2 kb in length. The synthesis of the Bβ chain is the rate-limiting step in the production of mature FI. The FGG is 8.4 kb long and has 10 exons. The γ-chain occurs in two isoforms (γ and γ'), which are produced by alternative splicing. The γ' isoform constitutes about 15% and contains an additional binding site for FXIII and for thrombin.

Congenital Afibrinogenemia

It is an autosomal recessive condition that has been shown to be due to defective FI synthesis. The majority of mutations found to date are in FGA. These mutations are mainly deletions, frameshift, nonsense or splicing mutations and several recurrent mutations have been detected, including an 11 kb deletion in the FGA gene and a donor splice mutation in intron 4 + 1 G > T in FGA.

Dysfibrinogenemia

Overall 300 abnormal FIs have been described and over 100 different structural defects identified. These are mainly associated with missense mutations affecting FI structure or function. The majority (180) of these mutations are in FGA of which 74 are at (Aα 16). Twenty-seven mutations have been reported in the FGB and 75 in the FGG of which 25 affect γ 275. These mutations affect regions associated with all aspects of FI function.

Management

A suggested amount of FI required is: Dose (g) = Desired increment in gL^{-1} × plasma volume, where the plasma volume is 0.07 × (1 – hematocrit) × weight (kg). Therefore, to raise the FI concentration by 1 gL^{-1} a dose of about 30 mg kg^{-1} would be required.

Although cryoprecipitate is a good source of FI it should not usually be used, as it is not virally inactivated. Fibrin glue and tranexamic acid may be useful to treat superficial wounds or following dental extraction and mucosal bleeding. Its use may, however, increase the risk of thrombosis and should be used with caution.

Spontaneous Bleeding

Afibrinogenemia

Fibrinogen concentrate is the treatment of choice for significant bleeding. The FI level should be maintained above 1 gL^{-1} until hemostasis is secure and above 0.5 gL^{-1} until wound healing is complete. Antifibrinolytic agents may be useful for mucosal bleeding and estrogen/progesterone preparations have been used in menorrhagia.[5]

Dysfibrinogenemia

The abnormal FI in the patient may be dysfunctional and may interfere with the function of infused FI. Raising the measured FI level in the patient to 1 gL^{-1} may, theoretically, not provide adequate hemostasis. With these considerations in mind, patients who are bleeding are likely to require FI concentrate although in some cases topical fibrin glue or tranexamic acid may be sufficient for superficial or mucosal bleeding. The functional FI level should be raised to 1 gL^{-1} above baseline level and the clinical response observed.

Surgery

Afibrinogenemia

It is recommended that FI levels are increased to 1 gL^{-1} and maintained at this level until hemostasis is secure and above 0.5 gL^{-1} until wound healing is complete.

Dysfibrinogenemia

Patients with a known bleeding phenotype should be treated similar to afibrinogenemia while patients with a thrombotic phenotype should be treated with compression stockings and low-molecular weight heparin (LMWH).

Pregnancy

Afibrinogenemia

Prophylaxis with FI concentrate is reported to improve pregnancy outcome and prevent postpartum hemorrhage. [3,4]

Dysfibrinogenemia

During delivery it should be assumed that the neonate has dysfibrinogenemia and invasive monitoring and procedures should be avoided, particularly if the family phenotype is of bleeding. Women with a personal or family history of thrombosis should be offered antenatal prophylaxis with LMWH.

FACTOR II — PROTHROMBIN DEFICIENCY

Molecular Biology

Prothrombin (FII) is a 72 kDa single chain glycoprotein which is synthesized by hepatocytes. It is one of the vitamin K-dependent coagulation factors and requires post-translational carboxylation to become functionally active. Prothrombin consists of four domains—Gla domain, kringle 1 and kringle 2 domains and a serine protease domain. FXa activates prothrombin on the surface of platelets in the presence of FV and calcium. During cleavage of prothrombin the activation peptide fragment 1 + 2 is released.

Incidence

Prothrombin deficiency is probably the rarest inherited bleeding disorder with an estimated prevalence of 1:2 000 000 in the general population. As with many rare hemostatic disorders the mode of inheritance is autosomal recessive. Till 2004 only 26 cases of prothrombin deficiency and 22 cases with other prothrombin abnormalities had been described in the world literature.[6]

Clinical Phenotypes

Two clinical phenotypes are recognized—hypoprothrombinemia (type I deficiency), in which prothrombin antigen and activity levels are reduced concomitantly, and dysprothrombinemia (type II deficiency) in which prothrombin activity is reduced but antigen levels are normal. Occasional combined defects (compound heterozygotes) have also been reported. Hemarthrosis and muscle hematomas are the most frequent severe bleeding manifestations in hypoprothrombinemia.[6] Intracranial bleeding, mucosal bleeding and life-threatening umbilical bleeding are rare.[7]

Diagnosis

PT and APTT may be prolonged in FII deficiency. A specific FII assay may therefore be required in the presence of clinical suspicion or appropriate a family history and normal screening tests. The one-stage clotting assay employing thromboplastin and based on the PT is suitable and is the most widely used technique.

In hypoprothrombinemia results of all assays are reduced essentially in parallel.[6] It has been reported that in homozygous individuals for hypoprothrombinemia, FII activity levels were 9-16 U dL^{-1} by PT based assay, compared with levels of 43-75 U dL^{-1} in heterozygous subjects. Normal subjects related to these kindreds and unrelated normal subjects had FII levels in the range 84-130 U dL^{-1}.[6] In dysprothrombinemias FII activity levels were 26-49 U dL^{-1}. The diagnosis of mild prothrombin deficiency may be especially difficult in premature or young neonates where vitamin K deficiency may complicate assessment.

Molecular Defects

Prothrombin is encoded by a gene on chromosome 11. To date at least 32 different mutations have been identified. Seventeen missense mutations have been described in dysprothrombinemia. The mutations in hypoprothrombinemia are also predominantly missense, although nonsense mutations have also been found. In dysprothrombinemia the mutations result in amino acid substitutions within the cleavage sites for FXa and the serine protease region of prothrombin, whereas the mutations in hypoprothrombinemia are often close to the Gla and kringle domains and the A chain.

Management

Treatment Options

Prothrombin complex concentrates are treatment of choice. The majority of these products are 3-factor concentrates containing therapeutic quantities of FII, FIX and FX.[8] The 4-factor concentrates, which in addition contain FVII, are also available.[8] In the absence of these virally inactivated fresh frozen plasma (FFP) is an alternative source of prothrombin.

Bleeding and Surgery

It is estimated that 1 unit of prothrombin will raise the plasma prothrombin level by 1 IU dL^{-1}. 20-30 IU dL^{-1} of prothrombin is thought to be required for normal hemostasis and doses of 20-30 IU kg^{-1} have been used previously and seem to be effective. Higher doses may, however, be required in the event of life-threatening bleeding or major surgery, and monitoring of prothrombin levels should be performed. The half-life of prothrombin is around 72 hours, which facilitates relatively infrequent dosing, usually every 2-3 days.

Pregnancy

It is difficult to make firm recommendations on pregnancy management due to lack of published data but it would seem reasonable to increase the prothrombin level to above 25 IU dL^{-1} prior to delivery.

Children

The use of prophylaxis in children should be based on the frequency and type of bleeding. Where recurrent joint bleeding is a feature prophylaxis should be used to prevent the development of a chronic arthropathy.

FACTOR V DEFICIENCY

Molecular Biology

Clotting FV is a large glycoprotein of MW 249 kDa encoded by a gene on chromosome 1, which is synthesized by hepatocytes and megakaryocytes. Platelets contain approximately 20% of total circulating FV. FV is activated by thrombin and the resulting heterodimer FVa acts as a cofactor for FXa in the conversion of prothrombin to thrombin. Till 2004, 26 separate mutations have been characterized.[9] Twelve of these are located in the exon 13, which encodes the entire B domain.

Clinical Phenotype

Hereditary FV deficiency is a very rare autosomal recessive condition. The prevalence of the homozygous state is approximately 1 per million.[10] It has been reported that in homozygote individuals FV levels range from < 1 to 10 U dL^{-1} with a normal range of 71-125 U dL^{-1}.[11] Homozygous deficiency is associated with a moderately severe bleeding disorder.[11] It usually presents in childhood with easy bruising and mucous membrane bleeding, in particular epistaxes and oral cavity bleeding. Gastrointestinal bleeding and hematuria may occur rarely. Postoperative, postdental extraction and postpartum bleeding have been reported.

Diagnosis

The FV deficiency is associated with prolongation of both the PT and APTT but a normal TT. Both PT and APTT are corrected by mixing with normal plasma. Deficiency of FV is confirmed by performing a prothrombin time-based FV assay or by immunological assessment of FV levels. Individuals with reduced FV levels should also have a FVIII assay performed to exclude combined FV and FVIII deficiency.

Management

The only blood product available for FV replacement is FFP. It is recommended that a virally inactivated preparation is used[1] preferably sourced from a country that has no reported case of variant CJD in its donor population or BSE in its cattle.

Spontaneous Bleeding Episodes

The minimum circulating level of FV that has to be achieved for effective hemostasis is 15 U dL^{-1} [12] and the doses of 15-20 mL kg^{-1} have been used. Use of agents such as tranexamic acid, recombinant activated factor VII (rFVIIa) and platelets should also be considered.

Surgery

FFP should be administered if excessive bleeding occurs. In patients with partial deficiency of FV and in patients with levels of < 1 U dL^{-1}, FFP should be administered immediately prior to the procedure. FFP dosages should be those recommended for bleeding episodes.

Pregnancy

In patients with < 1 U dL^{-1} of FV, it is recommended that the administration of FFP at the dosage suggested above for surgery as soon as the patient is in established labor, with close monitoring of FV levels.

Neonates

Administration of virucidally treated FFP at a dose of 15-20 mL kg^{-1} is recommended in neonates and platelets transfusion provide an alternative source.

COMBINED DEFICIENCY OF FACTORS V AND FVIII

Molecular Biology

Combined FV and FVIII deficiency is a rare autosomal recessive disorder which usually arises as a consequence of consanguinity.[13] Studies of the inheritance pattern indicated that it is due to a single gene defect rather than due to coinheritance of separate defects of the FV and FVIII genes. This has been confirmed, the gene located on the long arm of chromosome 18 which encodes a resident protein of the endoplasmic reticulum, the golgi intermediate compartment, termed the ERGIC-53 protein.[14] This protein has been identified as playing a major role in intracellular trafficking of certain proteins including FV and FVIII.[15] Defective ERGIC-53 function results in disturbance of the passage of the factors through the cell and impaired release into the circulation. A number of different mutations have been described in this gene leading to combined FV and FVIII deficiency.[14]

Clinical Phenotype

Although mild bleeding symptoms such as easy bruising and epistaxes are not uncommon in affected individuals, circulating levels of FV and FVIII are usually sufficient to prevent more severe spontaneous bleeding episodes. However, bleeding is common following surgery, dental extraction and trauma; menorrhagia and postpartum hemorrhage are commonly seen in affected women.[16]

Diagnosis

The combined deficiency disorder is associated with a prolongation of both the PT and APTT, with the APTT prolongation disproportionate to that of the PT. Both test times are corrected by mixing studies using normal plasma. APTT-based activity assays and antigen assays reveal levels of between 5 and 20 IU dL^{-1} for both FV and FVIII.[13]

Management

Bleeding Episodes

Spontaneous bleeding episodes occurring in patients with combined FV and FVIII deficiency should be treated with both FVIII concentrates and FFP (as a source of FV). For minor bleeding episodes FVIII levels should be raised to at least 30 IU dL^{-1} and to at least 50 IU dL^{-1} for more severe bleeds with rFVIII concentrate being the treatment of choice. As for patients with FV deficiency, FFP should be administered in order to increase the FV level to at least 25 U dL^{-1}.

Surgical Procedures

These should be covered with FVIII concentrates administered 12 hourly to maintain FVIII levels above 50 IU dL^{-1} and 12 hourly FFP to achieve minimum levels of FV of 25 U dL^{-1} until wound healing is established.

Pregnancy

FV levels in pregnancy do not consistently increase or decrease whereas FVIII levels will increase throughout pregnancy. Any possible bleeding is therefore likely to be dependent on the FV level during labor and delivery. FV levels should be maintained above the hemostatic level of 15 U dL^{-1} during labor.

Neonates

Affected babies should receive oral vitamin K and go on to receive vaccinations.

FACTOR VII DEFICIENCY

Molecular Biology

Factor VII is a vitamin K-dependent glycoprotein with a MW of approximately 50 kDa and circulates in plasma in two forms — the majority in a single chain inactive form with a concentration of 10 nmoles L^{-1} (0.5 µg mL^{-1}) and a much smaller amount (approximately 10-110 pmoles L^{-1}) as the active two-chain form. The FVII gene maps to chromosome 13 at 13q34, spans approximately 12 kb of DNA and consists of nine exons encoding a mature protein of 406 amino acids.

Factor VII deficiency is the most common of the 'rare inherited coagulation disorders'. Severe FVII deficiency (FVII: C < 2 IU dL^{-1}) has an estimated prevalence of 1:300 000-1:500 000. FVII deficiency is inherited in an autosomal recessive manner and its frequency is significantly increased in countries where consanguineous marriage is practiced. The FVII mutation website (http://www.193.60.222.13/index.htm) lists 120 mutations throughout the FVII gene.

Plasma Factor VII Levels

Factor VII plasma levels are determined by both environmental and genetic factors with the latter accounting for up to one-third of the variation in plasma FVII. Amongst environmental factors, dietary fat intake and the levels of plasma triglycerides are positively correlated with FVII: C levels but age, obesity, diabetes and in women the use of sex hormones can all influence FVII levels.

Six polymorphisms within the human F7 gene have been shown to affect both plasma FVII: C levels and plasma VIIa levels.[17] Of these the most important is the Arg353Gln polymorphism within exon 7, which affects approximately 20% of the UK population. Heterozygosity for this polymorphism is associated with an approximately 25% reduction in FVII: C and VII:Ag levels and homozygosity leads to approximately 50% reduction in circulating plasma FVII.

Clinical Phenotype

Epistaxes, gum bleeding, menorrhagia and other mucous membrane-type bleeding are common. Menorrhagia and chronic iron deficiency are frequently seen in women with FVII deficiency. In patients with severe FVII deficiency (FVII: C < 2 IU dL^{-1}), bleeding into the central nervous system is common and reported in between 15 and 60% of cases.[18]

Diagnosis

The diagnosis of FVII deficiency is suspected following the finding of a prolonged PT, which corrects, unless an inhibitor is present, in a 50:50 mix with normal plasma. It is important to exclude vitamin K deficiency or other acquired causes of a clotting disorder before the diagnosis of FVII deficiency is made.

Functional FVII Assays

Functional FVII activity (FVII: C) is measured using a one-stage PT-based assay. Blood samples for determination of FVII: C should not be stored at 4°C because this can lead to cold activation of FVII and lead to substantial overestimation of the true FVII level.[19]

Immunological FVII assays FVII antigen (FVII:Ag) is frequently measured using an enzyme-linked immunosorbent assay (ELISA) or immunoradiometric assay (IRMA). Such assays can detect as little as 0.01 IU dL^{-1} of FVII. Immunological assays should not be used in preference to a functional FVII assay.

Management

Current therapeutic options to manage patients with FVII deficiency include fibrinolytic inhibitors, plasma, intermediate purity FIX concentrates (prothrombin complex concentrates), FVII concentrates and rFVIIa. Plasma FVII has a short *in vivo* half-life of approximately 5 hours although this may be shorter during a bleeding episode.[20]

Acute Bleeding Episodes

Efficient hemostasis can be achieved with levels of FVII: C in the range of 10-15 IU dL^{-1}. rFVIIa is the recommended choice for patients with FVII deficiency requiring replacement therapy.

Surgery

Doses of FVII concentrate ranging from 8 to 40 U kg^{-1} every 4-6 hours have been successfully used.[21] Doses of rFVIIa ranging from 14-30 ug/kg was given at 2-3 hours intervals for the first 24 hours followed by longer intervals (3-8 hours) for the remaining postoperative period.

Pregnancy

Continuous infusion of rFVIIa has been used in patients with FVII deficiency to provide hemostatic cover for an elective cesarean section.[22] An initial bolus or rFVIIa of 13.3 µg kg^{-1} followed by a continuous infusion initially at a rate of 3.3 µg kg^{-1} hour^{-1} for 48 hours and then at 1.66 µg kg^{-1} hour^{-1} for a further 48 hours is recommended.

Neonates

Cranial ultrasound should be undertaken in severely affected neonates because of the increased risk of intracranial hemorrhage and prophylaxis may be necessary although even with appropriate replacement therapy, hemorrhage may occur.

FACTOR X DEFICIENCY

Molecular Biology

The gene for FX is 22 kb long and located at 13q34-ter and encodes a 59 kDa protein. FX synthesis occurs in the liver and following secretion into plasma, circulates at a concentration of 10 µg mL^{-1} as a two-chain molecule. Activation of FX–FXa occurs during the initiation of coagulation by a complex consisting of tissue factor, FVIIa, calcium ions and a suitable phospholipids membrane. However, activation can also take place through FIXa, FVIIIa, calcium ions and acidic phospholipid surfaces.

Severe (homozygous) FX deficiency is inherited as an autosomal recessive disorder with an incidence of 1:1-000-000 in the general population. The prevalence of heterozygous FX deficiency is about 1:500, but individuals are usually clinically asymptomatic.[23] 45 mutations within the FX gene have been reported.[24]

Clinical Phenotype

Patients with severe deficiency [FX activity (FX:C) < 1 IU dL^{-1}] may present with umbilical-stump and mucosal-type bleeding, epistaxis, menorrhagia, recurrent hemarthrosis, severe postoperative hemorrhage. Moderately affected patients (FX: C 1-5 IU dL^{-1}) may bleed only after hemostatic challenge, e.g. trauma or surgery. Mild FX deficiency (FX: C 6-10 IU dL^{-1}) may experience easy bruising or menorrhagia.

Diagnosis

The diagnosis of FX deficiency is suspected following the finding of a prolonged PT and APTT which corrects, unless an inhibitor is present, in a 50:50 mix with normal plasma. The diagnosis of FX deficiency is confirmed by measuring plasma FX levels using either of these — the one-stage PT- and APTT-based assays or a chromogenic assay or Russell viper venom (RVV) assay or an immunological assay. It is important to exclude vitamin K deficiency or other acquired causes of a clotting disorder before the diagnosis of FX deficiency is made.

Management

Current therapeutic options to manage patients with FX deficiency include fibrinolytic inhibitors, plasma, intermediate purity FIX concentrates (prothrombin complex concentrates) and rVIIa. The biological half-life of FX is 20-40 hours,[25] so an adequate level can be achieved with repeated infusions. Factor levels of 10-20 IU dL^{-1} are generally sufficient for hemostasis, even in the immediate postoperative period.[26]

Acute Bleeding

No specific concentrates are available and prothrombin complex concentrates are the treatment of choice at the doses of 30 units kg^{-1} administered twice weekly. In cases where these are not available or are contraindicated, FFP can be used at doses of 20 mL kg^{-1} followed by 3-6 mL kg^{-1} twice daily. rVIIa has been used successfully to treat acquired FX deficiency secondary to amyloidosis.[27] In women with menorrhagia, tranexamic acid 15 mg kg^{-1} 8 hourly may be effective when taken for the duration of the menstrual period.

Surgery

It has been successfully performed following infusion of either FFP or PCCs. In the case of FFP, a level of 35 U dL^{-1} was achieved prior to surgery and FX levels were maintained above 20 U dL^{-1} in the postoperative period with no bleeding reported.[26]

Pregnancy

Women with severe FX deficiency and a history of adverse outcome in pregnancy may benefit from aggressive replacement therapy.

Neonates

In neonates it is similar to FVII deficiency.

FACTOR XI DEFICIENCY

Molecular Biology

Factor XI is a dimeric serine protease whose function in the coagulation pathway was recently clarified. Thrombin may activate FXI and thereby recruits the 'intrinsic' pathway of coagulation.[28] Factor XI deficiency is an autosomally inherited condition described in all racial groups, but in general, the incidence of severe deficiency (FXI: C level < 10 U dL^{-1}) is very low (estimated at 1:1 million).[29]

The FXI gene is 23 kb in length. In the Ashkenazi Jewish population most FXI deficiency is related to two mutations. Type II, a stop codon in exon 5, and type III, a missense mutation in exon 9. These mutations occur in equal frequency in Jews leading to type II homozygotes who typically have undetectable FXI levels and a more severe bleeding phenotype; type III homozygotes who have a low level of FXI (about 10 U dL^{-1}) while compound heterozygotes have levels and clinical expression between these two.[30] Several other mutations such as C128X in exon 5 have been described.

Clinical Phenotype

Bleeding occurs in people with heterozygous deficiency and is not related to the FXI: C level.[31] Bleeding is most commonly provoked by injury or surgery from the mouth, nose and genitourinary tracts. Women with FXI deficiency (including heterozygotes) are at risk of menorrhagia[32] and bleeding in relation to childbirth.

Diagnosis

The diagnosis depends upon determination of a FXI levels. Data from published studies suggest that most widely used APTT reagents will have prolonged APTT results in samples from patients with FXI below 20-25 U dL^{-1}, whereas there is a more mixed pattern of normal and abnormal results when FXI is in the region 25-60 U dL^{-1}. The lower limit of normal range for FXI activity is probably between 60 and 70 U dL^{-1}.

Management

Spontaneous Bleeding

It does not usually occur in FXI deficiency.

Surgery

For patients with severe deficiency, FXI levels of > 30 U dL^{-1} are considered hemostatic for minor surgery and > 45 U dL^{-1} for major surgery. In practise one should aim to obtain FXI levels in the region of 70 U dL^{-1} prior to major surgery. FXI has a half-life of approximately 52 ± 22 hours and daily dosing may not, therefore, be necessary. People with mild FXI deficiency are more difficult to manage because of the variability and unpredictability of the bleeding tendency. Oral tranexamic acid, with or without a virally inactivated FFP should be considered. For major surgery in younger people factor concentrates may be required.

Pregnancy

For women with FXI levels between about 15 and 70 U dL^{-1} and a significant bleeding history tranexamic acid is often used for 3 days with the first dose being administered during labor. For women with severe FXI deficiency (FXI: C < 10-20 U dL^{-1}) FXI concentrate should be given during labor.

Neonates

No instances of neonatal intracranial hemorrhage resulting from FXI deficiency have been reported.

FACTOR XIII DEFICIENCY

Factor XIII (fibrin stabilizing factor) deficiency inherited (autosomal recessive) or acquired is a very rare bleeding disorder. The estimated prevalence is one case per 1 million.

Clinical Phenotype

Patients with FXIII < 1 U dL^{-1} are at greatest risk from severe spontaneous bleeding. Those with levels between 1 and 4 U dL^{-1} are likely to have moderate or severe bleeding. Occasionally patients with levels above 5 U dL^{-1} may bleed.[33] Umbilical bleeding, which occurs a few days after birth, is reported in 80% of cases. Patients experience a lifelong tendency to severe bruising, muscle hematomas (32%), hemarthroses (24%), intracranial hemorrhage (30%), miscarriages, postnatal bleeding, delay in healing of wounds and bleeding after surgery and trauma.[34]

Diagnosis

The range of FXIII activity within the normal population is very wide, ranging from 53.2 to 221.3% (mean ± SD: 105 ± 28.56%), of the standard normal plasma value.[34] The bleeding time, PT and APTT are normal. The clot solubility test is a qualitative screening test in which test plasma is clotted with calcium, thrombin or a combination of both and exposed to a chemical challenge, which lyses the clot unless sufficient FXIII dependant cross-linking has occurred. The clot may be lysed with 5 mol L^{-1} urea, 2% acetic acid, 1% mono-chloroacetic acid or similar.

Several types of FXIII activity assay have been reported. These are based on the cross-linking of glycine-ethylester into a specific peptide[35] or on incorporation of an amine substrate into FI,[36] both of which employ thrombin activation of FXIII. ELISA assays have been used to determine antigenic levels of FXIII, but are not widely available.

Management

The FXIII has a long circulating half-life of 7-10 days.[33] It has been suggested that levels of 3-10 U dL^{-1} are sufficient to prevent spontaneous hemorrhage.[33] This appears to prevent recurrent clinical problems and bleeding episodes.

Acute Bleeding Episodes

Whole blood, FFP, stored plasma and cryoprecipitate have all been used successfully in treatment and are adequate sources of FXIII. Plasma-derived FXIII concentrates are superior to FFP or cryoprecipitate as these provide reliable and high concentrations of FXIII in minimum volume have fewer contaminating substances, and are virally inactivated.[37] It is recommended that 10 units kg^{-1} body weight be given at intervals of 4 weeks. Platelets contain FXIII, and in a hemorrhagic emergency platelet transfusions may be helpful.[38]

Surgery

Adults should receive 10–20 units kg^{-1} immediately before the operation and ideally, the plasma levels monitored. Further treatment can be given if necessary to keep the level in the normal range for the following 5 days or until the wound has healed completely.

Pregnancy

All severely affected women should be started on monthly infusions of FXIII concentrate from the time of diagnosis and these should be continued throughout pregnancy.

Neonates

All neonates (and older children) who have been diagnosed as having a FXIII level of < 3 U dL^{-1} should commence treatment with prophylactic FXIII concentrate 10 U kg^{-1} given once every 4 weeks.

TAKE HOME MESSAGE

Deficiencies of rare coagulation factors (FII, FV, FV + FVIII, FVII, FX, FXI, FXIII) that cause bleeding disorders are inherited as autosomal recessive traits and are rare. As a consequence of the rarity of these deficiencies, the type and severity of bleeding symptoms, the underlying molecular defects, and the actual management of bleeding episodes are not as well established as for hemophilia A and B. The study of the genetic basis of these disorders could represent an important tool for prevention through prenatal diagnosis. Patients with rare coagulation disorder and clinically significant manifestations are usually homozygous or compound heterozygous. Out of the various RCDs most severe diseases are factor X and factor II deficiencies. For the remaining defects only a minority of patients, even those with unmeasurable plasma levels, had life-endangering hemorrhages or musculoskeletal disabilities as a consequence of hemarthroses and hematomas. The relatively mild severity of clinical manifestations in recessive coagulation disorders commands safety as the primary criterion in the choice of replacement material for treatment. Hence, virally inactivated plasma and factor concentrates should be the products of choice.

REFERENCES

1. Peyvandi F, Asselta R, Mannucci PM. Autosomal recessive deficiencies of coagulation factors. Rev Clin Exp Hematol 2001;5:369-88.
2. Lak M, Keihani M, Elahi F, Peyvandi F, Mannucci PM. Bleeding and thrombosis in 55 patients with inherited afibrinogenemia. Br J Haematol 1999;107:204-06.
3. Goodwin TM. Congenital hypofibrinogenemia in pregnancy. Obstet Gynecol Surv 1989;44:157-61.
4. Kobayashi T, Kanayama N, Tokunaga N, Asahina T, Terao T. Prenatal and peripartum management of congenital afibrinogenemia. Br J Haematol 2000; 109:364-66.
5. Rizk DE, Kumar RM. Congenital afibrinogenemia: Treatment of excessive menstrual bleeding with continuous oral contraceptive (letter). Am J Hematol 1996;52:237-38.
6. Girolami A, Scarano L, Saggiorato G, Girolami B, Bertomoro A, Marchiori A. Congenital deficiencies and abnormalities of prothrombin. Blood Coagul Fibrinolysis 1998;9:557-69.

7. Strijks E, Poort SR, Renier WO, Gabreels FJ, Bertina RM. Hereditary prothrombin deficiency presenting as intracranial haematoma in infancy. Neuropediatrics 1999;30:320-24.
8. UKHCDO. Guidelines on the selection and use of therapeutic products to treat haemophilia and other hereditary bleeding disorders. Haemophilia 2003;9:1-23.
9. Peyvandi F, Duga S, Akhavan S, Mannucci PM. Rare coagulation deficiencies. Haemophilia 2002;8:308-21.
10. Girolami A, De Marco L, Dal Bo Zanon R, Patrassi G, Cappellato MG. Rarer quantitative and qualitative abnormalities of coagulation. Clin Haematol 1985;14:385-411.
11. Lak M, Sharifian R, Peyvandi F, Mannucci PM. Symptoms of inherited factor V deficiency in 35 Iranian patients. Br J Haematol 1998;103: 1067-69.
12. Peyvandi F, Mannucci PM. Rare coagulation disorders. Thromb Haemost 1999;82:1207-14.
13. Seligsohn U. Combined factor V and factor VIII deficiency. In: Savidge G (Eds) Factor VIII – von Willebrand Factor. New York: CRC, 1989.
14. Nichols WC, Terry VH, Wheatley MA, et al. ERGIC-53 gene structure and mutation analysis in 19 combined factors V and VIII deficiency families. Blood 1999;93:2261-66.
15. Moussalli M, Pipe SW, Hauri HP, Nichols WC, Ginsburg D, Kaufman RJ. Mannose-dependent endoplasmic reticulum (ER)-Golgi intermediate compartment-53-mediated ER to Golgi trafficking of coagulation factors V and VIII. J Biol Chem 1999;274:32539-42.
16. Seligsohn U, Zivelin A, Zwang E. Combined factor V and factor VIII deficiency among non-Ashkenazi Jews. N Engl J Med 1982;307:1191-95.
17. Perry DJ. Factor VII deficiency. Br J Haematol 2002;118:689-700.
18. Ragni MV, Lewis JH, Spero JA, Hasiba U. Factor VII deficiency. Am J Hematol 1981;10:79-88.
19. Kitchen S, Malia RG, Preston FE. A comparison of methods for the measurement of activated factor VII. Thromb Haemost 1992;68:301-05.
20. Lindley CM, Sawyer WT, Macik BG, et al. Pharmacokinetics and pharmacodynamics of recombinant factor VIIa. Clin Pharmacol Ther 1994;55:638-48.
21. Greene WB, McMillan CW. Surgery for scoliosis in congenital factor VII deficiency. Am J Dis Child 1982;136:411-13.
22. Jimenez-Yuste V, Villar A, Morado M, et al. Continuous infusion of recombinant activated factor VII during cesarean section delivery in a patient with congenital factor VII deficiency. Haemophilia 2000;6:588-90.
23. Graham JB, Barrow EM, Hougie C. Stuart clotting defect:II. Genetic aspects of a new hemorrhagic state. J Clin Invest 1957;36:497-503.
24. Uprichard J, Perry DJ. Factor X deficiency. Blood Rev 2002;16:97-110.
25. Roberts HR, Lechler E, Webster WP, Penick GD Survival of transfused factor X in patients with Stuart disease. Thromb Diath Haemorrh 1965;13:305-13.
26. Knight RD, Barr CF, Alving BM. Replacement therapy for congenital factor X deficiency. Transfusion 1985;25:78-80.
27. Boggio L, Green D. Recombinant human factor VIIa in the management of amyloid-associated factor X deficiency. Br J Haematol 2001;112:1074-5.
28. Broze GJ Jr, Gailani D. The role of factor XI in coagulation. Thromb Haemost 1993;70:72-74.
29. Peyvandi F, Lak M, Mannucci P. Factor XI deficiency in Iranians: Its clinical manifestations in comparison with those of classic hemophilia. Haematologica 2002;87:512-14.

30. Hancock JF, Wieland K, Pugh RE, et al. A molecular genetic study of factor XI deficiency. Blood 1991;77:1942-48.
31. Bolton-Maggs PH, Young Wan-Yin B, McCraw AH, Slack J, Kernoff PB. Inheritance and bleeding in factor XI deficiency. Br J Haematol 1988;69:521-28.
32. Leiba H, Ramot B, Many A. Heredity and coagulation studies in ten families with factor XI (plasma thromboplastin antecedent) deficiency. Br J Haematol 1965;11:654-65.
33. Anwar R, Minford A, Gallivan L, Trinh CH, Markham AF. Delayed umbilical bleeding—a presenting feature for factor XIII deficiency: Clinical features, genetics, and management. Pediatrics 2002;109:E32.
34. Anwar R, Miloszewski KJ. Factor XIII deficiency. Br J Haematol 1999;107:468-84.
35. Fickenscher K, Aab A, Stuber W. A photometric assay for blood coagulation factor XIII. Thromb Haemost 1991;65:535-40.
36. Kohler HP, Ariens RA, Whitaker P, Grant PJ. A common coding polymorphism in the FXIII A-subunit gene (FXIIIVal34Leu) affects cross-linking activity. Thromb Haemost 1998;80:704.
37. Board PG, Losowsky MS, Miloszewski KJ. Factor XIII: Inherited and acquired deficiency. Blood Rev 1993;7:229-42.
38. Wagner B, Seyfert UT, Gosse M, Wenzel E, Fickenscher K, Ruhl HG. Determination of factor XIII activity by a new photometric assay in plasma and platelets of healthy blood donors. Thromb Res 1994; 74:169-74.

Chapter 2

Autologous Stem Cell Transplantation for Multiple Myeloma

Kevin W Song

SUMMARY

Autologous stem cell transplantation (ASCT) for multiple myeloma is well established as standard treatment for eligible patients. Until recently efforts were focused on optimizing the conditioning chemotherapy and the number of transplant required to achieve the best response to improve survival for as many eligible patients as possible. With the advent of novel agents, particularly lenalidomide and bortezomib, recently the focus has shifted to how to integrate these agents into the transplant procedure to obtain the best response. Data is maturing in the use of novel agents as a part of induction therapy, clearly demonstrating the advantage of this approach. Other areas of research include integrating novel agents into the conditioning regimens and as a part of maintenance/consolidation. Coupled with these therapeutic advances is an increasing understanding of the biology of the malignant cells which has led to improvements in prognostication. Future advances in ASCT in myeloma will be in determining how to most effectively utilize novel agents; tailoring the approach to the biology of the malignancy that the individual suffers from; and the cost and convenience of the treatments. What is uncertain is whether ASCT will remain the standard of care in the future. This will be determined by the continued progress in the development of novel agents in the battle against myeloma and the willingness of the physician to offer and patients to accept ASCT with its toxicities as the number of therapeutic options and the duration of survival increase.

KEYWORDS

Multiple myeloma, Autologous stem cell transplant, Novel agents

INTRODUCTION

Multiple myeloma is currently the most common indication for autologous stem cell transplantation (ASCT) in North America and Europe. The foundations for ASCT were first established in the 1980's by McElwain and Powles, but ASCT truly became established as standard treatment for myeloma after the Intergroup Francais du Myelome (IFM) published their landmark article in the New England Journal of Medicine demonstrating its superiority compared to more traditional cytotoxic chemotherapy dosing.[1,2] Since that time, many advances in the treatment of myeloma have been made leading to changes in practice and more recently reexamination of the role of ASCT. This review will attempt to address recent progress in myeloma and the role of ASCT as a treatment.

NOVEL AGENTS

Until recently, treatment of myeloma was centered upon the optimal use of cytotoxic agents (e.g. melphalan and cyclophosphamide) and corticosteroids (e.g. prednisone and dexamethasone). Over the past 10 years, newer agents have been introduced into the treatment of myeloma leading to a paradigm shift. The first of these agents, thalidomide, was demonstrated to be effective in heavily pretreated myeloma patients by Singhal et al.[3] For patients with myeloma, thalidomide is felt to act via an immunomodulatory mechanism with a different side-effect profile compared to cytotoxic drugs. Thalidomide was shortly followed by bortezomib, the first drug in its class, whose mechanism of action is through proteosome inhibition.[4] More recently lenalidomide, an analogue of thalidomide with more potent antimyeloma activity has been integrated into clinical practice.[5] The advent of these novel agents have led to improved overall survival as demonstrated by several groups.[6,7] Although these drugs have demonstrated their efficacy for myeloma in general, recent research forays have been into integrating these drugs with transplantation as an overall treatment strategy to improve outcome.

INDUCTION AND STEM CELL MOBILIZATION

At diagnosis, the majority of patients require treatment of their myeloma for immediate control of symptoms and to reduce tumor burden. As a part of the initial evaluation an assessment has to be made to determine eligibility for ASCT. This evaluation will influence the initial treatments and the overall treatment philosophy. For patients who are eligible for ASCT, the consideration is to choose an induction regimen which will be highly effective yet, not compromise stem cell collection. Although many different regimens have been used as initial treatment of newly diagnosed transplant eligible patients with myeloma, until recently, VAD (vincristine, adriamycin, dexamethasone) or similar dexamethasone based regimens were universally used. It was believed that dexamethasone would give the most rapid reduction of tumor mass and symptom control without toxicity to stem cells. The use of stem cell toxic chemotherapy such as melphalan was avoided. Such induction regimen achieved response rates of between 40-60% although a complete remission was rarely achieved. Induction treatment was to establish control the disease while the major bulk of the antimyeloma effect was left to the high-dose chemotherapy. The landmark trial by the IFM published in 1996 revealed that a CR rate of 20-30% was achievable with a single ASCT.[2] This trial also demonstrated that the level of response was predictive of overall survival.

With the advent of novel drugs, newer induction regimens, incorporating these drugs are being assessed. This strategy is being investigated in the hopes of producing a higher response rate as well as a deeper response pretransplant, possibly resulting in a higher overall response rate post-transplant. The high post-transplant response rate would hopefully translate into improved progression free and overall survival. Thalidomide being the first of the novel drugs being generally available for myeloma, led to it being used in combination with dexamethasone as induction treatment. Although increased response rated were noted, a randomized trial by Macro et al failed to demonstrate an improvement in the post-transplant response rate.[8] The IFM is currently assessing one of the most promising regimens, bortezomib in combination with dexamethasone.[9] This combination given for 4 cycles is being compared to VAD for 4 cycles in a randomized trial prior to proceeding to transplant. Improved remission rates have been achieved both pre- and post-transplant compared to the standard arm (> VGPR 46.7%/18.6% and 71.8%/51%, P = < 0.0001/< 0.0001). Importantly stem cell collection has not been compromised (although there was a trend towards lower CD34 positive cells collected in the bortezomib arm) and 97% of enrolled patient were able to have adequate stem cells collected. Post-ASCT, response rates have improved demonstrating the persisting effect of the induction regimen. At this time although progression free survival is superior in the bortezomib arm, improvement in overall survival has not yet been demonstrated. Importantly, fewer patients required proceeding to a second ASCT for failing to achieve at least a VGPR with the first ASCT in the bortezomib plus dexamethasone arm. The Gruppo Italiano Malattie Ematologiche Ddell'Adulto (GIMEMA) is currently studying the combination of thalidomide, bortezomib and dexamethasone versus thalidomide and dexamethasone.[10] At their interim analysis, similar to the IFM, an improvement in remission pre- and post-ASCT has been found for the bortezomib containing regimen. At this time, survival results have not yet been presented. A notable induction regimen is the use of lenalidomide in combination with dexamethasone. In addition to the convenience of being oral chemotherapy, this combination has been found to be highly effective in newly diagnosed patients leading to its recommended use by the group at the Mayo Clinic.[11,12] At this time, it is uncertain if this regimen will result in deeper post-transplant remissions or improved survival. What has been well recognized is that the use of lenalidomide prior to stem cell collection hampers stem cell collection, leading to the recommendation that collection be done within 6 months of initiation of treatment with lenalidomide and the use of cyclophosphamide as priming.[13] The recent availability of AMD3100 gives another option for patients who fail to mobilize stem cells for ASCT.[14] One of the most interesting regimens being studied is the combination of lenalidomide and bortezomib. Small studies have reported responses approaching 100%.[15] These initial investigations examining the use of novel drugs as induction treatment prior to stem cell collection and transplant are laying the groundwork for future regimens. What is safe to say at this time is that VAD as induction is being supplanted by induction regimens which incorporate novel agents. In doing this higher pretransplant response rates will hopefully translate into higher post-transplant response-rates and longer progression free and overall survival. It is likely that the ideal induction regimen will be determined to have a combination of the major classes of drugs currently in use for myeloma (immunomodulatory, proteosome inhibitor, glucocorticoid, cytotoxic) attenuating efficacy with the ability to collect stem cells. Given the cost of the novel agents, what is unknown is if there is a subgroup of patients with myeloma who will not have substantial benefit from novel agents and may be treated with the less costly older agents.

CONDITIONING

Since the mid-1990's there has been a universal acceptance of melphalan 200 mg/m^2 as the conditioning regimen for ASCT. A randomized trial by the IFM demonstrated the superiority of this regimen over melphalan 140 mg/m^2 combined with radiation.[16] Patients who received radiation had more treatment related morbidity and extended follow-up has revealed that overall survival was superior for patients who received melphalan alone. Although most centers now use melphalan alone as conditioning, there have been reports of possible improvement in survival using busulfan as a part of the conditioning regimen.[17] At this time, it is less likely that there will be significant efforts in developing a combination of cytotoxic agents as conditioning chemotherapy regimens as the focus will begin to move towards integrating novel agents. Recently, investigations into the incorporation of the novel drugs in the conditioning regimen have been presented. Lonial et al have looked at using bortezomib peritransplant.[18] They found that bortezomib in addition to high-dose melphalan followed by stem cell infusion resulted in an impressive post-ASCT response rate without increase in toxicity. Currently, the IFM is also looking into a similar strategy where bortezomib is given before and shortly after stem cell infusion.[19] Response rates have been encouraging with 66% of patients achieving a VGPR or better post-transplant. Likewise, toxicity has not been found to be increased. How these results will alter practice is not yet certain, as it remain unknown if the improvements will be additive to the advances made in the area of induction treatment.

SINGLE VERSUS TANDEM

The IFM initially demonstrated the superiority of a single ASCT compared to conventional chemotherapy.[2] This was confirmed by the MRC although there were other studies, which did not.[20] As these studies were ongoing, the group in Arkansas pioneered the use of tandem transplants for myeloma.[21] In a randomized study the IFM demonstrated the superiority of tandem transplants over a single transplant.[22] Patient were randomly assigned to receive one transplant using melphalan 140 mg/m^2 with TBI or two transplants using melphalan 140 mg/m^2 for the first transplant followed by melphalan 140 mg/m^2 with TBI. Subgroup analysis revealed that the benefit was most pronounced in patients who had achieved at least a PR but not a VGPR. Similar results were produced by other groups. At this time, most centers have adopted the policy of offering a second transplant to patients who have achieved a partial remission but not a VGPR. With the promise of superior induction regimen, leading to improved response rates post first transplant, the percentage of patient offered a second transplant to consolidate the first transplant will likely diminish. Initial reports from the IFM has demonstrated such a result.[9] What is currently unknown is if this will result in an improved overall survival. The role of tandem transplants may become less relevant with the strategy of improving remission rate with induction chemotherapy.

SECOND TRANSPLANTS

Patients are sometimes offered a second transplant after relapsing from the first. Based upon the data from the Royal Marsden Hospital this strategy seems to be most effective for those who have had a prolonged remission after the first.[23] Importantly, if a patient has a prolonged first remission they seem to do just as well regardless of whether they received a second ASCT or nontransplant based therapy. It is also helpful to know that patients with a short remission from a first transplant are unlikely to benefit from a second transplant. This result is suggestive that a long first remission is a marker of prognosis for future outcome irrespective of treatment. This is likely representative of patients who have biologically more responsive disease and are likely to do well with conventional therapy as well. Whether a second transplant should ever be offered and the minimum time interval of first remission required is determined by the institution and their support of a second transplant. At this time, most centers recommend that a second transplant be considered only if the remission has been at least 2-3 years.[24]

MAINTENANCE AND CONSOLIDATION

Previously, interferon has been investigated as maintenance therapy for myeloma. Meta-analysis demonstrated a marginal benefit but interferon was not widely used given the significant toxicity.[25] Corticosteroids have also demonstrated modest benefit as maintenance but it also has not been widely accepted due to toxicity.[26] More recently thalidomide has been assessed as maintenance post-ASCT in several trials. The IFM randomized 597 patients post-transplant to no maintenance (arm A), pamidronate (arm B) or pamidronate plus thalidomide (arm C).[27] The 3-year event free survival was significantly higher in arm C (52%) compared to arm B (37%) and arm A (36%) ($p < 0.009$). Overall survival at 4 years was also superior in arm C (87%) compared to arm B (74%) and arm C (77%). Importantly, patients who had achieved a VGPR post-ASCT did not derive benefit from thalidomide maintenance. The result of this subanalysis is suggestive that thalidomide post-ASCT has a consolidative effect to patients with suboptimal results post-ASCT rather than a broad maintenance effect for all patients. Spencer et al also examined thalidomide use post-ASCT.[28] Similar to the IFM study, progression free and overall survival were superior in the thalidomide group. In their study, patients who had a VGPR or better also had benefit. These results are encouraging in that some form of maintenance treatment is beneficial to patients with myeloma. Acceptance of maintenance will be dictated by the ability to tolerate side-effects and the cost of the drug. Maintenance and consolidation treatment using lenalidomide post-ASCT is currently being studies by a number of groups.

ARE THERE PATIENTS WHO SHOULD NOT BE OFFERED ASCT?

Although there is clear benefit of ASCT for the majority of patients who suffer from myeloma, retrospective reports have suggested that there are a minority who may not benefit. A report by the IFM examined survival of patients post-ASCT based upon the level of their β2M and the presence of chromosome 13 abnormalities by fluorescence *in situ* hybridization (FISH).[29] What they found was that those with a β2M ≥ 2.5 and a chromosome 13 abnormality did poorly with a median survival of 25.3 months from diagnosis. Although a small number of patients, eight patients with these 2 risk factors and with an IgA isotype had a median survival of 11.7 months. These results were highly suggestive that a group of patients did poorly with short survival in-spite of have an ASCT. With further investigations on genetic aberrations in myeloma, recurring cytogenetic abnormalities detectable by FISH were found to be prognostic of outcome in patient with myeloma treated with conventional therapy.[30] The IFM has analyzed the influence of FISH testing in almost 1000 patients who received ASCT.[31] Patients with t(4;14) and del 17p had worse prognosis. A subgroup analysis of 100 patients with t(4;14) stratified based upon β2M and hemoglobin, revealed that those with t(4;14), an elevated β2M > 4 mg/L and hemoglobin < 100 g/L did particularly poorly with an EFS of 11 months and overall survival of 19 months. The other groups had superior survival although it still remained inferior to patients without t(4;14). What this implies is that there continues to remain significant heterogeneity even in patients with a poor risk karyotype by FISH. With the advent of novel drugs, the improvement in their survival may be due to the novel drugs and ASCT is likely having little impact in their outcome. This has led to questions regarding the benefit of high-dose melphalan in certain risk groups. The recent "Risk-Adapted Therapy (mSMART)" consensus statement by the Mayo group suggests that patients with high-risk myeloma can have stem cells collected, but no recommendation is made as to when they should (if ever) receive an ASCT. At this time, the community of physicians treating myeloma remains hesitant to recommend that certain groups of patients should never be offered ASCT partially because of the high tolerability of the procedure but also because of the fear of loosing one option in the treatment of this incurable disease. Regardless, recent improvements in overall survival of patients are primarily due to the use of novel agents.[6]

Patients with renal failure remain a particularly difficult group of patients to treat. Patients who present with renal failure now have an improved chance of recovering their renal function with the novel agents, particularly bortezomib which can produce rapid control of the myeloma.[32,33] Regardless, irreversible renal damage is not uncommonly encountered in patients with myeloma. It is recognized that treatment related morbidity and mortality will be significantly higher compared to patients with normal renal function.[34] Regardless patients with a good performance status may derive significant benefit and lower doses of melphalan may help attenuate the risk.[35]

CONCLUSION

Optimizing delivery of high-dose chemotherapy in patients with myeloma was the primary area of advance until the past decade. With the advent of novel agents, future research will be in determining how to most effectively integrate these agents before, during and after the transplant. The development of induction regimens have been the primary focus over the past several years. With maturation of this body of data it has become clearly evident that novel agents should be used prior to transplant. Further research is required in integrating these drugs in the peri-transplant and post-transplant setting. What will determine how novel agents are used in the future will be a combination of efficacy, convenience and cost. Regardless, the availability of novel agents has fortunately resulted in a paradigm shift from which there is no returning. Although the use of ASCT for myeloma remains well established, the increase in therapeutic options is leading to questions regarding its use for all patients with myeloma. There remains much to investigate regarding the role of ASCT in the treatment of patients with myeloma.

TAKE HOME MESSAGE

Previously, investigations into ASCT for myeloma centered upon the optimization of delivering high-dose chemotherapy as conditioning for myeloma. This centered on the knowledge that options were limited and the greatest survival benefit would be derived from the best possible response obtained with high-dose chemotherapy. These investigations determined the optimal conditioning regimen and the number of ASCT that could be tolerated and lead to benefit. With the advent of novel agents, there is an increased focus on the induction treatment to derive the best possible response prior to ASCT which may promote the highest rates of remission post-transplant. There is also an increased focus on the use of novel agents as a part of the conditioning regimen and as consolidation/maintenance. Regardless of this research, it has yet to be determined if any of these modifications will lead to a "cure" of myeloma. The cost of these novel agents and their side-effects profile will serve as limitations to the ability to use them ubiquitously. For this reason, further research is required to determine how to optimally use these agents to derive the most benefit yet be as cost-effective and convenient as possible. Risk stratification will guide the use of ASCT and the novel agents so that patients with higher risk disease may receive the most effective agents early, before their overall status compromises the benefit that can be derived. For patients with better risk myeloma, less intensive treatment may lead to the same survival benefit without the increased risk of more intensive treatment. As available option to treat myeloma increase, the importance of ASCT for all patients and subgroups of patients with myeloma is becoming less firm.

REFERENCES

1. McElwain TJ, Powles RL. High-dose intravenous melphalan for plasma-cell leukaemia and myeloma. Lancet 1983;2(8354):822-24.
2. Attal M, Harousseau JL, Stoppa AM, et al. A prospective, randomized trial of autologous bone marrow transplantation and chemotherapy in multiple myeloma. Intergroupe Francais du Myelome. N Engl J Med 1996;335(2):91-97.
3. Singhal S, Mehta J, Desikan R, et al. Antitumor activity of thalidomide in refractory multiple myeloma. N Engl J Med 1999;341(21):1565-71.
4. Richardson PG, Barlogie B, Berenson J, et al. A phase 2 study of bortezomib in relapsed, refractory myeloma. N Engl J Med 2003;348(26):2609-17.
5. Richardson PG, Blood E, Mitsiades CS, et al. A randomized phase 2 study of lenalidomide therapy for patients with relapsed or relapsed and refractory multiple myeloma. Blood 2006;108(10): 3458-64.
6. Kumar SK, Rajkumar SV, Dispenzieri A, et al. Improved survival in multiple myeloma and the impact of novel therapies. Blood 2008;111(5): 2516-20.
7. Kastritis E, Zervas K, Symeonidis A, et al. Improved survival of patients with multiple myeloma after the introduction of novel agents and the applicability of the International Staging System (ISS): An analysis of the Greek Myeloma Study Group (GMSG). Leukemia 2009;23(6): 1152-57.
8. Macro M, Divine M, Uzunhan Y, et al. Dexamethasone + Thalidomide (Dex/Thal) Compared to VAD as a Pre-Transplant Treatment in Newly Diagnosed Multiple Myeloma (MM): A Randomized Trial. Blood (ASH Annual Meeting Abstracts); 2006;108(11):57.
9. Harousseau JL, Mathiot C, Attal M, et al. Bortezomib/dexamethasone versus VAD as induction prior to autologous stem cell transplantion (ASCT) in previously untreated multiple myeloma (MM): Updated data from IFM 2005/01 trial. ASCO Annual Meeting Abstracts 2008;26: abstr 8505.
10. Cavo M, Testoni N, Terragna C, et al. Superior Rate of Complete Response with up-Front Velcade-Thalidomide-Dexamethasone Versus Thalidomide-Dexamethasone in Newly Diagnosed Multiple Myeloma is not Affected by Adverse Prognostic Factors, Including High-Risk Cytogenetic Abnormalities. Blood (ASH Annual Meeting Abstracts) 2008;112(11):1662.
11. Dispenzieri A, Rajkumar SV, Gertz MA, et al. Treatment of newly diagnosed multiple myeloma based on Mayo Stratification of Myeloma and Risk-adapted Therapy (mSMART): Consensus statement. Mayo Clin Proc 2007;82(3): 323-41.
12. Lacy MQ, Gertz MA, Dispenzieri A, et al. Long-term results of response to therapy, time to progression, and survival with lenalidomide plus dexamethasone in newly diagnosed myeloma. Mayo Clin Proc 2007;82(10): 1179-84.

13. Kumar S, Dispenzieri A, Lacy MQ, et al. Impact of lenalidomide therapy on stem cell mobilization and engraftment post-peripheral blood stem cell transplantation in patients with newly diagnosed myeloma. Leukemia 2007;21(9): 2035-42.
14. Kumar S, Giralt S, Stadtmauer EA, et al. Mobilization in myeloma revisited: IMWG consensus perspectives on stem cell collection following initial therapy with thalidomide-, lenalidomide-, or bortezomib-containing regimens. Blood 2009;114(9): 1729-35.
15. Richardson P, Lonial S, Jakubowiak A, et al. Lenalidomide, Bortezomib, and Dexamethasone in Patients with Newly Diagnosed Multiple Myeloma: Encouraging Efficacy in High-Risk Groups with Updated Results of a Phase I/II Study. Blood (ASH Annual Meeting Abstracts) 2008;112(11):92.
16. Moreau P, Facon T, Attal M, et al. Comparison of 200 mg/m^2 melphalan and 8 Gy total body irradiation plus 140 mg/m^2 melphalan as conditioning regimens for peripheral blood stem cell transplantation in patients with newly diagnosed multiple myeloma: Final analysis of the Intergroupe Francophone du Myeloma 9502 randomized trial. Blood 2002;99(3): 731-35.
17. Blanes M, de la Rubia J, Lahuerta JJ, et al. Single daily dose of intravenous busulfan and melphalan as a conditioning regimen for patients with multiple myeloma undergoing autologous stem cell transplantation: A phase II trial. Leuk Lymphoma 2009;50(2): 216-22.
18. Lonial S, Kaufman J, Torre C, et al. A Randomized Phase I Trial of Melphalan + Bortezomib as Conditioning for Autologous Transplant for Myeloma: The Effect of Sequence of Administration. Blood (ASH Annual Meeting Abstracts) 2008;112(11): 3332.
19. Roussel M, Huynh A, Moreau P, et al. Bortezomib (BOR) and High Dose Melphalan (HDM) as Conditioning Regimen Before Autologous Stem Cell Transplantation (ASCT) for De Novo Multiple Myeloma (MM): Final Results of the IFM Phase II Study VEL/MEL. Blood (ASH Annual Meeting Abstracts) 2008;112(11):160.
20. Child JA, Morgan GJ, Davies FE. et al. High-dose chemotherapy with hematopoietic stem-cell rescue for multiple myeloma. N Engl J Med 2003;348(19): 1875-83.
21. Barlogie B, Jagannath S, Desikan KR, et al. Total therapy with tandem transplants for newly diagnosed multiple myeloma. Blood 1999;93(1): 55-65.
22. Attal M, Harousseau JL, Facon T, et al. Single versus double autologous stem-cell transplantation for multiple myeloma. N Engl J Med 2003;349(26): 2495-502.
23. Alvares CL, Davies FE, Horton C, et al. The role of second autografts in the management of myeloma at first relapse. Haematologica 2006;91(1): 141-42.
24. San-Miguel J, Harousseau JL, Joshua D, Anderson KC. Individualizing treatment of patients with myeloma in the era of novel agents. J Clin Oncol 2008;26(16): 2761-66.
25. Greipp PR, San Miguel J, Durie BG, et al. International staging system for multiple myeloma. J Clin Oncol 2005;23(15): 3412-20.
26. Berenson JR, Crowley JJ, Grogan TM, et al. Maintenance therapy with alternate-day prednisone improves survival in multiple myeloma patients. Blood 2002;99(9): 3163-68.
27. Attal M, Harousseau JL, Leyvraz S, et al. Maintenance therapy with thalidomide improves survival in patients with multiple myeloma. Blood 2006;108(10): 3289-94.
28. Spencer A, Prince HM, Roberts AW, et al. Consolidation therapy with low-dose thalidomide and prednisolone prolongs the survival of multiple myeloma patients undergoing a single autologous stem-cell transplantation procedure. J Clin Oncol 2009;27(11): 1788-93.
29. Facon T, Avet-Loiseau H, Guillerm G, et al. Chromosome 13 abnormalities identified by FISH analysis and serum beta-2-microglobulin produce a powerful myeloma staging system for patients receiving high-dose therapy. Blood 2001;97(6):1566-71.

30. Fonseca R, Blood E, Rue M, et al. Clinical and biologic implications of recurrent genomic aberrations in myeloma. Blood 2003;101(11):4569-75.
31. Avet-Loiseau H, Attal M, Moreau P, et al. Genetic abnormalities and survival in multiple myeloma: The experience of the Intergroupe Francophone du Myelome. Blood 2007;109(8):3489-95.
32. Dimopoulos MA, Kastritis E, Rosinol L, et al. Pathogenesis and treatment of renal failure in multiple myeloma. Leukemia 2008;22(8):1485-93.
33. Chanan-Khan AA, Kaufman JL, Mehta J, et al. Activity and safety of bortezomib in multiple myeloma patients with advanced renal failure: A multicenter retrospective study. Blood 2007;109(6):2604-06.
34. San Miguel JF, Lahuerta JJ, Garcia-Sanz R, et al. Are myeloma patients with renal failure candidates for autologous stem cell transplantation? Hematol J 2000;1(1): 28-36.
35. Raab MS, Breitkreutz I, Hundemer M, et al. The outcome of autologous stem cell transplantation in patients with plasma cell disorders and dialysis-dependent renal failure. Haematologica 2006;91(11):1555-58.

Chapter 3

Role of Autologous Stem Cell Transplantation in Hematological Malignancies

Lalit Kumar, Deepak Dabkara, Ajay Gogia, Deepanjan Panda

SUMMARY

High dose chemotherapy followed by autologous stem cell transplantation (ASCT) has been in use since past two decades. Its role has been clearly defined in young patients of multiple myeloma without significant co-morbidities and chemosensitive relapse Hodgkin's and non-Hodgkin's lymphoma. For many other hematological and solid malignancies single center data is promising. This is also being explored for a number of nonmalignant conditions particularly autoimmune diseases. While the morbidity and mortality of ASCT has come down significantly in the past decade, relapse continues to be a major cause of failure. Identification of patients at high-risk of relapse and use of novel approaches to reduce the relapse risk are likely to be areas of research in future studies.

KEYWORDS

Autologous stem cell transplantation, Acute myeloblastic leukemia, Hodgkin's lymphoma, Non-Hodgkin's lymphoma, Multiple myeloma

INTRODUCTION

Autologous stem cell transplantation (ASCT) is currently a standard treatment for young patients of multiple myeloma without major co-morbidities, Hodgkin's and non-Hodgkin's lymphoma with chemo-sensitive relapse and high-risk/advanced neuroblastoma. In addition, ASCT is being used for treatment of acute myeloid leukemia, poor risk/relapsed germ cell tumors and many other solid tumors. The morbidities and mortality due to ASCT have come down significantly in the past few years due to improved supportive care, use of peripheral blood derived stem cells (in place of bone marrow) and proper case selection. We here review role of ASCT in hematological malignancies.

EVALUATION

Potential recipients of ASCT are evaluated for the underlying disease (remission status) and for any major organ dysfunction. This includes assessment of cardiac, renal, lung and liver function. Evaluation for viral infections (hepatitis B and C, CMV, etc.) is also done. Patients with moderate to severe major organ dysfunction or those with active infection are at high risk for transplant-related complications or reactivation of infection and are not suitable candidates for ASCT. It is important to carefully record details of chemotherapeutic drugs received in past and any history of major infection such as fungal/tubercular and allo-immunization to platelets.[1]

Stem Cell Mobilization

For ASCT, peripheral blood stem cells are harvested as a routine, rarely in a few patients bone marrow harvest may need to be done due to technical reasons or if PB stem cells collection is not adequate. For this purpose, PB stem cells have to be mobilized from the BM. This is done by giving to patient granulocyte colony-stimulating factor (G-CSF) in a dose of 10 μg/kg/day in 2 divided doses, subcutaneously for 4-5 days. On day 5-6, PB stem cells are collected by leukapheresis using an apheresis (cell separator) machine. A PB-stem cell harvest contains substantially more CD34+ cells and 10 times more lymphocytes than a BM harvest. The recovery of neutrophil and platelet numbers is quicker in recipients of PB-derived stem cells than in those receiving BM. Neither anesthesia nor hospitalization is required. Once harvested, the PB stem cells are cryopreserved at – 80°C using 7.5% dimethyl sulphoxide (DMSO) or liquid nitrogen.[2] The patient is then administered high dose chemotherapy (HDCT). Depending upon the half-life of the chemotherapeutic drugs used, the PB stem cells can be re-infused either after 24 hours (melphalan) or a longer interval (5-7 days).

The precise number of PB stem cells (mononuclear cells) required is not known. In practice, for BM, approximately 3×10^8 nucleated cells/kg of the recipient's body weight and for PB 5×10^8 mononuclear cells/kg or $\geq 2 \times 10^6$/kg CD34+ cells (marker for stem cells) are harvested.

Some centers use cyclophosphamide 2-4 Gm/m^2 followed by G-CSF. Patient is monitored daily with blood counts. Once total WBC count is about 2000/cmm, stem cell harvest is initiated and continued on alternate day basis till target number of stem cells is collected. In most patients 1-2 harvests may be adequate, about 10-20% of patients may need ≥ 3 harvests to achieve the target number. Recently, Stiff et al (2009) have reported use of Plerixafor, (a bicyclam molecule which is a reversible inhibitor of hemopoietic stem cell adhesion to stromal cells mediated through CXCR4 binding to stromal derived factor -1-α) with G-CSF for mobilization of stem cells in patients of NHL and myeloma who were heavily pretreated. Adequate number of stem cells (2×10^6/kg) could be achieved in 96% of patients.[3] This molecule may be of value in patients who are heavily pre-treated and in whom adequate number of stem cells is not mobilized with G-CSF alone.

The primary concern with autologous HSCT is relapse due to re-infusion of malignant cells along with progenitor cells. Various methods including *in vitro* treatment with chemotherapeutic drugs or monoclonal antibodies have been used to remove the contaminating tumor cells (purging). Retrospective analyses suggest that purging leads to decreased rates of relapse in patients with acute myeloblastic leukemia (AML) and non-Hodgkin lymphoma (NHL).

PREPARATORY REGIMEN

Prior to ASCT, the patient's own BM is destroyed by giving high dose chemotherapy (HDCT) with or without total body irradiation (TBI). This is done to (i) eradicate the malignant cells (cytoreduction) and to (ii) possibly to create space (niche) within the BM microenvironment to allow engraftment of stem cells. For autologous transplantation immunosuppression is not required and the preparatory regimen is used to provide maximum dose intensity with a goal of eradicating the malignancy. In earlier period, most patients have received cyclophosphamide and TBI (Cy-TBI) as the preparatory regimen. Fractionation of TBI (total dose 1200-1500 cGy) was used to reduce toxicity to the normal tissues. A combination of busulphan (4 mg/kg/day × 4 days; total 16 mg/kg) and cyclophosphamide (60 mg/kg/day × 2 days; total 120 mg/kg; Bu-Cy2) is effective for allogeneic and autologous SCT, and has been popular in the past two decades. The same regimens are used for autologous SCT.

For patients of myeloma, high dose melphalan 200 mg/m^2 is currently the standard. For patients with Hodgkin's and non-Hodgkin's lymphoma – BEAM (BCNU, etoposide, cytosine arabinoside and melphalan) or CVB (cyclophosphamide, VP-16 (etoposide) and BCNU) are commonly used. Radiation based preparatory regimens[4] used earlier are no longer popular in view of long-term toxicity of radiation.

STEM CELL INFUSION

After completion of the preparatory regimen, there is a 24-48 hours period (called rest period) prior to infusion of the stem cells. For patients undergoing ASCT the stem cells are removed from the deep freezer, thawed at room temperature in a water bath and re-infused into the patient. Some patients may experience nausea, dizziness or a suffocating feeling—all side-effects related to the use of DMSO for cryopreservation of stem cells. These patients require strict isolation after infusion (transplantation) of the stem cells.

Most centers use prophylactic antibiotics (quinolones—ciprofloxacin), antifungals (oral fluconazole or itraconazole) and antiviral drugs (oral acyclovir).

Complications Following ASCT

In addition to infections secondary to severe myelosuppression a number of other complications can occur (Table 3.1).

Table 3.1. Complications of autologous stem cell transplantation

• **Acute**
  − Infection
  − *Regimen-related complications*
    ♦ Gastrointestinal: Nausea/vomiting, diarrhea, mucositis:
    ♦ Pulmonary and cardiac disease
    ♦ Hemorrhagic cystitis disease
    ♦ Veno-occlusive disease
• **Late**
  − Relapse
  − Sterility
  − Myelodysplasia/Secondary leukemia

Infections

Infections can be divided into three categories based on the time of their occurrence after transplant. In the first 30 days, most bacterial infections are due to chemotherapy-induced neutropenia. Fungal infections tend to occur during the first 3-4 months after SCT. The commonly encountered organisms include *Candida species (C. albicans and C. tropicalis)* and *Aspergillus*. The risk of *Pneumocystis carinii*-induced interstitial pneumonia may be reduced to < 10% by chemoprophylaxis with oral trimethoprim–sulphamethoxazole given 2-3 times per week, starting after engraftment (when the neutrophils are >1000/cmm) and continued for 6-12 months. In patients allergic to sulphamethoxazole, pentamidine (300 mg) once a month can be given. In ASCT patients risk of bacterial infections diminishes with hematopoietic recovery. However, recovery of humoral and cell-mediated immunity may take 3-12 months; therefore, such patients may be at risk for viral infections, particularly *Varicella zoster*. Reactivation of *Mycobacterium tuberculosis* infection can also occur infrequently.

Mucositis

Oral mucositis is common in the second week after ASCT. Patients with grade III-IV oral mucositis may need parenteral opioids for pain relief and parenteral alimentation to maintain an adequate calorie intake. Spielberger et al in a randomized trial reported the use of recombinant human keratinocyte growth factor (pelifermin) to decrease mucosal injury. Both severity (grade III-IV, 63% *vs* 98%, p< 0.001) and the median duration of mucositis (6 days *vs* 9 days, p< 0.01) were significantly less in the group receiving pelifermin compared with placebo.[5]

In another study, the severity of oral mucositis was reduced following administration of amifostine in myeloma patients who underwent ASCT using highdose melphalan for conditioning.[6]

Pulmonary Complications

Diffuse pulmonary hemorrhage manifests as dyspnea (92%), fever (67%), cough (56%), hemoptysis (15%) and hypoxia. Pulmonary infiltrates are seen on chest X-ray and CT scan during the first 30 days after ASCT. This syndrome is probably related to pulmonary injury due to HDCT and is most frequently seen in patients who receive autologous HSCT. The condition seems to respond to corticosteroids.[1]

Engraftment Syndrome

A clinical picture similar to capillary leak syndrome may occur during the second or third week following engraftment. It is characterized by excessive weight gain, ascites and edema (similar to noncardiogenic pulmonary edema) and is associated with kidney and liver abnormalities, suggesting a common injury to multiple organs. The pathogenesis of this disorder is poorly understood; a pivotal contribution by circulating leukocytes is a possibility.[7] Treatment with prophylactic steroids may prevent the engraftment syndrome.

Hemorrhagic Cystitis

This occurs most often following the use of preparatory regimens containing ifosphamide or cyclophosphamide, which cause marked chemical inflammation of the bladder mucosa. Infection with a virus (polyoma, BK virus or adenovirus) has also been implicated. Its incidence varies from 7% to 70%. Mild cystitis (grade I, dysuria and microscopic hematuria) is self-limiting and occurs early (during or immediately after conditioning) and can be prevented with diuresis and 2-mercaptoethane sulphonate (Mesna). However, overt cystitis (grade > II, gross hematuria, clot retention, urinary tract obstruction and impairment of renal function) is clinically more important. This occurs late and has a protracted course requiring regular bladder irrigation and repeated cystoscopy, and is a cause of substantial morbidity. A variety of uroprotective measures including alkaline diuresis, frequent voiding, urethral catheterization and bladder irrigation and the use of Mesna reduces the risk of hemorrhagic cystitis.[8]

Veno-occlusive Disease

Veno-occlusive disease of the liver is a common regimen-related toxicity characterized by jaundice (serum bilirubin > 2 mg/dl), tender hepatomegaly, ascites and unexplained weight gain (> 2% of baseline body weight) within 20 days of HSCT.[9] The incidence varies from 15% to 25%, being lower in autologous compared with allogeneic SCT. The median time of onset is day 8-10 post-transplant (generally before day 21). The course may range from mild, reversible disease to severe disease associated with multi-organ failure with a poor prognosis. It occurs due to injury to the sinusoidal endothelial cells and hepatocytes with subsequent damage to the zone 3 central veins of the hepatic acinus. Early changes include deposition of fibrinogen, factor VIII and fibrin within the venular walls and sinusoids. As the process of venular micro-thrombosis, fibrin deposition, ischemia and fibrinogenesis advances, widespread zonal disruption leads to portal hypertension, hepatorenal syndrome, multiorgan failure and death.

Patients with elevated transaminases prior to ASCT, and those with persistent fever during the cytoreductive phase are at high-risk for developing severe disease. Management of mild/moderate disease requires fluid restriction and diuretics. Treatment of severe disease is unsatisfactory. Therefore, efforts have been directed towards its prevention by using drugs that interrupt the coagulation cascade or those that diminish the influence of thrombogenic factors. Richardson et al reported the use of defibrotide, a single-strand polydeoxyribonucleotide with fibrinolytic, antithrombotic and anti-ischemic properties. Complete resolution of severe disease was seen in 36% with a 35% survival at day 100. 27 Younger age, autologous HSCT and abnormal portal flow predicted survival whereas busulphan-based conditioning and encephalopathy predicted a worse outcome. Similar results with defibrotide have also been reported in children.[10]

CLINICAL RESULTS

Acute Myeloblastic Leukemia (AML)

Following induction chemotherapy 60-75% of patients with AML achieve complete remission (CR) (Table 3.2). This is followed by 3-4 cycles of consolidation chemotherapy with high dose cytosine arabinoside (15-18 g/m^2). AML is a heterogeneous disease with widely different risk for relapse following standard treatment. Cytogenetic abnormality and time to achieve CR are two important prognostic factors. In addition, age and a variety of molecular markers have been defined.[11] Table 3.3 gives various cytogenetic abnormalities. Morra et al[12] for the Italian Society of Hematology and Italian Group for Bone Marrow transplantation have recently described guidelines for clinical management of AML patients

Table 3.2: Response criteria in acute myeloid leukemia[12]

Response criterion	Neutrophils (ul)	Platelets (ul)	BM Blasts (%)	Other
Morpholgical CR	>1000	>100,000	<5	Transfusion Independent No EMD
Cytogenetic CR	>1000	>100,000	<5	Cytogenetics Normal, no EMD
Molecular CR	>1000	>100,000		Molecular negative NO EMD
Partial remission	>1000	>100,000	5-25	Blasts < 5%, if Auer rods positive

EMD—extramedullary disease, BM—bone marrow, CR—complete remission

Table 3.3: Cytogenetic molecular risk in acute myeloid leukemia

Risk	Pattern
Low risk	Inv (16)/ t (16;16); CBFB/MYH11
	* t (8;21); AML1/ETO
	Normal karyotype: NPM+,FLT3–
	Normal karyotype: CEBPA+
Intermediate	+8 (isolated)
	t (9; 11)
	Normal karyotype
High	Complex karyotype
	–7/7q;5/5q–
	t (11q21-23)/MLL;MLLampl; CALM/AF10
	Inv (3)/ t (3;3)
	t (6;9)
	t (9;22)
	t (8;16); inv (8)
	t (3;5)
	Normal karyotype: FLT3+

* Core binding factors leukemia, in the absence of KIT mutations

(other than acute promyelocytic leukemia). These are summarized in Tables 3.3 and 3.4 Breems et al in a prospective randomized trial evaluated role of autologous SCT vs chemotherapy for AML patients less than 60 years of age in CR1. patients who achieved CR after two courses of induction chemotherapy and who were not eligible for an HLA matched sibling transplant were randomized after a third consolidation cycle of chemotherapy to either autologous SCT or no further treatment.

No significant difference was observed in disease-free survival and overall survival between the two arms.[13]

Acute Promyelocytic Leukemia (APML)

AML with t (15;17) (q22;q12) is a molecularly defined disease entity. Current treatment strategies based on all transretinoic acid and anthracycline based induction, anthracycline based consolidation and maintenance therapy without any transplantation results in excellent CR (up to 90%) and overall survival (up to 85%). Even in high-risk subsets of APML the relapse rates does not exceed 20-25%. Hence stem cell transplant has no role in consolidation in first line treatment of APML. Nonrandomized studies show that autologous SCT can offer an effective salvage treatment when performed in second molecular remission.[14]

Autologous HSCT could be considered in AML patients in first complete remission, poor risk category, if HLA-matched sibling donor is not available. For patients with normal cytogenetics, allogeneic HSCT should be considered if the patient requires 2 cycles to achieve complete remission. Karyotypes (> 3 abnormalities), have poor CR and leukemia-free survival (LFS) rates with chemotherapy and should be

Table 3.4: Indications for HSCT in acute myeloid leukemia (AML)[12]

Myeloablative allogeneic SCT from a fully matched sibling donor	In CR1 to (i) All children with intermediate to high-risk cytogenetics (ii) To all adults with high-risk cytogenetics, under age 55 years without major co-morbidities (iii) To adults under 40 years without severe comorbidities, with intermediate cytogenetics with the exception of NPM1 mutant and FLT3 –ITD negative cases (iv) Achievement of CR1 after 2 courses of induction chemotherapy irrespective of cytogenetic risk. Provided they are under 55 years and do not have severe comorbidities.
Allogeneic SCT from an unrelated donor	All adults in CR1 under 30 years of age, (i) with high-risk cytogenetics, (ii) achieved CR after second course. Not recommended for patients above 50 years who achieved CR. Children with (i) AML-M7, (ii) complex cytogenetics, monosomy 7, (iii) a high level of MRD measured by flow cytometry after consolidation chemotherapy.
Alternative donors (e.g. mismatched-related, cord blood)	(i) At a center with active programme for adults without related or unrelated donor but have high-risk cytogenetics (ii) Children who are candidates for transplant as above but lack a donor.
Allogeneic SCT with RIC regimen	High-risk patients aged > 55 years OR with severe comorbidities.
Autologous peripheral blood SCT	Favorable (Low-risk): CR1: Not recommended CR2: Allogeneic SCT is choice, if match is not available or if allo-SCT can not be carried out due to practical reasons then autologous SCT can provide effective therapy. For patients aged < 60 years, eligible for high dose chemotherapy but who are not candidate for allogeneic SCT from a fully matched donor or lack a donor. Not recommended for children with Down syndrome. Time for transplant should be done within 6 months of achieving CR.

SCT—stem cell transplantation, MRD—minimal residual disease, RIC—reduced intensity transplant

considered for allogeneic HSCT. Many investigators prefer to transplant patients with intermediate risk cytogenetics such as +8, –Y, +6, Del 12p, normal karyotype if an HLA-identical sibling is available. Patients in the second CR or those with an untreated relapse can be cured with allogeneic HSCT with 3-year LFS rates of 22-30%. About 10-20% of patients with primary chemorefractory AML can be salvaged with allogeneic HSCT.

Thus, allogeneic SCT from an HLA-identical sibling remains treatment of choice for young patients with high-risk cytogenetics in CR1. Next best option is unrelated matched donor transplant. For those not having match, autologous SCT would be a reasonable option.

Acute Lymphoblastic Leukemia (ALL)

About 80% of children with good risk ALL are now cured with standard chemotherapy. Therefore, allogeneic HSCT is usually reserved for (i) children < 15 years of age with cytogenetic abnormalities such as t(4;11) and Philadelphia (Ph) chromosome, t (9;22), (ii) children in the second or third remission and (iii) young adults between 15 and 21 years of age who have a high leukocyte count at diagnosis and have the Ph chromosome. Such patients are considered at high-risk for relapse with standard chemotherapy. The best results for allogeneic SCT in ALL are reported in children and adults in first remission; the LFS is 60% and 52% respectively.[15] Allogeneic HSCT might also cure a proportion of patients (15%) with ALL in whom remission could not be achieved with conventional chemotherapy.[15]

Results with autologous SCT are not superior to chemotherapy alone in patients with high-risk ALL. For adult patients with Ph+ ALL, early allogeneic SCT from a sibling donor is the treatment of choice; 27-65% of patients in first CR achieve long-term survival. Survival decreases to 17% and 5% for those undergoing HSCT in the second and third remission, respectively. For Ph+ ALL, the current recommendation is to give induction chemotherapy with imatinib followed by allogeneic SCT if an HLA-identical match is available. Dhedin et al have reported results of an individual data based overview of three trials from the LALA Group. With intent to treat analysis, investigators compared 175 patients (age 15 to 50 years old without HLA identical sibling or 15-55 years age group with high-risk ALL) from the ASCT arm with 174 patients in the chemotherapy arm. ASCT was associated with a lower cumulative incidence of relapse (66% vs 78% at 10 years, p<.05) without significant gain in disease-free or overall survival.[16] A recent study by the PETHEMA group has compared the outcome of intensive chemotherapy, allogeneic or autologous SCT as post-remission treatment for 106 children with very high-risk ALL (age < 1 year, WBC $\geq 30 \times 10^9/l$ in B lineage ALL, $\geq 100 \times 10^9/L$ in T lineage ALL or t (9;22), t (4;11) or other 11q23 rearrangements and patients without these criteria but slow (> 25% blasts in bone marrow at day 35) response to induction therapy. Overall 100 (94%) patients achieved CR. Intention to treat analysis showed no difference in disease-free survival (DFS): Donor vs no donor, (45% vs 45%) and overall survival (48% vs 51%). Between autologous vs chemotherapy — DFS 44% vs 60% and OS-45% vs 57%. This study failed to prove better outcome with allogeneic SCT compared to autologous SCT and intensive chemotherapy.[17]

Myelodysplastic Syndrome (MDS)

Allogeneic HSCT is the treatment of choice for patients with International Prognostic Scoring System (IPSS) intermediate-2 and high-risk MDS. However, its use is limited because of the higher median age of patients at the time of diagnosis (70 years). For the small number of eligible patients, myeloablative allogeneic HSCT results in long-term EFS in 32-54%. Experience with reduced intensity conditioning HSCT in patients > 50 years of age is encouraging. In the CIBMTR study, in 384 patients > 50 years of age who received an HLA-identical sibling HSCT, the 3-year probabilities of survival were 32% and 39% with myeloablative and reduced intensity conditioning, respectively.[15] Autologous HSCT can be considered in selected patients who achieve CR following induction chemotherapy and do not have an HLA-identical donor. In a prospective study by de Witte et al 36 of 59 patients (61%) without a donor received autologous HSCT in their first CR. The 4-year DFS rates in patients with or without a donor were 31% and 27%, respectively.[18]

Chronic Myeloid Leukemia (CML)

Imatinib mesylate is now the treatment of choice for all newly diagnosed CML patients. It achieves complete cytogenetic response (Ph–metaphases) in 50-75% of patients at 12 months. Currently, allogeneic HSCT is considered for patients (i) who fail to achieve complete hematological remission after 3 months of imatinib therapy, (ii) who fail to achieve complete cytogenetic response after 12-18 months of imatinib therapy, (iii) who relapse after an initial response, and (iv) with advanced disease (accelerated phase/blast crisis). Many investigators also prefer to transplant younger patients (< 20-30 years of age), if an HLA-identical sibling is available. For CML patients in the chronic phase, following allogeneic HSCT, the 5-year LFS is > 50%.[15] Similar results have been reported from India.[19] In patients with accelerated phase and blast crisis, allogeneic HSCT results in DFS rates of 15-25% and <15% respectively.[15] CML appears to be most susceptible to the GVL effect. Patients who relapse after allogeneic HSCT can be treated successfully using donor lymphocyte infusion (DLI) without pretransplant conditioning. For patients with molecular or cytogenetic relapse of CML, the CR rate is 85-90%. These observations have led to the use of nonmyeloablative or less intensive allotransplants, especially for patients > 45 years of age. Patients may engraft with mixed chimerism which gradually converts to full donor chimerism with the use of DLI.

Chronic Lymphocytic Leukemia (CLL)

The median age at presentation of CLL patients is 65 years, 40% are < 60 years of age and 12% are < 50 years of age. A number of single center studies have reported the results of autologous SCT in younger patients with high-risk CLL. Treatment-related mortality is low (1-5%) with CR in 12-67% of patients. Allogeneic HSCT in CLL is associated with significant morbidity and mortality due to regimen-related toxicity, GVHD and Infection.[20] Recently, HSCT with reduced intensity conditioning has also been performed. In the CIBMTR study, among 949 patients who underwent HSCT for CLL, the 3-year probabilities of survival were 77% after autologous HSCT, 50% after allogeneic HSCT with myeloablative conditioning and 53% after HLA-identical Sibling SCT with reduced intensity conditioning.[15] At present, the experience with HSCT is small but it appears that allogeneic SCT could be considered in selected young patients using reduced intensity conditioning.[21]

Hodgkin Lymphoma (HL)

HDCT supported with autologous SCT is currently considered the standard of care for relapsed HL or HL refractory to primary chemotherapy. In the CIBMTR study, among the 5,219 patients receiving autotransplants for HD between 1998 and 2006, the 3-year probabilities of survival were 78% ± 1%, 69% ± 1%, and 49% ± 3% for patients in complete remission, in partial remission, and with chemoresistant disease, respectively.[15]

Currently, there is no evidence to suggest that autologous SCT is superior to conventional chemotherapy for patients with advanced HL responding to frontline therapy.

Allogeneic SCT for HD is generally performed in patients who experience disease relapse after receiving multiple lines of therapy or who have refractory disease and an available HLA-matched donor. The use of reduced-intensity conditioning regimens in these heavily pretreated patients allows for a graft-versus lymphoma effect with less regimen-related toxicity. Among 297 patients receiving HLA-matched SCT for HD between 1998 and 2006, the 3-year probabilities of survival were 39% ± 5% with myeloablative conditioning regimens and 38% ± 5% with reduced-intensity conditioning regimens. The corresponding probabilities of survival in the 138 recipients of unrelated donor HCT were 35% ± 7% and 46% ± 8%[15].

The EBMT collected data on 94 patients who received reduced intensity allogeneic SCT for HL. Nearly 50% had a failed previous autologous SCT. The 3-year overall, progression-free survival and transplant-related mortality rates were 45%, 35% and 18%, respectively. There appears to be evidence for a GVL effect in these studies[22] however, at present, allogeneic SCT for HL must be considered experimental.

Non-Hodgkin Lymphoma

Autologous SCT is currently recommended for the treatment of patients with diffuse large B cell who have relapsed and have achieved a second

CR or good partial response following salvage chemotherapy. Lazarus et al for the Center for International Blood and Marrow Transplant Research (CIBMTR) has analyzed the results of patients reported to CIBMTR between 1990 and 2000. They compared autologous HCT (Bone marrow/ peripheral blood) outcome in 805 NHL patients aged ≥ 55 years to 1949 NHL patients < 55 years according to histology (indolent vs aggressive (follicular grade III, DLBC, immunoblastic lymphoma). For indolent histology, DFS and OS rates at 5 years favored younger patients, 37% vs 29% and 60% vs 54%, respectively. Transplant related mortality (TRM) was 8% vs 7% (p = ns). Similarly, for aggressive histology corresponding DFS and OS rates at 5 years were superior in younger patients 32% vs 19% and 47% vs 30%, respectively. TRM rates were significantly lower in younger patients (9% vs 15%). In aggressive histology group, apart from age, poor performance status, pretransplant chemoresistant disease, > 12 months interval between diagnosis and transplant and use of purging were associated with higher TRM. For the indolent histology patients significant co-variates for increased TRM included-use of BM rather than PB as the graft source, and TBI containing regimen.[23] Higher TRM has also been reported for patients > 55 years with aggressive histology in the European Group for Blood and Marrow transplantation (EBMT) data.[24]

Mantle cell NHL is an incurable B cell NHL with a median survival of 3 to 5 years. Results of CHOP (cyclophosphamide, adriamycin, vincristine and prednisolone) or similar regimens as front line therapy are poor, with a complete remission rates being achieved in < 25% of patients and responses lasting a median of 1 to 2 years. Recently with use of front line Rituximab (anti CD 20 monoclonal antibody) and hyper CVAD (hypercyclophosphamide, vincristine, adriamycin and dexamethasone) chemotherapy regimen higher CR rates were obtained. Use of ASCT in first remission resulted in the actuarial PFS and OS rates of 39% and 61%, respectively at median follow-up of six years in a recent study from MD Anderson Cancer Center.[25] Similar results have been reported by the Nordic lymphoma group (Geisler et al 2008); In this study, following rituximab based induction therapy and ASCT, among 60 patients at a median follow-up of 3.8 years, estimated overall, event-free and progression-free survival rates at six years were 70%, 56%, and 66%, respectively.[26] These results suggest that rituximab may be included both in induction therapy and in the preparatory regimens during the front line ASCT for mantle cell NHL.

Role of rituximab has also been demonstrated in relapsed/progressive aggressive CD20+ve NHL by the Dutch-Belgium Hematology – Oncology Cooperative Group (HOVON) in a prospective randomized trial. In this study, patients were randomized to receive DHAP (dexamethasone, Ara-C and cisplatin) — VIM (etoposide, ifosfamide and methotrexate) — DHAP chemotherapy with or without rituximab. This was followed by ASCT. At a median follow-up of 24 months, there was a significant difference in failure free survival (50% vs 24%, p < .001), and progression-free survival (52% vs 31%, p <. 002) in favor of rituximab arm.[27]

Limited data is available on the role of ASCT in Peripheral T cell lymphomas (ALK negative anaplastic large cell NHL, PTCL unspecified, angio-immunoblastic, nasal type extranodal NK/T cell, hepatosplenic and adult T cell leukemia/lymphoma) — a small subgroup of aggressive NHL histological subtypes. Preliminary, single center studies indicate long-term outcome for patients transplanted in first CR or PR. This is one area which needs further exploration.[28,29]

The consensus is that not all patients with aggressive lymphoma benefit when HSCT is incorporated into the frontline treatment. Patients with a high-risk International Prognostic Index (IPI) score seem to benefit from HDCT and HSCT as frontline treatment.[30-31] Most failures after autotransplants are due to relapse. Though the relapse rate is lower with allogeneic HSCT, the beneficial effect is negated by the high transplant-related mortality.

Transplantation for follicular lymphoma (FL) is generally reserved for patients with recurrent or aggressive disease. In the CIBMTR study among the 1,726 patients receiving an autotransplant for FL between 2000 and 2006, most had chemosensitive disease. The 3-year probabilities of survival were 73% ± 1% and 53% ± 5% for patients with chemosensitive and chemoresistant disease, respectively. Similar to CLL and HD, the use of reduced-intensity conditioning regimens is increasing for patients with FL. Among 641 patients with chemosensitive FL undergoing HLA-matched sibling HCT between 1998 and 2006, the 3-year probabilities of survival were 67% ± 3% and 71% ± 3% for those receiving myeloablative and reduced-intensity conditioning regimens, respectively. Corresponding probabilities in the 115 patients with chemoresistant FL were 70% ± 6% and 50% ± 8%.[15]

Autologous SCT as first line therapy for follicular (FL) NHL remains controversial. In multicentric, randomized French study 172 previously untreated FL patients were randomized for either immuno-chemotherapy (conventional) or high dose therapy followed by purged ASCT. Conditioning was performed with TBI and cyclophosphamide. At a median follow-up of 9 years, overall survival (OS) was similar in both arms, 76% vs 80% (HDCT). The 9-year progression-free survival (PFS) was higher in the ASCT than the chemotherapy group, 64% vs 39%, p.004. A PFS plateau was observed in the ASCT arm after 7 years. Secondary malignancies were more frequent in the ASCT arm, p < .01. The occurrence of a PFS plateau suggests that a subgroup of patients might have their FL cured by ASCT. TBI based regimen and purged BM may possibly be responsible for higher risk of secondary malignancies in ASCT arm.[32]

A number of strategies have been attempted to reduce post ASCT relapse. These include-induction of GVHD like reaction (using cyclosporine),[33] rituximab, interferon-alfa, interleukin-2 (as immuno-therapy) with hypothesis that immunotherapy early post-transplant might be effective in eliminating lymphoma cells that survived the preparatory regimen or that were infused with the stem cells, and thereby reducing relapse. However, no significant effect on PFS or OS has been observed in these studies.[34]

Multiple Myeloma

During the past decade, a number of randomized and nonrandomized studies in a large number of patients have confirmed that treatment with HD melphalan 200 mg/m^2 followed by ASCT is associated with CR rates of 40-60% with improved overall and event-free survival.[35] Transplant results from our center have been reported recently.[3] Following ASCT-79.6% of patients responded; complete response-36%, very good partial response-29.6%, and partial response-13.9%. CR rate was higher for patients with chemosensitive disease; 33 of 66 patients (50.0%) achieved CR compared to 7 of 42 patients (14.3%) with progressive disease, p < .01. Grade III-IV mucositis was the major regimen related toxicity. At a median follow-up of 70 months, the median overall and event-free survival is 71 and 42 months, respectively. Estimated overall and event-free survival at 60 months is 54.4% ± 0.05% (SE) and 49.3% ± 0.05 (SE), respectively. OS was significantly better for patients with pretransplant chemosensitive disease and those who achieved complete response following SCT.[36]

Higher CR rates achieved with SCT are possibly main mechanism responsible for superior outcome with ASCT compared to conventional chemotherapy.[37] The data on the effectiveness of ASCT in patients > 65 years of age and those with end-stage renal disease is limited. Higher VGPRs and CRs obtained with newer drugs, e.g. lenalidomide, bortezomib based combinations have led to the debate about the need of ASCT. It is arguable that with ASCT, these VGPR could not only be converted into higher CR rates but also duration of response is likely to be longer (depth).

Double or Tandem Transplant

A second autologous transplant within 1-6 months of recovery from the first transplant has been attempted to improve the CR rates and survival. Barlogie et al[38] first developed this concept of a second transplant. Non-randomized studies from their group and others reported a higher CR rate, improved overall and event-free survival with double transplant compared with single transplant. Attal et al for the French Group reported results of a first randomized trial; overall and event free survival was superior with double transplant compared to single transplant.[39] In this study, patients with less than a very good partial response (< 90% response) benefited more from a second transplant; overall survival of 11% at 7 years in the group receiving single vs 43% in the group receiving double transplant (p < 0.001). The benefit was not so significant (p = 0.70) among patients who had very good partial response (≥ 90% response) or CR after the first transplant.[39]

Kumar et al have most recently reported results of a meta-analysis of six randomized trials. Response rate was significantly better with double transplant (risk ratio = 0.79, 95% CI = 0.67 to 0.93 but with significantly higher increase in mortality (risk ratio = 0.79, 95% CI = 1.05 to 2.79). Overall survival was not improved for patients treated with tandem transplants.[40] Thus, presently, double transplant should be considered as an experimental approach for younger patients who achieve less than a very good PR with the first transplant or have high-risk features.

Allogeneic BMT

Allogeneic BMT has the potential to eradicate the myeloma clone due to graft *vs* myeloma effect. However, the role of conventional allogeneic BMT in myeloma remains limited due to (i) high transplant-related mortality from severe graft *vs* host disease (GVHD), (ii) availability of HLA-identical sibling donor in one third of patients, and (iii) age (median age at diagnosis is 55-58 years, about 5-10% of patients are young). Gahrton et al *for the European Bone Marrow transplant Registry (EBMT)* compared the outcome of patients transplanted between 1983-93 and 1994-98. The median overall survival was 10 months in the initial period and 50 months in the later period. This improvement was due to significant reduction in transplant-related mortality in the later period. During the past decade, a number of studies have explored the role of nonmyeloablative (mini-transplant or reduced intensity transplant (RIC) allogeneic transplantation from an HLA-identical sibling donor. Initially, ASCT followed by mini allotransplants is associated with a decreased risk of acute and chronic GVHD resulting in reduced transplantation-related mortality (15-20%). This approach allows transplant even for older patients up to 65 years of age.

Crowley et al for the EBMT registry have recently reported the outcomes of patients who underwent allograft using RIC with myeloablative conditioning (MAC). In a data set of 320 RIC and 196 MAC allografts performed between 1998 and 2002, RIC patients were older (51 vs 45 years), had progressive disease (28% vs 21%) and more had received a prior transplant (76% vs 11%). In addition, there was a longer time to transplantation and an increased use of peripheral blood and T-cell depletion. For RIC and MAC, respectively, the nonrelapse mortality (NRM) at 2 years was 24% and 37% (P = .002); overall survival, 38.1% and 50.8% (not significant [ns]); and progression-free survival (PFS), 18.9% and 34.5% (P = .001). On multivariate analysis, RIC was associated with a reduction in NRM (HR, 0.5), but this was offset by an increase in relapse risk (HR, 2.0).[42] Most recently, Rotta et al for the Seattle group have reported the long-term results on 102 patients who underwent initially autograft followed by RIC allgraft from an HLA-identical sibling. For conditioning, total body irradiation (TBI) – 2 Gys with or without fludarabine was used. Cyclosporin or tacrolimus plus mycophenolate mofetil was used for GVHD prophylaxis. 42% of patients developed grade II-IV acute GVHD and 74% had extensive chronic GVHD. Five-year nonrelapse mortality was 18% due to GVHD/infections. Among 95 patients with detectable disease-59 achieved CR. Five-year overall and progression-free survival was 64% and 36%, respectively.[43]

Donor lymphocyte infusions (DLI) have been shown to be effective for the treatment of relapsed myeloma after allogeneic stem cell transplantation. Molecular CR can be obtained in a relatively high proportion of myeloma patients who have achieved clinical CR after allogeneic transplantation.[44] Thus, the high morbidity and mortality associated with allogeneic SCT precludes its routine use and presently this treatment must be considered experimental. However, by virtue of the graft vs myeloma effect, allogeneic transplant results in cure in some patients and may be worth considering in young patients with high-risk myeloma who have an HLA-identical sibling donor.

Maintenance Therapy

To improve progression-free and overall survival, a number of nonrandomized and randomized studies have explored the role of maintenance therapy after induction therapy and/or stem cell transplant. Interferon-α, steroids (prednisolone or dexamethasone) with or without thalidomide have been used. Maintenance with Interferon-α was associated with modest benefit in progression-free survival but minimal improvement in overall survival.[45] However, in view of the toxicity and cost, this is no longer used. One randomized study compared 10 mg vs 50 mg oral prednisolone given on alternate days. There was significant improvement in the overall and event-free survival in the group receiving 50 mg prednisolone. However, the side-effects of long-term steroid therapy (e.g. weight gain, hyperglycemia, proximal myopathy, increased risk of infectious complications, osteoporosis, avascular necrosis, mood changes, etc.) preclude its routine use.[46] Results of three randomized studies are summarized in Table 3.5. Barlogie et al[47] used a complex protocol involving induction therapy, double ASCT, consolidation therapy and interferon-α plus dexamethasone maintenance (total therapy 2). Thalidomide was given from beginning of treatment until relapse or toxicity. In the IFM-99-02 trial,[48] patients with standard risk (β2 microglobulin < 3 mg/l), and/or no deletion 13 by FISH) were randomly assigned after double ASCT to receive (i) no further treatment or (ii) pamidronate or (iii) pamidronate + thalidomide. Recently, Spencer et al have reported results of an Australian study where patients after upfront ASCT were randomized to receive maintenance therapy with corticosteroids alone or corticosteroids plus thalidomide.[49]

We prefer to use low dose thalidomide (50 mg daily) for one year in patients who achieve CR or VGPR after transplant. This is an area which needs to be studied further. Although timing of ASCT in myeloma does not have a significant impact on overall survival outcomes for patients with multiple myeloma, transplant as initial treatment is preferred because it may prolong time in remission and avoid risk of myelodysplasia from conventional alkylating agent therapy.

Table 3.5: Maintenance therapy: Randomized studies

Author (ref)	# Pts (transplant)	Thalidomide Dose	Duration	PFS	OS	PN Grade 3-4 (%)
Barlogie et al[47]	668 (double)	Start = 400 mg/day	From onset until relapse	56% vs 44% @ 5 yr	65% vs 65% @ 5 yr	27
IFM 99-0[48]	597 (double)	200 mg/day (median)	Until relapse or toxicity (median 15 months)	52% vs 36% or 37% @ 3 yr	87% vs 74% or 77% @ 4 yr	7
Australian study[49]	243 (single)	200 mg/day	12 months	42% vs 23% @3 yr, p < .001	86% vs 75% @ 3 yr p < .004	10

CR—complete remission, PFS—progression-free survival, OS—overall survival, yr-year, PN—peripheral neuropathy @-at

CONCLUSION

Outcome of patients with hematological malignancies has improved significantly during the past two decades. This progress has been a result of better supportive care, improved understanding of the biology of disease and SCT and use of stem cell transplantation in proper perspective. While prospective, randomized trials have clearly defined the role of autologous SCT in multiple myeloma, and in salvage of patients with Hodgkin's and non-Hodgkin's lymphoma with chemosensitive relapse, its place need to be defined in upfront treatment for both poor risk Hodgkin's and poor risk, aggressive NHL. Presently, autolgous SCT appear to have limited role in myelodysplastic syndrome and chronic lymphocytic leukemia. It is likely that many novel targeted therapies, monoclonal antibodies and signal transduction inhibitors may be added in near future in management of above conditions. These developments along with risk stratification may allow/redefine the place of high dose chemotherapy and autologous stem cell transplantation and may provide the basis for individualized and tailored treatment.

REFERENCES

1. Kumar L. Haemopoietic stem cell transplantation: Current status. Nat Med J India 2007;20(3):128-37.
2. Raju GM, Kochupillai V, Kumar L. Storage of haemopoietic stem cells for autologous bone marrow transplantation. Natl Med J India 1995;8:216-21.
3. Stiff P, Micallef I, McCarthy P, Magalhaes-Silverman M, et al. Treatment with plerixafor in non-Hodgkin's lymphoma and multiple myeloma patients to increase the number of peripheral blood stem cells when given a mobilizing regimen of G-CSF: Implications for the heavily pretreated patient. Biol Blood Marrow Transplant. 2009 15(2):249-56.
4. Delgado FG, Maloney DG, Press OW, et al. Autologous stem cell transplantation for non-Hodgkin's lymphoma: Comparison of radiation based and chemotherapy —only preparative regimens. Bone Marrow transplant 2001;28:455-61.

5. Spielberger R, Stiff P, Bensinger W, et al. Palifermin for oral mucositis after intensive therapy for hematologic cancers. N Engl J Med 2005;352:1264-65.
6. Spencer A, Horvath N, Gibson J, et al. Australasian Leukemia and Lymphoma Group. Prospective randomised trial of amifostine cytoprotection in myeloma patients undergoing high-dose melphalan conditioned autologous stem cell transplantation. Bone Marrow Transplant 2005;35:971-77.
7. Mossad S, Kalaycio M, Sobecks R, Pohlman B, Andresen S, Avery R, et al. Steroids prevent engraftment syndrome after autologous hematopoietic stem cell transplantation without increasing the risk of infection. Bone Marrow Transplant 2005;35:375-81.
8. Leung AY, Mak R, Lie AK, Yuen KY, Cheng VC, Liang R, et al. Clinicopathological features and risk factors of clinically overt haemorrhagic cystitis complicating bone marrow transplantation. Bone Marrow Transplant 2002;29:509-13.
9. McDonald GB, Hinds MS, Fisher LD, Schoch HG, Wolford JL, Banaji M, et al. Veno-occlusive disease of the liver and multiorgan failure after bone marrow transplantation: A cohort study of 355 patients. Ann Intern Med 1993;118:255-67.
10. Corbacioglu S, Greil J, Peters C, Wulffraat N, Laws HJ, Dilloo D, et al. Defibrotide in the treatment of children with veno-occlusive disease (VOD): A retrospective multicentre study demonstrates therapeutic efficacy upon early intervention. Bone Marrow Transplant 2004;33:189-95.
11. Breems DA and Lowenberg B. Autologous stem cell transplantation in the treatment of adults with acute myeloid leukemia. Brit J Haematol 2007;130: 825-33.
12. Morra E, Barosi G, Bosi A, et al. Clinical management of primary non-acute promyelocytic leukemia acute myeloid leukemia: Practice Guidelines by the Italian Society of Hematology, the Italian Society of Experimental Hematology, and the Italian Group for Bone Marrow Transplantation. Haematologica 2009; 94(1):102-12.
13. Breems DA, Boogaerts MA, Dekker AW, et al. Autologous bone marrow transplantation as consolidation therapy in the treatment of adult patients under 60 years with acute myeloid leukemia in first complete remission: A prospective randomized Dutch-Belgian haemato-Oncology Co-operative Group (HOVON) and Swiss Group for Clinical Research (SAKK) trial. Br J Haematol 2005;128:59-65.
14. De Botton S, Fawaz A, Chevret S, et al. Autologous and allogeneic stem cell transplantation as salvage treatment of acute promyelocytic leukemia initially treated with all transretinoic acid: A retrospective analysis of the European acute promyelocytic leukemia group. J Clin Oncol 2005;23:120-26.
15. Pasquini M. CIBMTR summary slides 2005. CIBMTR (Centre for International Blood and Marrow Transplant Research) Newletter 2006;12:5-8.
16. Dhedin N, Dom,bert H, Thomas X, et al. Autologous stem cell transplantation in adults with acute lymphoblastic leukemia in first complete remission: Analysis of the LALA-85,97 and 94 trials. Leukemia 2006;20:336-44.
17. Ribera JM, Ortega JJ< Oriol A, et al. Comparison of intensive chemotherapy, allogeneic or autologous stem cell transplantation as postremission treatment for children with very high-risk acute lymphoblastic leukemia: PETHEMA ALL-93 trial. J Clin Oncol 2007;25:16-24.
18. de Witte T, Suciu S, Verhoef G, Labar B, Archimbaud E, Aul C, et al. Intensive chemotherapy followed by allogeneic or autologous stem cell transplantation for patients with myelodysplastic syndromes (MDSs) and acute myeloid leukemia following MDS. Blood 2001;98:2326-31.
19. Saikia TK, Parikh PM, Tawde S, Amare-Kadam PS, Rajadhyaksha S, Chhaya S. Allogeneic blood stem cell transplantation in chronic myeloid leukaemia-chronic phase following conditioning with busulphan and cyclophosphamide: A follow-up report. Natl Med J India 2004;17:71-73.

20. Crawley C, Szydlo R, Lalancette M, Bacigalupo A, Lange A, Brune M, et al. Outcomes of reduced-intensity transplantation for chronic myeloid leukemia: An analysis of prognostic factors from the Chronic Leukemia Working Party of the EBMT. Blood 2005;106:2969-76.
21. Gribben JG, Zahrieh D, Stephans K, Bartlett-Pandite L, Alyea EP, Fisher DC, et al. Autologous and allogeneic stem cell transplantations for poor-risk chronic lymphocytic leukemia. Blood 2005;106:4389-96.
22. Peggs KS, Hunter A, Chopra R, Parker A, Mahendra P, Milligan D, et al. Clinical evidence of a graft-versus-Hodgkin's-lymphoma effect after reduced-intensity allogeneic transplantation. Lancet 2005;365:1934-41.
23. Lazarus HM, Carreras J, Boudreau C, et al. Center For International Blood and Marrow Transplant Research (CIBMTR). Influence of age and histology on outcome in adult non-Hodgkin lymphoma patients undergoing autologous hematopoietic cell transplantation (HCT): A report from the Center for International Blood and Marrow Transplant Research (CIBMTR). Biol Blood Marrow Transplant 2008;14(12):1323-33.
24. Sweetenham JW, Pearce R, and Philip T, et al. High dose therapy and autologous bone marrow transplantation for intermediate and high grade non Hodgkin's lymphoma in patients aged 55 years and over. Results from the European group for bone marrow transplantation. The EBMT Lymphoma Working party, bone Marrow Transplant 1994;14:981-87.
25. Tam CS, Bassett R, Ledesma C, et al. Mature results of the MD Anderson Cancer Center risk-adapted transplantation strategy in mantle cell lymphoma. Blood 2009;113(18):4144-52.
26. Geisler CH, Kolstad A, Laurell A, et al. Long-term progression free survival of mantle cell lymphoma after intensive front line immunochemotherapy with *in vivo* purged stem cell rescue: A nonrandomized phase 2 multicenter study by the Nordic Lymphoma group. Blood 2008;112:2687-93.
27. Vellenga E, van Putten WL, van 't Veer MB, et al. Rituximab improves the treatment results of DHAP-VIM-DHAP and ASCT in relapsed/progressive aggressive CD20+ NHL: A prospective randomized HOVON trial. Blood 2008;111(2):537-43.
28. Chen AI, McMillan A, Negrin RS, et al. Long-term results of autologous hematopoietic cell transplantation for peripheral T cell lymphoma: The Stanford experience. Biol Blood and Marrow trans 2008;14:741-47.
29. Paolo C, Lucia F and Anna D, et al. Hematopoietic stem cell transplantation in peripheral T cell lymphomas. Leuk and Lymphoma 2007;48(8):1496-1501.
30. Strehl J, Mey U, Glasmacher A, et al. High dose chemotherapy followed by autologous stem cell transplantation as first line therapy in aggressive non-Hodgkin's lymphoma: A meta-analysis. Haematologica 2003;88:1304-15.
31. Schmitz N, Buske C and Gisselbrecht, C, et al. Autologous stem cell transplantation in lymphoma. Sem Hematol 2007;44:234-45.
32. Gyan E, Foussard C, Bertrand P, et al. Groupe Ouest-Est des Leucémies et des Autres Maladies du Sang (GOELAMS). High-dose therapy followed by autologous purged stem cell transplantation and doxorubicin-based chemotherapy in patients with advanced follicular lymphoma: A randomized multicenter study by the GOELAMS with final results after a median follow-up of 9 years. Blood 2009;113(5):995-1001.
33. Bolaños-Meade J, Garrett-Mayer E, Luznik L, et al. Induction of autologous graft-versus-host disease: Results of a randomized prospective clinical trial in patients with poor risk lymphoma. Biol Blood Marrow Transplant. 2007;13(10):1185-91.
34. Thompson JA, Fisher RI, Le Blanc M, et al. Total body irradiation, etoposide, cyclophosphamide and autologous peripheral blood stem cell transplantation followed by randomization to therapy with interleukin-2 versus observation for

patients with non-Hodgkin's lymphoma: Results of a phase III randomized trial by the Southwest Oncology Group (SWOG 9438). Blood 2008;111:4048-54.
35. Kumar L, Vikram P, Kochupillai V. Recent advances in the management of multiple myeloma. Natl Med J India 2006;19:80-89.
36. Kumar L, Ghosh J, Ganessan P, Gupta A, Hariprasad R, Kochupillai V. High-dose chemotherapy with autologous stem cell transplantation for multiple myeloma: What predicts the outcome? Experience from a developing country. Bone Marrow Transplant 2009;43:481-89.
37. Harousseau JL, Attal M, and Loiseau HA. The role of complete response in myeloma. Blood 2009, (Epub ahead of print).
38. Barlogie B, Jagannath S, Vesole DH, et al. Superiority of tandem autologous transplantation over standard therapy for previously untreated multiple myeloma. Blood 1997;89:789-93.
39. Attal M, harousseau JL, Facon T, et al. Single versus double autologous stem cell transplantation for multiple myeloma. N Eng J Med 2003;349:2495-2502.
40. Kumar A, kharfan-darbaja MA, Glasmachar A and Djulbegovic B. Tandem versus single autologous hematopoietic cell transplantation for the treatment of multiple myeloma: A systemic review and meta-analysis. J Natl Cancer Inst 2009; 101:100-06.
41. Gahrton G, Svensson H, cavo M, et al. Progress in allogeneic bone marrow and peripheral blood stem cell transplantation for multiple myeloma: A comparison between transplants performed between 1983-93 and 1994-98 at European Group for Blood and Marrow Transplantation centres. Br J Haematol 2001;113:209-16.
42. Crawley C, Iacobelli S, Björkstrand B, et al Reduced-intensity conditioning for myeloma: Lower nonrelapse mortality but higher relapse rates compared with myeloablative conditioning. Blood 2007;109(8):3588-94.
43. Rotta M, Storer BE, Sahebi F, et al. Long-term outcome of patients with multiple myeloma after autologous hematopoietic cell transplantation and nonmyeloablative allografting. Blood 2009;113(14):3383-91.
44. Kröger N, Badbaran A, Lioznov M, Post-transplant immunotherapy with donor-lymphocyte infusion and novel agents to upgrade partial into complete and molecular remission in allografted patients with multiple myeloma. Exp Hematol 2009;37(7):791-8. Epub 2009 May 31.
45. Myeloma Trialist's Collaborative Group. Interferon as therapy for multiple myeloma: An individual patient data overview of 24 randomized trials and 4012 patients. Br JHaematol 2001;113:1020-34.
46. Berenson JR, Crowley JJ, Grogan TM, Zangmeister J, Briggs AD, Mills GM, et al. Maintenance therapy with alternate-day prednisone improves survival in multiple myeloma patients. Blood 2002;99:3163-68.
47. Attal M, Harousseau JLLeyvraz S, et al. Maintenance therapy with thalidomide improves survival in multiple myeloma patients. Blood 2006;108(10):3289-94.
48. Barlogie B, Tricot G, Anaissie E, et al. Thalidomide and hematopoietic-cell transplantation for multiple myeloma. N Engl J Med 2006;354:1021-30.
49. Spencer A, Prince HM, Roberts AW, et al Consolidation therapy with low dose thalidomide and prednisolone prolongs the survival of multiple myeloma patients undergoing a single autologous stem-cell transplantation procedure J Clin Oncol 2009;27:1788-93.

Note: Part of this review has been taken from a previously published article Kumar L. Haemopoietic stem cell transplantation: Current status. Nat Med J India 2007;20(3): 128-37.

Chapter 4

Evidence-based Management of Fever in the Neutropenic Patient

Matthew D Seftel

SUMMARY

The febrile neutropenic episode (FNE) is a medical emergency, primarily because of the attendant risks of severe infection and mortality. Infection, particularly bacterial in nature, is the most important cause of FNE, although other causes exist, depending on host, disease, and therapy related factors. As the spectrum of pathogens varies depending on both the clinical and geographic circumstances, the provision of universal recommendations for antimicrobial therapy is challenging. However, there are unifying principles in the management of FNE that are helpful in guiding therapeutic decisions. Using a case-based approach in a patient with acute leukemia, the following controversies regarding the management of FNE are discussed: The role of prophylactic antibacterial antimicrobials, the management of febrile patients in the out-patient setting, and the choice of initial antimicrobials.

KEYWORDS

Fever, Infection, Neutropenia, Cancer

Case: A 43-year-old man with newly diagnosed acute myeloid leukemia (AML) develops an oral temperature of 39.1°C on day 14 of his first cycle of remission induction chemotherapy. He has no significant past medical history. Antileukemic therapy consisted of daunorubicin and cytarabine ("7 plus 3"). He was not receiving granulocyte colony stimulating factor (GCSF) therapy. His prophylactic antimicrobials consist of daily oral ciprofloxacin, acyclovir, and fluconazole.

INTRODUCTION

According to widely used clinical guidelines, fever is defined as single temperature of > 38.3°C (101.3°F), or > 38.0°C (100.4°F) that continues for more than one hour.[1] There are some important caveats when using this definition during clinical assessments of patients: Firstly, some neutropenic patients with infection may not develop fever, especially patients tasking corticosteroids or antipyretics, or patients whose clinical infection is paradoxically heralded by hypothermia. Neutropenic patients with concomitant mucositis may have a disproportionately elevated oral temperature, resulting in a false positive documentation of systemic fever.[2]

In patients with mucositis, measurement of temperature by other means is recommended, such as via the tympanic route. Neutropenia is defined by an absolute neutrophil count (ANC) of less than $0.5 \times 10^9/l$ or an ANC of $> 0.5 \times 10^9/l$ and $<1.0 \times 10^9/l$ with a predicted drop to less than $0.5 \times 10^9/l$.[1]

Data on management of FNE are largely focused on patients who have received myelosuppressive chemotherapy for malignant conditions rather than on individuals who have neutropenia from other conditions such as congenital neutropenia, aplastic anemia, and autoimmune disease. There are major differences between the latter group of "benign" neutropenic conditions and that of the neutropenia from myelosuppressive chemotherapy. Systemic chemotherapy agents, particularly in high doses, result in concomitant mucosal damage and exfoliation; this increases the risk of microbial translocation through a compromised gastrointestinal tract, may predispose to herpes simplex virus infection, and may hamper adequate enteral nutrition. The effect of concomitant mucositis is seen most obviously in patients undergoing remission induction therapy for acute leukemia such as the case under discussion, and in patients undergoing myeloablative blood and marrow transplantation (BMT). Apart from mucositis, oncology patients may have disrupted integument (e.g. from concomitant surgery, radiation, or the underlying tumor itself), indwelling medical equipment [e.g. central venous access devices (CVADs) and intra-cisternal reservoirs] and be may taking other therapeutic agents that suppress immunity such as corticosteroids or monoclonal antilymphocyte antibodies. In diseases that primarily cause hematopoietic failure, particularly the leukemias, there may already profound quantitative and qualitative defects in phagocytic function even before chemotherapy is administered.

In the era of myelosuppressive systemic chemotherapy, FNE is a common complication. The frequency of FNE depends on the nature of the disease being treated, the choice of therapeutic regimen, as well as host factors that may influence innate immunity. For the "7 plus 3" regimen, FNE is virtually universal,[3-6] with an infection-related mortality risk in the region of 11 to 15.6%.[4,5]

INITIAL MANAGEMENT

The primary step in the management of a patient with suspected FNE is a detailed history and physical examination, with specific and careful attention to the presence of tachypnea, tachycardia, hypotension, and possible sources of infection. Particular attention should be paid to indwelling devices such as CVADs and urinary catheters. Laboratory analyses are essential in order to document the presence and degree of neutropenia, coincident cytopenias, and to establish whether complications have ensued, such as electrolyte deficiencies and renal or hepatic compromize. Specimens for blood cultures should be obtained from both peripheral blood and central venous access devices and inoculated into both aerobic and anaerobic media. Chest radiography should be performed when respiratory symptoms are present. However, whether a chest X-ray is indicated in the absence of thoracic symptoms or signs remains arguable.[1] Serum lactic acid may be a useful marker severity of the FNE, particularly whether patients are at risk of progressing to septic shock.[7]

> He reports a four day history of diffuse oral ulceration with progressive difficulty eating and drinking. He also reports a one day chills and rigors. He has no known drug allergies. Physical examination reveals an alert man with a pulse of 108/minute, supine blood pressure of 102/72 mm Hg, and respiratory rate of 24/min. Significant orthostatic hypotension is present, with a drop in blood pressure to 82/58 mm Hg on standing. Oxygen saturation is 95% in room air. There is no sinus tenderness. A tunneled CVAD is present in the left subclavian vein; the tunnel and exit site are free of signs of infection. Oropharyngeal region reveals extensive mucositis, with several areas of ulceration. Respiratory, cardiovascular, and abdominal examinations are unremarkable. No rashes are noted.
> Relevant laboratory tests reveal an absolute neutrophil count of $0.1 \times 10^9/l$, with platelet count of $8 \times 10^9/l$ and hemoglobin of 104g/l. Serum creatinine was 131umol/l. Blood cultures were drawn from both the CVAD and a peripheral venous site. He was given a 1000 ml intravenous saline bolus.

RISK STRATIFICATION

Patients with FNE are heterogeneous with respect to their risk of serious adverse outcomes. An ability to stratify patients based on level of infection-related risk would allow selected patients to receive oral antimicrobials and/or out-patient based therapy for their FNE.[6] The 2002 IDSA guidelines list a group of conditions that predict low-risk for severe infection, hence allowing delivery of out-patient based care.[1] Key criteria that would permit safe out-patient therapy include: Duration of neutropenia that is expected to be short (less than five days); absence of hemodynamic instability; organ failure, or pneumonia; a compliant individual; immediate access to medical care available in the event of clinical deterioration; the presence of an informed caretaker in order to monitor the patient.[1]

Alternatively, a weighted scoring system devised by Multinational Association for Supportive Care in Cancer (MASCC)[8] is a validated method for predicting risk of serious infection-related events. A score of ≥ 21 using the MASCC scoring system is indicative of "low-risk" status, and has been shown to predict patients who can be discharged early and subsequently receive oral antimicrobials at home. The MASCC score is available via the IDSA guidelines,[1] and more recently has become available for use on software for desktop and handheld computers.[10] For the AML patient described above, the MASCC score was 18. Not surprisingly, he would thus be classified as being "high-risk" for serious complications from FNE.[8]

INITIAL ANTIBACTERIAL THERAPY

Empirical antimicrobials are indicated in the initial management of patients with FNE. Choice of antibiotic should be guided by a detailed clinical assessment of the patient as well as knowledge of the local institution's and region's spectrum of pathogens and their respective antibiotic sensitivities. In the era of widespread use of CVADs and fluoroquinolone prophylaxis, gram-positive organisms are currently the predominant group recovered in blood cultures specimens.[1,3-5] However, the relatively high frequency of gram-positive bacteria is not uniform: In a recent study from Israel, gram-negative bacteria continue to be the more frequently detected pathogens.[11] Thus, knowledge of local epidemiology is an important element in deciding on initial antibacterial therapy.

For selected "low-risk" patients, (as described in the section on risk stratification) the oral antibiotic regimens supported by published evidence include amoxicillin-clavulanate in combination with ciprofloxacin,[12-14] and more recently, single agent moxifloxacin.[15] A meta-analysis of randomized trials comparing oral versus intravenous treatment for FNE in cancer patients supports the efficacy of oral antibiotics. Specifically, mortality and treatment failure rates were similar.[16] An important caveat is that the clinical trials that evaluated the safety and effectiveness of these oral antibiotics in low-risk patients specifically excluded patients already receiving fluoroquinolone prophylaxis. In addition, out-patient management still requires that patients be carefully evaluated on a daily basis, have easy access to hospital care if needed, are adherent to a therapeutic plan, and have sufficient support while taking antibiotic treatment at home. In many jurisdictions, it is possible that these conditions for safe out-patient antibiotic management cannot be met, and such patients would then require in-patient care.

For patients at high-risk of infection-related complications, including those already receiving antibiotic prophylaxis, the IDSA guidelines of 2002 recommend one of three choices: Dual therapy with an extended spectrum penicillin with an aminoglycoside; monotherapy with a carbapenem (imipenem, meropenem), or a fourth generation cephalosporin (cefepime). Vancomycin is recommended only in selected in four specific clinical circumstances: (i) CVAD related cellulitis or bacteremia; (ii) known colonization with penicillin- and/or cephalosporin-resistant pneumococci or methicillin-resistant *Staphylococcus aureus*; (iii) documentation of gram-positive bacteremia prior to further identification and susceptibility testing; (iv) hemodynamic compromise.[1] Since, the time of the widely used IDSA 2002 recommendations, several published studies support that modifications to these recommendations may be needed; such studies are discussed below.

Choice of Initial β-lactam Agent

In an attempt to clarify the best choice of initial anti-pseudomonal β-lactam agent, Paul et al[17] conducted a systematic review and meta-analysis of randomized trials that compared anti-pseudomonal β-lactam agents administered as empirical monotherapy for febrile neutropenia, with or without vancomycin. The authors found that cefepime was associated an increase risk of all-cause mortality, while the carbapenem antibiotics were associated with fewer treatment modifications (including addition of glycopeptides) compared to ceftazidime or other comparators. However, adverse events were more frequent with the carbapenem group, including a 94% increase in the risk of pseudomembranous colitis. Concerns about the safety of cefipime have continued to be raised. Another meta-analysis of randomized trials compared cefepime with other beta-lactam antibiotics: In the 57 trials analysed, all-cause mortality was higher with cefepime [risk ratio (RR) 1.26, 95% Confidence interval (CI) 1.08-1.49]. However, there were no significant differences in treatment failure, secondary infection, or adverse events.[18] Possible explanations for the excess mortality in the cefepime treated patients included the possibility of an unrecognized adverse event such as neurotoxicity, or the possibility that cefepime has suboptimal antimicrobial efficacy *in vivo* despite apparent efficacy *in vitro*.[18] The Food and Drug administration (FDA) issued an early communication that articulates concern about the safety of cefepime.[19] The controversy about cefepime remains an active one, and further communication about the safety of this drug is eagerly awaited. Until then, it is prudent for prescribers to be aware of the potential risks of cefepime, including the need for dose adjustments in renal impairment, and, wherever possible, to consider alternative antimicrobials.[20]

Piperacillin-tazobactam was not specifically recommended as a first line agent for in the 2002 IDSA guidelines.[1] However, there is increasing evidence that piperacillin-tazobactam is an excellent choice as first line antibacterial therapy.[17,21,22] In the multicenter trial by Bow et al, 528 patients undergoing chemotherapy for leukemia or BMT who experienced FNE were randomized to pipercillin-tazobactam or cefepime as initial therapy. Resolution of fever at 72 hours occurred in 57.7% and 48.3%, respectively. The trial demonstrated noninferiority for piperacillin-tazobactam at all time points studied. In multivariate analysis, piperacillin-tazobactam was independently associated with treatment success (odds ratio, 1.65; 95% CI, 1.04-2.64).[21]

Regarding the use of ceftazidime as monotherapy, the activity of this third generation cephalosporin may be incomplete against the *viridans streptococci* group. This is in contrast to other β-lactam agents such as piperacillin-tazobactam and the carbapenems.[1] *Viridians streptococci* are capable of causing a rapidly progressive sepsis syndrome; thus, appropriate treatment of this organism needs to be timely.[23] If the probability of recovering *viridans streptococci* is high, such as in situations of oropharyngeal mucositis, the addition of vancomycin to ceftazidime is recommended.

Aminoglycosides

Whether aminoglycoside use (in addition to β-lactam anti-pseudomonal agents) is required has been a matter of debate. As described by the 2002 IDSA guidelines, the advantage of dual β-lactam-aminoglycoside therapy rests in potential synergy between these agents and the reduction of emergent drug resistant strains during treatment.[1] However, arguments against the use of such combination therapy include a heightened risk of renal impairment.[1] Since the publication of the 2002 IDSA recommendations, Paul et al analyzed 47 randomized controlled trials of β-lactam monotherapy versus β-lactam-aminoglycoside combination therapy in the treatment of patients with FNE;[24] there was no difference in all cause mortality. However, for the outcome of treatment failure, there was a significant advantage with monotherapy. This advantage appeared to be isolated to trials that had compared different β-lactams, where the monotherapy arm generally used a broad spectrum β-lactam agent such as a carbapenem, piperacillin-tazobactam, or ceftazidime. Adverse events were significantly more common in the combination treatment group. Overall, there does not appear to be an advantage in treatment with β-lactam-aminoglycoside combination therapy as compared to β-lactam monotherapy.

Empirical Use of Glycopeptides

Based on the increasing prevalence of vancomycin resistant pathogenic bacteria, especially that of vancomycin resistant *enterococci* (VRE), the 2002 IDSA guidelines recommends the use of glycopeptide antibiotics such as vancomycin only in particular clinical scenarios, as listed earlier in this chapter.[1] Paul et al have demonstrated that empirical use of glycopeptides (compared to placebo or control) does not result in an improvement in all-cause mortality.[25] Not surprisingly, there is a greater need for antibiotic modifications in the control arm (RR 0.70, 95% CI 0.61-0.80), and secondary gram-positive bacterial infections are less frequent in the glycopeptide arm. Nephrotoxicity is more common with the addition of glycopeptides (RR 1.88, 95% CI 1.10-3.22). According to these data, the use of glycopeptides may be deferred until resistant gram-positive bacteria are identified. Several provisos to this advice exist. In centers with a high background incidence of penicillin resistant gram-positive cocci (especially *enterococci* and *viridans streptococci*), suspected or proven CVAD infection, known colonization with penicllin/cephalosporin resistant gram-positive organisms, and hemodynamic instability, the use of glycopeptides remains a potentially life-saving measure.[25,26] In an environment where there is a shifting spectrum of pathogens recovered in the neutropenic host, partnered with major changes in antibiotic sensitivities, the need for glycopeptides in the initial therapy of FNE is likely to evolve. It is thus necessary to regularly monitor clinical and microbiological outcomes in order to re-evaluate the need for frontline therapy with glycopeptides.

Role of Prophylactic Antibacterial Agents

The use of prophylactic antibacterials for the afebrile neutropenic cancer patient reduces the incidence of FNE. However, the risk of using such primary prophylaxis includes adverse events (e.g. hypersensitivity, myelosuppression), the generation of bacterial resistance in the host and surrounding environment, and the emergence of secondary fungal infections such as candidiasis. Furthermore, antibacterial prophylaxis was until recently thought not to offer a survival benefit.[1] Based on these significant limitations, the 2002 IDSA guidelines recommended against the generalized use of such prophylactic antibacterial agents, with the exception of the use of trimethoprim/sulphamethoxazole (TMP/SMX) for prevention of pneumocystis jirovecii infections. However, recent evidence suggests that antibacterial prophylaxis may reduce mortality, febrile events, and bacterial infections in selected patient groups.

As patients with acute leukemia or BMT recipients are expected to have a much higher risk of FNE, such patients stand to derive particular benefit from antibiotic prophylaxis.[27] A 2005 meta-analysis reviewed 95 trials, most of which had examined patients with hematological malignancy.[28] Fifty-two of these trials used quinolone prophylaxis. Antibiotic prophylaxis significantly decreased mortality compared with placebo or no treatment (RR 0.67, 95% CI, 0.55 to 0.81). When the analysis was restricted to studies of quinolone prophylaxis, all-cause mortality was reduced (RR, 0.52, 95% CI 0.35 to 0.77), as were infection-related mortality, fever, and infections. Following publication of this meta-analysis, at least two more randomized controlled trials in support of quinolone prophylaxis have been released. In a group of acute leukemia or BMT patients (whose neutropenia was expected to last more than seven days), levofloxacin prophylaxis, compared to placebo, resulted in a significant reduction in bacterial infections and febrile episodes [numbers needed to treat (NNT) 6 and 5, respectively]. There was also a reduction in death (NNT 43), although this last effect did not reach statistical significance (RR 0.54, 95% CI 0.25-1.16).[28]

Patients with lymphoma and solid tumors have a lesser degree and duration of chemotherapy related neutropenia. Hence, the benefits of primary antibacterial prophylaxis are likely to be smaller. In the SIGNIFICANT trial, Cullen et al exposed patients with these disease types to levofloxacin or placebo after chemotherapy.[29] Compared to placebo, bacterial infections and febrile episodes were significantly reduced (NNT 13 and 23, respectively), with no suggestion of improvement in all-cause mortality (relative risk reduction 0.67, 95% CI 0.32-1.38, NNT 138). In this study, hospitalizations were reduced by 27% (95% CI 10%-41%).

With the addition of these two recent publications that evaluated levofloxacin prophylaxis to the 2005 meta-analysis, the following conclusions can been made: In acute leukemia/BMT, the risk of death can be reduced with quinolone prophylaxis by 33% (95% CI 2-54%), NNT 55.[27] Febrile episodes are reduced by 22% (95% CI 17%-26%).[25]

In patients treated for solid tumors or lymphoma, quinolone prophylaxis reduces all-cause mortality by 49% (95% CI 3-73%).[25] As the overall incidence of infection related mortality in the solid tumor/lymphoma group is much lower, the number needed to prevent one death in the first month of therapy has been estimated to be 82. Febrile episodes are reduced by 26% (95% CI 20-43%). The estimated NNT to prevent one FNE is twenty-five.

A post-hoc analysis of the SIGNIFICANT trial suggested that the greatest benefit of quinolone prophylaxis is in cycle one of chemotherapy or in subsequent cycles only if FNE occurs with cycle one.[28] Thus, current evidence does offer support for the use of quinolone prophylaxis in solid tumor or lymphoma patients for cycle one of chemotherapy and on subsequent cycles only after a cycle one FNE.

It is important to account for the use of prophylactic myeloid colony stimulating factors (CSFs) that are now widely recommended in oncology patients receiving chemotherapy regimens whose likelihood of resulting in FNE is $\geq 20\%$.[6,29,30] These guidelines do not specify whether prophylactic antibiotics should be used or withheld. The use of CSFs may lessen the degree of benefit from prophylactic antibacterials.

Whether the combination of CSFs and quinolone antibiotics is more effective over either alone has not been extensively evaluated. In solid tumor patients scheduled to receive prophylactic quinolone antibiotics, the additional use of myeloid growth factors reduced febrile events in cycle one, but was later shown not to be cost-effective overall.[33,34] In a recent systematic review, Herbst et al compared the effectiveness of CSFs to antibiotics in cancer patients receiving chemotherapy. The authors found no evidence for or against antibiotics compared to myeloid growth factors for the prevention of infections in cancer patient.[35] A follow-up study published in abstract form used a Bayesian network analysis approach to compare two or more of the following four prophylactic measures: No prophylaxis, prophylaxis with antibiotics alone, prophylaxis using CSFs alone or dual prophylaxis using CSFs and antibiotics. In this analysis, the combination of antibiotics and CSFs was the superior strategy in the prevention of infections and infection-related mortality. Compared to antibiotics alone or CSF alone, clinically documented infections were significantly reduced (OR = 0.61, 95% CI 0.46-0.77).[36] This exploratory analysis supports the need for further clinical trials to examine the benefit of combination CSFs and prophylactic antibiotics versus either approach alone.

Regarding the potential development of antimicrobial resistance with antibacterial prophylaxis, Gafter-Gvili demonstrated that quinolone prophylaxis results in a small, statistically insignificant increase in colonization with quinolone resistant bacteria.[37] However, despite this observation, there in no evidence as yet to suggest that infections with quinolone-resistant organisms are increased. This meta-analysis supports the contention that the benefits of antibiotic prophylaxis are not outweighed by the risks of infection from antibiotic resistant bacteria. Future clinical trials, observational studies, and infection-control units should continue to monitor the incidence of quinolone resistant bacteria in an era of widespread use of quinolone antibiotics both within the oncology and BMT patient populations as well as in hospitals and communities in general.

Overall, in acute leukemia and BMT patients, the rational for use of prophylactic antimicrobials is strong, especially for the use of quinolones (rather than TMP/SMX). However, in patients with lymphoma and solid tumors, the evidence in favor of prophylactic antibiotics is less convincing, especially in an era where CSFs are used in highly myelosuppressive regimens.

> As initial therapy, intravenous piperacillin-tazobactam was commenced. Intravenous fluids were continued, and opioid analgesics were given for oral pain. Stenotrophomonas maltophilia was recovered from both central and peripheral venous culture bottles 24 hours after the initial testing. This organism was sensitive to both piperacillin-tazobactam and trimethoprim-sulphamethoxazole, but resistant to ciprofloxacin. The CVAD was removed. Fever defervesced after 96 hours of antimicrobial therapy (day 18 post-chemotherapy). Myeloid recovery occurred on day 23 post-chemotherapy. Piperacillin-tazobactam was continued for a total of 14 days. With knowledge of antibiotic sensitivities, the patient was discharged from hospital in complete remission, with a prescription to complete a further one week of oral amoxicillin-clavulanate.

CONCLUSION

Since the publication of the widely used IDSA guidelines in 2002, there have been several important randomized controlled trials and meta-analyses that influence clinical decision-making in the prevention and treatment of FNE. These data challenge our clinical strategies around the use of prophylactic antimicrobials and colony stimulating factors, the safety of oral antimicrobials for treatment of FNE, and the choice of initial antimicrobial therapy. The new version of the IDSA guidelines is expected to be published and disseminated in late 2009, and these guidelines are likely to reflect these changes in the evidence-based management of FNE.

REFERENCES

1. Hughes WT, Armstrong D, Bodey GP, et al. 2002 Guidelines for the use of Antimicrobial Agents in Neutropenic Patients with Cancer. Clin Infect Dis 2002;34:730-51.
2. Ciuraru NB, Braunstein R, Sulkes A, Stemmer SM. The influence of mucositis on oral thermometry: When fever may not reflect infection? Clin Infect Dis 2008;46:1859-63.
3. Madani TA. Clinical infections and bloodstream isolates associated with fever in patients undergoing chemotherapy for acute myeloid leukemia. Infection 2000; 28(6):367-73.
4. Cherif H, Kronvall G, Bjorkholm M, Kalin M, Hematol J. Bacteraemia in hospitalised patients with malignant blood disorders: A retrospective study of causative agents and their resistance profiles during a 14-year period without antibacterial prophylaxis 2003;4(6):420-26.
5. Hamalainen S, Kuittinen T, Matinlauri I, Nousiainen T, Koivula I, Jantunen E. Neutropenic fever and severe sepsis in adult acute myeloid leukemia (AML) patients receiving intensive chemotherapy: Causes and consequences. Leuk Lymphoma 2008;49:495-501.
6. Aapro MS, Cameron DA, Pettengell R, et al. EORTC guidelines for the use of granulocyte-colony stimulating factor to reduce the incidence of chemotherapy-induced febrile neutropenia in adult patients with lymphomas and solid tumours. Eur J Cancer 2006;42:2433-53.

7. Mato AR, Luger S, Alison LW, et al. Serum Lactic Acid (LA) as a Predictor of Septic Shock in Patients with Hematologic Malignancies (HM) Who Develop Febrile Neutropenia. ASH Annual Meeting Abstracts. Blood 2008;112:666.
8. Klastersky J, Paesmans M, Institut Jules Bordet, Centre des Tumeurs de l'Universite Libre de Bruxelles. Risk-adapted strategy for the management of febrile neutropenia in cancer patients. Support Care Cancer 2007;15:477-82.
9. Klastersky J, Paesmans M, Rubenstein EB, et al. The Multinational Association for Supportive Care in Cancer risk index: A multinational scoring system for identifying low-risk febrile neutropenic cancer patients. J Clin Oncol 2000;18: 3038-51.
10. Qx MD Hematology. Available at: http://www.qxmd.com/hematology/MASCC-Febrile-Neutropenia-Risk.php. Accessed February 27 2009.
11. Paul M, Gafter-Gvili A, Leibovici L, et al. The epidemiology of bacteremia with febrile neutropenia: Experience from a single center, 1988-2004. Isr Med Assoc J 2007;9:424-29.
12. Kern WV, Cometta A, De Bock R, Langenaeken J, Paesmans M, Gaya H. Oral versus intravenous empirical antimicrobial therapy for fever in patients with granulocytopenia who are receiving cancer chemotherapy. International Antimicrobial Therapy Cooperative Group of the European Organization for Research and Treatment of Cancer. N Engl J Med 1999;341:312-18.
13. Freifeld A, Marchigiani D, Walsh T, et al. A double-blind comparison of empirical oral and intravenous antibiotic therapy for low-risk febrile patients with neutropenia during cancer chemotherapy. N Engl J Med 1999;341:305-11.
14. Innes HE, Smith DB, O'Reilly SM, Clark PI, Kelly V, Marshall E. Oral antibiotics with early hospital discharge compared with in-patient intravenous antibiotics for low-risk febrile neutropenia in patients with cancer: A prospective randomised controlled single centre study. Br J Cancer 2003;89:43-49.
15. Sebban C, Dussart S, Fuhrmann C, et al. Oral moxifloxacin or intravenous ceftriaxone for the treatment of low-risk neutropenic fever in cancer patients suitable for early hospital discharge. Support Care Cancer 2008;16:1017-23.
16. Vidal L, Paul M, Ben dor I, Soares-Weiser K, Leibovici L. Oral versus intravenous antibiotic treatment for febrile neutropenia in cancer patients: A systematic review and meta-analysis of randomized trials. J Antimicrob Chemother 2004;54:29-37.
17. Paul M, Yahav D, Fraser A, Leibovici L. Empirical antibiotic monotherapy for febrile neutropenia: Systematic review and meta-analysis of randomized controlled trials. J Antimicrob Chemother 2006;57:176-89.
18. Yahav D, Paul M, Fraser A, Sarid N, Leibovici L. Efficacy and safety of cefepime: A systematic review and meta-analysis. Lancet Infect Dis 2007;7:338-48.
19. US Food and Drug Administration Center for Drug Evaluation and Research. Early communication about an ongoing safety review. Cefepime (marketed as Maxipime). Available at: http://www.fda.gov/Drugs/DrugSafety/Postmarket Drug Safety Information for Patients and Providers/Drug Safety Information for Heathcare Professionals/ucm070496.htm. Accessed August 4 2009.
20. Nguyen TD, Williams B, Trang E. Cefepime Therapy and All-Cause Mortality. Clin Infect Dis 2009.
21. Bow EJ, Rotstein C, Noskin GA, et al. A randomized, open-label, multicenter comparative study of the efficacy and safety of piperacillin-tazobactam and cefepime for the empirical treatment of febrile neutropenic episodes in patients with hematologic malignancies. Clin Infect Dis 2006;43:447-59.
22. Harter C, Schulze B, Goldschmidt H, et al. Piperacillin/tazobactam vs ceftazidime in the treatment of neutropenic fever in patients with acute leukemia or following autologous peripheral blood stem cell transplantation: A prospective randomized trial. Bone Marrow Transplant 2006;37:373-79.

23. Elting LS, Bodey GP, Keefe BH. Septicemia and shock syndrome due to viridans streptococci: A case-control study of predisposing factors. Clin Infect Dis 1992; 14:1201-07.
24. Paul M, Soares-Weiser K, Leibovici L. Beta lactam monotherapy versus beta lactam-aminoglycoside combination therapy for fever with neutropenia: Systematic review and meta-analysis. BMJ 2003;326:1111.
25. Paul M, Borok S, Fraser A, Vidal L, Cohen M, Leibovici L. Additional anti-Gram-positive antibiotic treatment for febrile neutropenic cancer patients. Cochrane Database Syst Rev 2005;(3):CD003914.
26. Tunkel AR, Sepkowitz KA. Infections caused by viridans streptococci in patients with neutropenia. Clin Infect Dis 2002;34:1524-29.
27. Leibovici L, Paul M, Cullen M, et al. Antibiotic prophylaxis in neutropenic patients: New evidence, practical decisions. Cancer 2006;107:1743-51.
28. Bucaneve G, Micozzi A, Menichetti F, et al. Levofloxacin to prevent bacterial infection in patients with cancer and neutropenia. N Engl J Med 2005;353:977-87.
29. Cullen M, Steven N, Billingham L, et al. Antibacterial prophylaxis after chemotherapy for solid tumors and lymphomas. N Engl J Med 2005;353:988-98.
30. Cullen MH, Billingham LJ, Gaunt CH, Steven NM. Rational selection of patients for antibacterial prophylaxis after chemotherapy. J Clin Oncol 2007;25:4821-28.
31. Smith TJ, Khatcheressian J, Lyman GH, et al. 2006 Update of Recommendations for the use of White Blood Cell Growth Factors: An Evidence-Based Clinical Practice Guideline. J Clin Oncol 2006;24:3187-205.
32. Kuderer NM, Dale DC, Crawford J, Lyman GH. Impact of primary prophylaxis with granulocyte colony-stimulating factor on febrile neutropenia and mortality in adult cancer patients receiving chemotherapy: A systematic review. J Clin Oncol 2007;25:3158-67.
33. Timmer-Bonte JN, de Boo TM, Smit HJ, et al. Prevention of chemotherapy-induced febrile neutropenia by prophylactic antibiotics plus or minus granulocyte colony-stimulating factor in small-cell lung cancer: A Dutch Randomized Phase III Study. J Clin Oncol 2005;23:7974-84.
34. Timmer-Bonte JN, Adang EM, Smit HJ, et al. Cost-effectiveness of adding granulocyte colony-stimulating factor to primary prophylaxis with antibiotics in small-cell lung cancer. J Clin Oncol 2006;24:2991-97.
35. Herbst C, Naumann F, Kruse EB, et al. Prophylactic antibiotics or G-CSF for the prevention of infections and improvement of survival in cancer patients undergoing chemotherapy. Cochrane Database Syst Rev 2009;(1):CD007107.
36. Herbst C, Naumann F, Herbst O, Bohlius J, Juni P, Engert A. Preventing Infections in Cancer Patients: Antibiotics, Hematopoetic Growth Factors or Both. A Network Analysis. ASH Annual Meeting Abstracts. Blood 2008;112:1315.
37. Gafter-Gvili A, Paul M, Fraser A, Leibovici L. Effect of quinolone prophylaxis in afebrile neutropenic patients on microbial resistance: Systematic review and meta-analysis. J Antimicrob Chemother 2007;59:5-22.

Chapter 5

Thrombin-activable Fibrinolysis Inhibitor (TAFI): An Important Contributor in the Fibrinolytic System

Arijit Biswas, Suhail Akhter, Renu Saxena

INTRODUCTION

Thrombin-activable fibrinolysis inhibitor (TAFI), also known as procarboxypeptidase B, is a plasma zymogen that potently inhibits fibrinolysis[1] when converted to an enzyme. The direct action of TAFI as an inhibitor of clot lysis involves removal of carboxy-terminals lysyl and arginyl residues from partially degraded fibrin.[2] Consequently, plasminogen binding sites are eliminated, and plasminogen activation and fibrinolysis are inhibited.[3] TAFI was first reported by Hendriks et al[4] who detected the presence of an unstable basic carboxypeptidase activity during blood coagulation. Campbell et al[5] confirmed these observation and named the enzyme as carboxypeptidase B. Eaton et al purified this protein, isolated its cDNA and deduced the amino acid sequence. The amino acid sequence turned out to be very much similar to pancreatic carboxypeptidase B. They therefore called it plasma procarboxypeptidase B (plasma proCPB). The binding of this proenzyme to plasminogen combined with the role of C-terminal lysine residues in the binding and activation of plasminogen suggested that this new basic carboxypeptidase may have a role in the fibrinolytic pathway.[5-11] The functional role of this enzyme was identified by Bajzar et al in 1995[12] when they found that the antifibrinolytic effect of thrombin was primarily due to the activation of a proenzyme which they called TAFI or Thrombin-activable fibrinolysis inhibitor. Amino acid sequencing of this proenzyme showed it to be identical[9,12,13] to plasma procarboxypeptidase B (plasma proCPB) identified earlier.

PROPERTIES OF TAFI

TAFI is synthesized as a 424 amino acid prepropeptide composed of a 22 amino acid signal peptide, a 92 amino acid activation peptide and a 309 amino acid catalytic domain.[11] The mature proCPU protein consists of 401 amino acids with a molecular weight of 45,999 Da. Upon glycosylation the molecular weight is increased to 60,000 Da as seen in a SDS-PAGE. The active TAFI has an apparent molecular weight of 35,000 Da. Boffa et al established and characterized a recombinant expression system for TAFI in mammalian cells.[13] The recombinant form of TAFI/TAFIa was found to be very similar to its plasma-derived counterpart with respect to its enzymatic and functional properties. They were also able to identify the thrombin cleavage site in TAFIa. In addition, analysis of the properties of the resultant mutants of TAFI/TAFIa allowed them to infer that certain arginine residues affect stability and define the relative roles of thermal instability and proteolytic cleavage of TAFIa in regulation of its enzymatic activity and ability to regulate fibrinolysis.

EPIDEMIOLOGICAL STUDIES AND TAFI

Several studies have reported a broad interindividual variation in the plasma TAFI concentration. Variations upto ten fold between the highest and the lowest levels of TAFI have been reported in certain populations. Bajzar et al[14] reported that the TAFI antigenic plasma concentration in pooled plasma from 60 donors was 4.4 ug/ml. Mosnier et al[15] reported a mean level of 15 ug/ml from 40 volunteers. Guo et al[16] found a mean level of 8.2 ug/ml from the pooled plasma of 80 volunteers. The largest of these studies by Stromqvist et al[17] reported an average of 13.4 ug/ml TAFI antigen levels in 479 healthy volunteers. However, in earlier studies the standardization of the assays or the use of different types of kits used was a critical issue. Since TAFI exists as two different isoforms (one which has Threonine at 325 position and the other which has Isoleucine at the same position), different kits showed different reactvities towards the different isoforms,[18-21] the variation in the levels of TAFI antigen across these studies was attributed to the difference in the type of kit as well as different modes of standardization (in cases where an in-house procedure and not a kit has been tried). More recently an antigen kit which is genotype independent, e.g. independent of increased or decreased reactivity towards 325 Thr/Ile and 147 Ala/Thr polymorphisms[22] has been developed. However, even with this kit TAFI antigen levels continues to show a large amount of interindividual variation in the general population. A comparatively lower level of interindividual variation has been observed when an activity based assay has been used (two to four fold). A low or high proCPU plasma concentration might, therefore, tip the balance between profibrinolytic and antifibrolytic pathways and thereby cause a predisposition to bleeding or thrombosis. Several epidemiological studies indicate that a relation between the plasma TAFI concentration and hemorrhagic or thrombotic tendency might exist. Studies on conditions like Deep Vein Thrombosis,[23,24] Stroke[25] and Coronary Artery diseases[26-28] have been contradictory as well as inconclusive. Elevated levels of plasma proCPU have been found in stroke patients.[29-36] Montaner et al[29] showed that TAFI Ag levels, measured within 24 hours of onset of the event, were increased in a small sample (n = 30) of elderly ischemic stroke patients. Santamarı́a et al[30] investigated 114 young (mean age 56 years) patients with ischemic stroke or transient ischemic attacks. TAFI levels, as measured within the first month after the event by an activity assay after full activation of TAFI with thrombin–thrombomodulin, were increased in patients compared with controls.

Leebeek et al[31] found increased functional TAFI levels, as determined by a clot lysis assay in 124 patients with a recent first episode of ischemic stroke. A subgroup of 36 patients was investigated at 3-month follow-up, and the results indicated that the finding was not attributable to an acute-phase response. Ladenval et al[33] found an increased level of TAFI antigen as well as TAFI activation peptide in a heterogenous stroke population. Biswas et al[32] found an increased level of TAFI antigen level in 120 Asian Indian stroke Patients.

SNPS IN THE TAFI GENE

The human TAFI gene is located on chromosome 13q14.11 and consists of 11 exons spanning approximately 48 kb.[34] Two polymorphisms in the coding sequence were first described: A 505 G > A substitution leading to an Ala- to Thr substitution at amino acid 147; and a C678T substitution leading to a silent polymorphism (Zhao et al, 1998). The promoter and the 3' UTR of the TAFI gene by PCR-SSCP and sequencing was carried out and seven new polymorphisms identified, 5 in the promoter (2599 C > G, 2345 2G > 1G, 1690 A > G, 1102 G > T and 438 G > A) and 2 in the 3'UTR (1542 C > G and 1583 T > A).[35] All of these polymorphisms are in strong linkage disequilibrium with each other and with the previously described functional Ala 147 Thr (505 A > G) polymorphism in the coding region of the gene. They generate 4 main haplotypes, accounting for 80% of all observed haplotypes. In univariate analysis, all polymorphisms have been associated with plasma TAFI antigen levels and, individually, contribute to a large fraction of plasma TAFI antigen levels, ranging from 20% to 52%. In a stepwise regression analysis including all polymorphisms, several combinations remain significantly and independently associated with plasma TAFI antigen levels; the 1542 C > G polymorphism associated with Ala 147 Thr, the 1583 T > A polymorphism, and the −2345 2G > 1G polymorphism explained 61.6%, 60.2% and 58.1% of the antigen variance, respectively. The polymorphisms that exhibit the highest R^2 in multivariate analysis include the 1542 C > G and the 147 Ala > Thr (= 505 A > G) polymorphisms. These findings clearly demonstrate that circulating levels of TAFI are strongly determined by polymorphic variations in the promoter and the 3'UTR of the TAFI gene. These results also suggest that the regulation of TAFI gene expression is complex and probably involves more than one single functional variant. There have been similar reports from the Brazilian[36] as well as African population[37] also which point to the presence of a quantitative trait loci in the TAFI gene involving these polymorphisms governing the TAFI levels. More number of polymorphisms have been discovered in this gene with similar effects. Most of these polymorphism studies were done in patients with myocardial infarction or arterial thrombosis or in the general control population. Only recently one study with stroke population has been reported from the Caucasian population.[33] Recently functional studies have demonstrated the importance of the 3'UTR polymorphisms in the regulation of TAFI antigen levels.[38] In the Asian Indian population Biswas et al[32] found an association of the TAFI antigenic levels with TAFI SNPS but no risk for stroke could be established for the SNPs.

INHIBITORS OF TAFI

Since zinc is an essential requirement for the catalytic action of TAFI therefore TAFI is sensitive to inhibition by chelating agents such as o-phenatroline and EDTA.[1,4,8] TAFI is also sensitive to dithiotheriotol and 2-mercaptoethanol, which reduce the disulfide bonds present in TAFI.[4,7] TAFI is also inhibited by chloromercurbenzoic acid probably due to the presence of a free cysteine reused in the enzyme.[4] The naturally occurring carboxypeptidase inhibitors derived form potato (PTCI) and leech (LCI) have been characterzied as inhibitors of TAFI. Potato tuber carboxypeptidase inhibitor (PTCI) is a 39 amino acid peptide frequently used as an inhibitors of CPU *in vitro* and *in vivo* experiment.

SUMMARY

Thrombin activatable fibrinolysis inhibitor [carboxypeptidase B2 (plasma), CPB] is a basic carboxypeptidase, which inhibits fibrinolysis by cleaving the C-terminal lysine residues on plasmin-modified partially degraded fibrin. An increasing number of studies are finding a role for this inhibitor in a large number of prothrombotic disorders like stroke and coronary artery disease. What makes this candidate even more interesting is that the antigenic levels of TAFI shows a stringent association with SNPs found mostly on the regulatory regions of the TAFI gene. Also the fact that there are potential inhibitors for this protein makes it an attractive target for future therapeutic practices. This review primarily elaborates on the past and present of TAFI in the context of disease associations.

TAKE HOME MESSAGE

TAFI is involved in the regulation of fibrinolysis and is therefore considered an attractive potential new drug target for the treatment of thrombotic disorders. This knowledge would prompt the generation of newer inhibitors in the next few years for the treatment of thrombotic disorders.

REFERENCES

1. Bajzar L, Manuel R, Nesheim ME. Purification and characterization of TAFI, a thrombin-activable fibrinolysis inhibitor. J Biol Chem 1995;270:14477-84.
2. Wang W, Boffa MB, Bajzar L, Walker JB, Nesheim ME. A study of the mechanism of inhibition of fibrinolysis by activated thrombin-activable fibrinolysis inhibitor. J Biol Chem 1998;273:27176-81.
3. Mosnier LO, von dem Borne PA, Meijers JC, Bouma BN. Plasma TAFI levels influence the clot lysis time in healthy individuals in the presence of an intact intrinsic pathway of coagulation. Thromb Haemost 1998;80:829-35.

4. Hendrinks D. Scharpe's, Van Sande M, et al. Characterization of carboxypeptidase in human serum distinct from carboxypeptidase N. J Clin Vhem Clin Biochem 1989;27:277-85.
5. Campbell W, Ikada H. An arginnie specific carboxypeptidase generated in blood during coagulation or inflammation which is unrelated to carboxypeptidase N or Its subunits. Biochem Biophys Res Commun 1989;162:933-39.
6. Campbell W, Yonezu K, Shinohara T. An arginine carboxypeptidase generated during coagulation is diminished or absent in patient with rheumatoid arthrist. J Lab Med 1990;155;610-12.
7. Hendriks D, Wang W, Scharpe S. Purification and characterization of a new arginnie carboxypeptidase in human serum Biohim Biophys Aeta 1990;1034: 86-92.
8. Hendrinks D, Wang W, van Sande M. Human serum carboxypeptidase U: A new kininase. Agents Action Suppl 1992;38:407-13.
9. Shinohara T, Sakurda C, Suzuki T, et al. Procarboxypeptidase R cleaves Bradykinin following activation. Int Arch Allergy Immunol 1994;103:400-04.
10. Kato K, Shinagawa, N, Hayakawa T, et al. Changes in arginine carboxypeptidase (CPR) activity in stressed rates. Pathophysiology 1994;1:131-36.
11. Eaton DL, Malloy, BE, Tsai SP. Isolation reocular cloning, and partial characterization of a novel carboxypeptidase B from human plasma. J Biot Chem 1991;266: 21833-38.
12. Bajzar L m, Manuel R, Nesheim ME. Purification and characterization of TAFI, a thrombin-activable fibribolysis inhibitor, J Biol Chem 1995;270:14477-84.
13. Boffa MB, Wang W, Bajzar L, Nesheim ME. J Biol Chem 1998;**273**:2127-35.
14. Bajzar, Nasheim ME; Tracy PB. The profibrino with effect of activated protein (in clots formed from plasma is TAFI-dependent. Blood 1996;88:2093-100.
15. Mosnier LO, Elisen MG, Bouma BN, et al. Protein c inhibitor regulates the thrombin – thrombomodulin complex in the up and down regulation of TAFI activation. Thromb Haemost 2001;86:1057-64.
16. Guo X, Morioka A, Kancko Y, et al. Arginnie carboxypeptidase U antigen levels in human plasma determined with sandwich. ELISA Microbiol Immunol 1999;43: 691-98.
17. Stromqvist M, Schatterman K Leurs J. Immunological assay for the determination of procarboxypeptidase U antigen levels in human plasma. Thromb Haemosr 2001;85:12-17.
18. Verdu J, Marco P, Benlloch S, Sanchez J, Lucas J. Thrombin activatable fibrinolysis inhibitor (TAFI) polymorphisms and plasma TAFI levels measured with an ELISA insensitive to isoforms in patients with venous thromboembolic disease (VTD). Thromb Haemost 2006;95(3):585-86.
19. Ceresa E, Brouwers E, Peeters M, Jern C, Declerck PJ, Gils A. Development of ELISAs measuring the extent of TAFI activation. Arterioscler Thromb Vasc Biol. 2006;26(2):423-28.
20. Frere C, Morange PE, Saut N, Tregouet DA, Grosley M, Beltran J, Juhan-Vague I, Alessi MC. Quantification of thrombin activatable fibrinolysis inhibitor (TAFI) gene polymorphism effects on plasma levels of TAFI measured with assays insensitive to isoform-dependent artefact. Thromb Haemost 2005;94(2):373-79.
21. Guimaraes AH, van Tilburg NH, Vos HL, Bertina RM, Rijken DC. Association between thrombin activatable fibrinolysis inhibitor genotype andlevels in plasma: Comparison of different assays. Br J Haematol 2004;124(5):659-65.
22. Gils A, Alessi MC, Brouwers E, Peeters M, Marx P, Leurs J, Bouma B, Hendriks D, Juhan-Vague I, Declerck PJ. Development of a genotype 325-specific proCPU/TAFI ELISA. Arterioscler Thromb Vasc Biol 2003;23(6):1122-27. Epub 2003 May 1.

23. Kostka H, Kuhlisch E, Schellong S, Siegert G. Polymorphisms in the TAFI gene and the risk of venous thrombosis. Clin Lab 2003;49(11-12):645-47.
24. Franco RF, Fagundes MG, Meijers JC, Reitsma PH, Lourenco D, Morelli V, Maffei FH, Ferrari IC, Piccinato CE, Silva WA Jr, Zago MA. Identification of polymorphisms in the 5′-untranslated region of the TAFI gene: Relationship with plasma TAFI levels and risk of venous thrombosis. Haematologica 2001;86(5): 510-17.
25. Montaner J, Ribo M, Monasterio J, Molina CA, Sabin AJ. Thrombin Activatable Fibrinolytic Inhibitor levels in the acute phase of ischemic stroke. Stroke 2003;34:1038-40.
26. Santamaria A, Martinez-Rubio A, Borrell M, Mateo J, Ortin R, Fontcuberta J. Risk of acute coronary artery disease associated with functional thrombin activatable fibrinolysis inhibitor plasma level. Haematologica 2004;89(7):880-81.
27. Schroeder V, Chatterjee T, Mehta H, Windecker S, Pham T, Devantay N, Meier B, Kohler HP. Thrombin activatable fibrinolysis inhibitor (TAFI) levels in patients with coronary artery disease investigated by angiography. Thromb Haemost 2002;88(6):1020-25.
28. Silveira A, Schatteman K, Goossens F, Moor E, Scharpe S, Stromqvist M, Hendriks D, Hamsten A. Plasma procarboxypeptidase U in men with symptomatic coronary artery disease. Thromb Haemost 2000;84(3):364-68.
29. Montaner J, Ribo M, Monasterio J, Molina CA, Sabin AJ. Thrombin Activatable Fibrinolytic Inhibitor levels in the acute phase of ischemic stroke. Stroke 2003;34:1038-40.
30. Santamaria A, Martinez-Rubio A, Borrell M, Mateo J, Ortin R, Fontcuberta J. Risk of acute coronary artery disease associated with functional thrombin activatable fibrinolysis inhibitor plasma level. Haematologica 2004;89(7):880-81.
31. Leebeek FW, Goor MP, Guimaraes AH, Brouwers GJ, Maat MP, Dippel DW, Rijken DC. High functional levels of thrombin-activatable fibrinolysis inhibitor are associated with an increased risk of first ischemic stroke. J Thromb Haemost. 2005;3(10):2211-18.
32. Biswas A, Tiwari AK, Ranjan R, Meena A, Akhter MS, Yadav BK, Behari M, Saxena R. Thrombin activatable fibrinolysis inhibitor gene polymorphisms are associated with antigenic levels in the Asian-Indian population but may not be a risk for stroke. Br J Haematol 2008;143(4):581-88.
33. Ladenvall C, Gils A, Jood K, Blomstrand C, Declerck PJ, Jern C.Thrombin activatable fibrinolysis inhibitor activation peptide shows association with all major subtypes of ischemic stroke and with TAFI gene variation. Arterioscler Thromb Vasc Biol 2007;27(4):955-62.
34. Boffa MB, TS Reid Joo E, Nesheim ME, Koschinsky ML. Characterization of the gene encoding human TAFI (thrombin-activable fibrinolysis inhibitor; plasma procarboxypeptidase B). Biochemistry 1999;38(20):6547-58.
35. Zhao L, J Morser, Bajzar L, Nesheim M, Nagashima M. Identification and characterization of two thrombin-activatable fibrinolysis inhibitor isoforms. Thromb Haemost 1998;80(6):949-55.
36. Henry M, H Aubert, Morange PE, Nanni I, Alessi MC, Tiret L, Juhan-Vague I. Identification of polymorphisms in the promoter and the 3′ region of the TAFI gene: Evidence that plasma TAFI antigen levels are strongly genetically controlled. Blood 2001;97(7):2053-58.
37. Franco RF, MG Fagundes, Meijers JC, Reitsma PH, Lourenço D, Morelli V, Maffei FH, Ferrari IC, Piccinato CE, Silva WA Jr, Zago MA. Identification of

polymorphisms in the 5'-untranslated region of the TAFI gene: Relationship with plasma TAFI levels and risk of venous thrombosis. Haematologica 2001;86(5): 510-17.
38. Frere C, Tregouet DA, Morange PE, Saut N, Kouassi D, Juhan-Vague I, Tiret L, Alessi MC. Fine mapping of quantitative trait nucleotides underlying thrombin-activatable fibrinolysis inhibitor antigen levels by a transethnic study. Blood 2006;108(5):1562-68.

Chapter 6
Pathobiology, Prognostication and Management of Low-risk Myelodysplastic Syndrome

HP Pati, Shyam Rathi

The myelodysplastic syndrome (MDS) is characterized by cytopenia (anemia, neutropenia and thrombocytopenia), with ineffective hematopoiesis and tendency for progression to leukemia. Management of MDS requires consideration of age, performance status and prognosis. Goal of therapy is to control symptoms due to cytopenia, minimize therapy related toxicity, improve overall survival and decrease progression to acute leukemia.

Advances in understanding of the pathogenic mechanism underlying MDS has generated novel strategies for management of this disease. For therapeutic decision assessment of prognosis is very important. The most common cause of death is not transformation of MDS to acute myeloid leukemia but rather complications associated with chronic cytopenia.[1]

PATHOBIOLOGY OF MYELODYSPLASTIC SYNDROME

MDS is considered to be a clonal disorder of stem cells. Defects within myeloid progenitors and bone marrow microenvironment, both contribute to abnormal apoptosis, accumulation of cells with mutated DNA and progression to acute myeloid leukemia.

Abnormal Apoptosis in the Bone Marrow

Apoptosis (programmed cell death) regulate the population of cells. The ratio of proapoptotic protein, e.g. p53, Bax, etc. to antiapoptotic protein, e.g. BCL-2 and BCL-XL regulate the rate of apoptosis.[2] TNF-α is well recognized as a cytokine promoter of apoptosis in erythroid cells in early stages of MDS. Overall in early stage MDS, rate of apoptosis is high. Use of growth factors such as erythropoiesis stimulating agents and G-CSF has been shown to decrease rate of apoptosis.

Epigenetic Alterations

The term epigenetics is the alterations of gene expression without altering the primary DNA sequence. The most studied epigenetic alterations in cancer are promoter hypermethylation and histone deacetylation. The role of promoter hypermethylation in low-risk MDS is not well studied while in high-risk MDS, hypermethylation of any of the tumor suppressor genes p15, HIC1, ER CDH1 is associated with adverse survival and increased risk of leukemia evolution.[3]

Genetic Alterations

MDS requires multiple hits and to date no single genetic lesion has been shown to be sufficient for developing the disease. Mutated N-RAS is identified in 6-48% (higher in patients with increase blast counts) and it correlates with increased risk of AML evolution.[4] The tumor suppressor gene TP53 is mutated in 8-14% of patients and is often associated with complex karyotype, resistance to chemotherapy and poor outcome. FLT3 mutations are found in < 1%, KIT mutation in 1.2% and MLL partial tandem duplications in 2.7% of MDS patients.[5]

Immune Mediated

A minority of MDS patients have hypocellular bone marrow and has a clear link to the HLA DR 15. Immunosuppressive therapy induces long lasting response in this subcategory.[6]

Pathogenesis of 5q⁻ Syndrome

In 5q⁻ syndrome commonly deleted segment is 31-32. There are 44 genes, out of which defect in RPS14 is found to be associated with block in erythroid maturation.[7] RPS 14 is a component of ribosomal 40s subunit, and interestingly another ribosomal gene RPS 19 is found to cause Diamond-Blackfan anemia.

PROGNOSIS ASSESSMENTS IN MDS

The French-American-British (FAB) and World health Organization (WHO) classification have been more useful for diagnosis than for determination of prognosis. Two most important scoring systems available for assessment of prognosis are international prognostic scoring system (IPSS)[8] and World Health Organization prognostic scoring system (WPSS).[9]

IPSS was derived from multivariable analysis of 816 patients with primary MDS. Patients who had received extensive chemotherapy and those with secondary MDS were excluded. Patients were stratified according to cytopenia, bone marrow blast percentage and cytogenetics (Tables 6.1 and 6.2).

Limitations of IPSS

1. Did not address other MDS subgroup like secondary MDS.
2. Included patients with blast count 20-30% which is now classified as acute leukemia.
3. Median time between symptoms and diagnosis is not mentioned.

Table 6.1: IPSS scoring [8]

Score value	Bone marrow blasts (%)	Karyotype	Cytopenias
0	< 5%	Normal, -Y, del 5q, del 20q	Nil /monocytopenia
0.5	5-10%	Others	Bi/pancytopenia.
1.0		Complex* and/ or chr 7 defects.	
1.5	11-20%		
2.0	21-30%		

*- Complex chromosomal defect: $\geq$ 3 chromosome abnormalities.

Table 6.2: Median survival and AML evolution with IPSS score

Prognostic score	Subgroups	Median AML transformation (yr)	Median survival (yr)	Median survival <60 (yr of age)	Median survival >60 (yr of age)
0	Low	9.4	5.7	11.8	4.8
0.5-1.0	Intermediate 1	3.3	3.5	5.2	2.7
1.5-2.0	Intermediate 2	1.1	1.2	1.8	1.1
$\geq$ 2.5	High	0.2	0.4	0.3	0.5

Table 6.3: WPSS[9] scoring

Variable	0	1	2	3
WHO category	RA, RARS, 5q⁻	RCMD, RCMD-RS	RAEB-1	RAEB-2
Karyotype	Good	Intermediate	Poor	
Transfusion requirement	No	Regular*	–	–

* Defined as $\geq$ 1 RBC unit/ 8 weeks. Karyotype Good- Normal,-Y, del5q, del20q. Poor- $\geq$ 3 chromosome abnormalities, chr 7 defects. Intermediate- Others.
RA: Refractory anemia, RARS: Refractory anemia with ringed sideroblast, 5q⁻ MDS with isolated del 5q, RCMD: Refractory cytopenia with multilinage dysplasia, RCMD-RS: RCMD with ringed sideroblast, RAEB-Refractory anemia with ringed sideroblast.

Table 6.4: Median survival according to WPSS

WPSS subgroups	Score	Median survival (months)
Very low	0	138
Low	1	63
Intermediate	2	44
High	3-4	19
Very high	5-6	8

4. Prognostic value of multilineage dysplasia compared to unilineage dysplasia was not addressed.
5. Blast percentage had been given more weightage than cytogenetics.

Malcovati[9] proposed new scoring system based on WHO classification, cytogenetics and transfusion requirements. This scoring system is more useful for patients with low risk MDS (Tables 6.3 and 6.4).

Other adverse prognostic factors in MDS are:
1. Transfusion dependence.[10]
2. Increased expression of Wilm's tumor gene.[11]

3. Mutations of the FLT3 gene.[12]
4. Abnormal localization of immature precursor (ALIP). [13]

TREATMENT MODALITY IN MDS

Treatment goals depend upon age of the patient, performance status and risk status (IPSS). The management objectives of these patients (NCCN guidelines) are (Fig. 6.1):[14]
1. Younger patients with good performance status and who are in IPSS low or int1 category should be considered for supportive or low intensity therapy like growth factor, low intensity chemotherapy, immunomodulator or immunosuppressive therapy.
2. Younger patients with good performance status, and who are in IPSS int2 or high-risk category should be considered for high intensity therapy like high dose chemotherapy or stem cell transplant.
3. Elderly patients (> 60 years) with good performance status and who are high or low-risk should be considered for low intensity therapy except for selected high-risk patients who could be candidate for high intensity therapy.
4. All patients with poor performance status should be considered for supportive therapy except for selected patients who could be candidate for low intensity therapy.

Therapeutic Options

1. Supportive care – Red cell transfusion, platelet transfusion and iron chelation.
2. Hematopoietic growth factors – Erythropoietin and G-CSF.
3. Immunosuppressive drugs – Anti-thymocyte globulin and cyclosporine.
4. Immunomodulatory drugs – Thalidomide and lenalidomide.
5. Hypomethylating agent – Azacitidine and decitabine.
7. Hematopoietic stem cell transplant.

Supportive Care

Due to advanced age of patients and chronicity of the disease, supportive care is central component to management of all types of MDS. Transfusion of RBCs is an integral component of supportive care for anemia of MDS, affording a transient relief of symptoms, improving quality of life and activities of daily living. There are no guidelines/target hemoglobin level or any optimal frequency of transfusion. Chronic transfusions are associated with clinical and economic consequences like poorer survival, blood product reactions, risk of infections transmission and iron overload.[15]

In patients with low or int1 risk, anticipated to have prolonged red cell transfusion, iron chelation should be considered after 20 transfusion or when serum ferritin > 2500 mcg/l.[14] The National Comprehensive Cancer Network (NCCN) MDS panel recommended deferoxamine SC

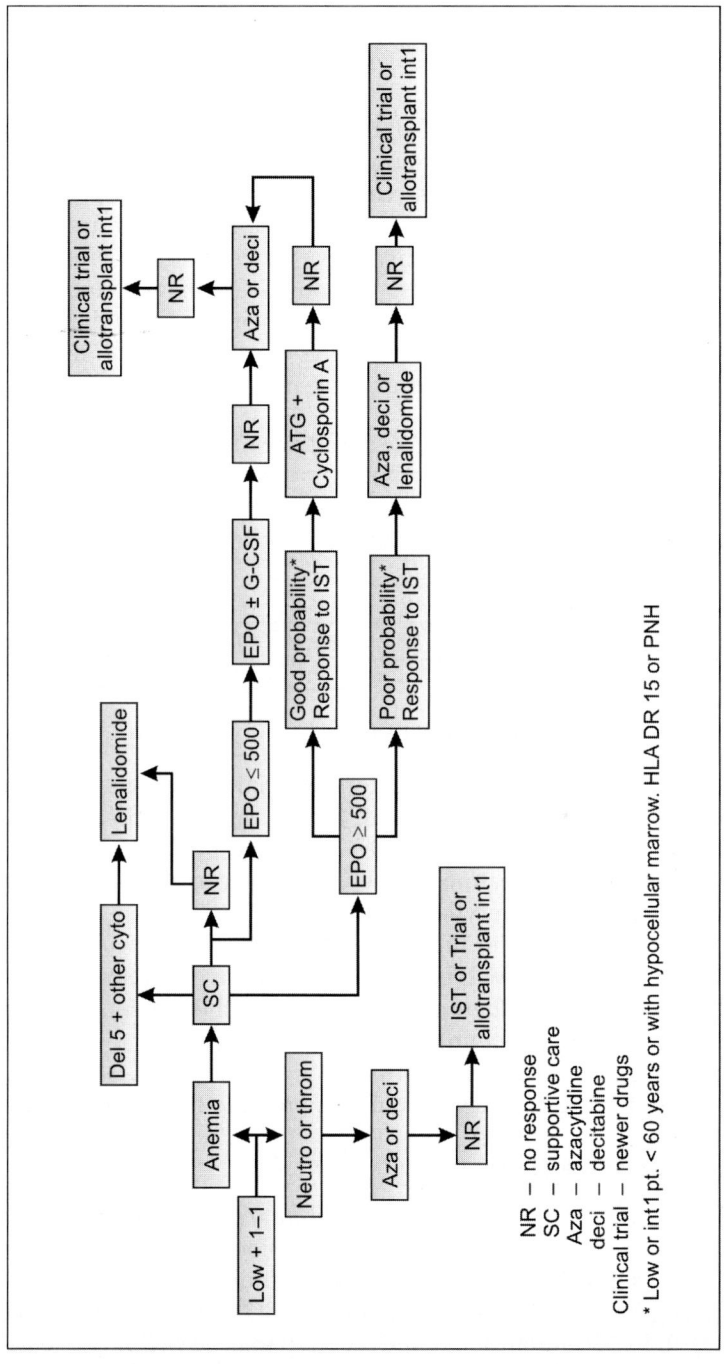

Fig. 6.1: NCCN guidelines (2009) for the treatment of MDS[14]

or deferasirox oral for iron chelation, aiming to decrease serum ferritin to < 1000 mcg/l. Long-term benefit of iron chelation includes improvement in survival.[16]

Hematopoietic Growth Factors

The rational for Erythropoietin (EPO) therapy is its potential for inhibition of apoptosis, enhancing differentiation of progenitor cells and stimulation of growth of hematopoietic cells. Until recently EPO is treatment of choice for low and int1 risk patients (except those with 5q-syndrome) due to its excellent safety and tolerability. EPO had synergistic effect when combined with G-CSF. EPO with or without G-CSF have demonstrated efficacy in improvement of quality of life and anemia.[11] From the analysis of 84 patients, Hellstrom and her colleague developed a risk model for predicting response to erythropoietin (Table 6.5). [17]

Table 6.5: Treatment response score[17]

Serum EPO	< 100	+2	Score > +1	Good response –74%
	100-500	+1		
	> 500	–3	Score = –1–+1	Intermediate response–23%
Transfusion	< 2 units/month	+2		
	> 2 units/month	–2	Score < –1	Poor response – 7%

CR—stable Hb > 11.5 g/dl.
PR—increase Hb > 1.5 g/dl or end of transfusion.

According to Parks et al,[18] the factors associated with good response to EPO include blast percentage < 10%, low or int1 IPSS score, RBC transfusion independence, serum EPO < 200 units/l, and shorter interval between diagnosis and treatment. There was no correlation of marrow dysplasia with response to erythropoietin.[18]

EPO is recommended in high doses of 40000 to 60000 units once a week. Response, if occurs, will be evident within 6 to 8 weeks. The drugs should be discontinued if there is no response by this time. Long lasting analogue of EPO (Darbepoetin) allows injections once in two or three weeks. Target goal for treatment with EPO is a hemoglobin level of 12 g/dl. Iron studies for its adequacy should be monitored throughout therapy.

Immunosuppressive Therapy

In a subset of MDS patients the clonal proliferation of T-lymphocytes has been demonstrated, and implicated in suppression of hematopoiesis. Pretreatment variables linked to response to immunosuppressive therapy include younger age (< 60 yr), shorter duration RBC transfusion dependence (< 6 months), hypocellular bone marrow (hypoplastic MDS), presence of PNH clone and HLA DR 15 phenotype (Table 6.6).[19] But as per a National Institute of Health (NIH) study,[6] only younger age, transfusion duration

Table 6.6: Predicting responsiveness to immunosupression in MDS[6]

HLA DR 15 status	Patient's age (yr) + duration of RCTD (months)		PPR
	HLA-DR 15 negative	HLA-DR 15 positive	
Age in years	> 57	> 71	Low (0-40%)
	≤ 57	≤ 71	High (41-100%)

RCTD—red cell transfusion dependence.
PPR—positive predictor of response.

and HLA DR 15 predict response. There is improvement of survival and decreased risk of leukemia transformation in responding patients.

Immunomodulatory Drugs

Thalidomide has antiangiogenic and anticytokine activity and therefore has a role in MDS. It has shown some activity in low-risk MDS. Also the low response rate is counter-balanced by adverse side effects, including neuropathy, sedation, fatigue and constipation.[20]

Lenalidomide, a thalidomide analogue is a more potent immunomodulator without the neurologic side effects, sedation and constipation. Myelosupression is dose limiting toxicity. It has remarkable activity in patients with 5q- syndrome. In a multicenter phase II trial of lenalidomide in 148 patients[21] with the 5q deletion with transfusion dependant low or int1 risk MDS, transfusion independence was achieved in 67%, and complete cytogenetic response achieved in 45% patients. Most common adverse effects were neutropenia (Grade III or IV in 55%) and thrombocytopenia (Grade III or IV in 44%). Degree of cytopenia is found to be a predictor of response. The 5q- syndrome is a unique subgroup in WHO classification, for which lenalidomide is drug of choice.

In another phase II trial[22] of lenalidomide in 214 transfusion dependant low or int1 risk MDS without 5q deletion, transfusion independence was achieved in 26% and > 50% reduction in transfusion was noted in 17%, yielding an overall response rate of 42%. Lenalidomide has some activity in high-risk MDS patients with deletion 5q. The US-FDA in December 2005 approved lenalidomide for treatment of low and Int 1 risk MDS with 5q deletion.

Hypomethylating Agent—Azacitidine and Decitabine

Epigenetic silencing—through promoter methylation of a number of genes, often predicts transformation to acute myeloid leukemia.[23] Methyltransferase inhibitor drugs are promising treatment modalities.[24]

In a phase III trial supporting drug approval, (CALGB (Cancer and leukemia group B study 9221) on 191 patients, azacitidine (75 mg/m^2 subcutaneously for 7 days in 28 day cycle) was compared with best supportive care.[25] In azacitidine arm, significant improvement in quality of life, higher response (60% versus 5%), delayed time to AML transformation or death

(21 months versus 12 months) was observed. Main side effects attributed to azacitidine were ≥ Grade 3 leukopenia (43%), granulocytopenia (58%), and thrombocytopenia (52%). Response to azacitidine was not affected by MDS subtypes.

In May 2004, US Food and Drug Administration (FDA) approved the use of azacytidine in the treatment of symptomatic patient with all FAB MDS subtypes including low and high-risk. Azacitidine is the first drug to prolong survival in high-risk MDS patients.

Azacitidine treatment prolongs overall survival (OS) in high-risk MDS patients compared with conventional care regimens (CCR) (supportive care, low dose cytosar or std CT): Results of the AZA- 001 phase III study (Table 6.7). [26]

Table 6.7: OS analyses by IPSS cytogenetic group

Group	Patients	AZA median (months)	CCR median (months)
Good	166/358-46%	Not reached	17.1
Intermediate	76/358-21%	26.3	17
Poor	100/358-28%	17.2	6

Mechanism of action of azacitidine has been observed to be cytotoxic at higher doses and inhibit DNA hypermethylation at lower doses. Azacitidine was approved at a dose schedule of 75 mg/m^2 per day for 7 days every 4 weeks. Three more cycle are to be given after achieving complete response.[27] Azacitidine has been shown to induce higher remission in cohort of high-risk MDS patients with chromosome 7 abnormality.[28]

In a phase II study of decitabine on 124 patients with intermediate or high-risk MDS treated with three different doses of decitabine, overall response rate was 72%. The median overall survival was 20 months.[29] Now azacitidine may be the new standard of care in high-risk MDS patient.

Allogenic Stem Cell Transplantation

Stem cell transplant is only potentially curative option but is available to < 10% of patients either because of age, comorbid condition, availability of matched relative and financial limitation. Allogeneic HSCT should be considered for patients who are < 60 years, HLA matched sibling available, good performance status and IPSS intermediate or high-risk. For low risk patients transplantation should be considered at the time of progression to high IPSS risk group.[30]

TAKE HOME MESSAGE

1. Advances in understanding of pathobiology of MDS leads to development of new treatment options.

2. IPSS and WPSS are important tool for assessing the prognosis.
3. Anemic patients with low erythropoietin level and low transfusion requirements should be treated with erythropoietin with or without GCSF.
4. Hypocellular MDS especially those with young age, hypocellular marrow, PNH clone and HLA DR 15 positive should be treated with immunosuppressive therapy.
5. Patient with 5q- syndrome should be treated with lenalidomide.
6. Hypomethylating agent or allogenic transplant should be reserved for patient refractory to primary therapy.

REFERENCES

1. Bowen DT, et al. Treatment strategies and issues in low-intermediate1 risk myelodysplastic syndrome patients. Sem Oncol. 2005;32(Suppl 5) S16-S23.
2. Parker J, et al. Low-risk' myelodysplastic syndrome is associated with excessive apoptosis and an increased ratio of proversus anti-apoptotic bcl-2-related proteins. Br J Haematol 1998;103:1075.
3. Aggerholm A, et al. Promoter hypermethylation of p15INK4B, HIC1, CDH1, and ER is frequent in myelodysplastic syndrome and predicts poor prognosis in early-stage patients. Eur J Haematol 2006;76:23.
4. Padua R, et al. RAS, FMS and p53 mutations and poor clinical outcome in myelodysplasias: A 10- year follow-up. Leukemia 1998;12:887.
5. Bacher U, et al. A comparative study of molecular mutations in 381 patients with myelodysplastic syndrome and in 4130 patients with acute myeloid leukemia. Haematologica 2007;92:744.
6. Sloand E, et al. Factor affecting response and survival in patients with myelodysplasia treated with immunosuppressive therapy. JCO2008:26;2505-11.
7. Ebert B, et al. An erythroid differentiation signature predicts response to lenalidomide in myelodysplastic syndrome. PLoS Med 2008;5:e35.
8. Greenberg P, et al. International scoring system for evaluating prognosis in myelodysplastic syndromes. Blood 1997:89;2079-88.
9. Malcovati L, et al. Time dependant prognostic scoring system for predicting survival and leukemic evolution in myelodysplastic syndromes. JCO 2007:23; 3503-10.
10. Balducci L, et al. Transfusion independence in patients with myelodysplastic syndromes: Impact on outcome and quality of life. Cancer 2006:106;2087.
11. Cilloni D, et al. Significant correlation between the degree of WT1 and IPSS. JCO 2003:21;1988.
12. Georgiou G, et al. Serial determinations of FLT3 mutations in myelodysplastic syndrome patients at diagnosis, follow-up or acute myeloid leukemia transformation: Incidence and their prognostic significance. BJH 2006:134;302.
13. Verburgh E, et al. Additional prognostic value of bone marrow histology in patients subclassified according to the international prognostic scoring system for myelodysplastic syndrome. JCO 2003:21;273.
14. Myelodysplastic syndrome v.1.2009. NCCN clinical practice guidelines in oncology.
15. Takatoku, et al. Retrospective nationwide survey of Japanese patients with transfusion dependant MDS and aplastic anemia. Highlight the negative impact of iron overload on morbidity and mortality. Eur JH 2007;109:4586.

16. Rose C, et al. Positive impact of iron chelation therapy on survival in regularly transfused MDS patients. A prospective study. ASH.abstract.2007:110;249.
17. Hellstrom-Lindberg E, et al. A validated decision model for treating the anemia of myelodysplastic syndrome with erythropoietin + granulocyte colony-stimulating factor: Significant effect on quality of life. BJH 2003:120;1037-46.
18. Parks, et al. Predictive factors of response and survival in myelodysplastic syndrome treated with erythropoietin and G CSF: The GFM experience. Blood 2008:111;574-82.
19. Sunthararajah Y, et al. A simple method to predict response to immunosuppressive therapy in patients with myelodysplastic syndrome. Blood 2003:102;3025.
20. Bouscary D, et al. A non-randomized dose-escalating phase II study of thalidomide for the treatment of patients with low-risk myelodysplastic syndrome: The Thal-SMD-2000 trial of the groupe Francais des Myelodysplatsies. BJH.2005:131;609.
21. List A, et al. Lenalidomide in the myelodysplastic syndrome with chromosome 5q deletion. NEJM 2006:355;1456.
22. Raza A, et al. Phase II study of lenalidomide in transfusion dependant low-risk and intermediate-1 risk myelodysplastic syndrome with karyotypes other than deletion 5q. Blood 2008:111;86.
23. Herman JG, et al. Gene silencing in cancer in association with promoter hypermethylation. N Engl J Med 2003;349:2042-54.
24. List A, et al Methyltransferase inhibitors changing the treatment algorithm for myelodysplastic syndrome. Cancer Control 2004;11 (suppl 6):16-19.
25. Silverman LR, et al. Randomized controlled trial of azacitidine in patients with the myelodysplastic syndrome: A study of cancer and leukemia group B. J Clin Oncol 2002;20:2429-40.
26. Fenaux P, et al. Azacitidine treatment prolong overall survival (OS) in high-risk MDS patients compared with conventional care regimens (CCR): Results of the AZA- 001 phaseIII study. Blood 2007;110 Abstract:817.
27. Kaminskas E, et al. Approval summary: Azacitidine for treatment of myelodysplastic syndrome subtypes. Clin Cancer Res 2005;11:3604-08.
28. Lim A, et al. Outcomes of MDS patients with chromosome 7 abnormalities treated with 5-azacitidine. Blood 2007;110 Abstract:4615.
29. Kantarjian H, et al. Survival and efficacy of decitabine in myelodysplastic syndromes, analysis of 5-day IV dosing regimen. Blood 2007:110:42a; abstract 115.
30. Cutler C, et al. A decision analysis of allogeneic bone marrow transplantation for the myelodysplastic syndromes: Delayed transplantation for low-risk myelodysplasia is associated with improved outcome. Blood 2004;104:579.

Chapter 7

Antiphospholipid Syndrome—Recent Insights

Ashok Kumar, Hemant Gopal

SUMMARY

Antiphospholipid syndrome (APS) is characterized by the presence of antiphospholipid (aPL) antibodies and clinical features of vascular thrombosis and recurrent fetal loss. The aPL do not target the phospholipids directly but a large number of other molecules among which the principal antigenic target is a phospholipid binding plasma protein- β_2 GP-1. APS can exist as primary APS or it may be secondary to other autoimmune conditions, most notably SLE. Hemostatic alterations lead to thrombotic and less commonly, hemorrhagic complications in various organs. The criteria for the diagnosis of APS have been revised in 2006 and comprise clinical evidence of vascular thrombosis or fetal loss and repeated presence of lupus anticoagulant, anticardiolipin antibodies or anti-β2-GP1 antibodies 12 weeks apart. Aspirin and hydroxychloroquine may be protective against development of both venous and arterial thrombosis. APS patients who have had an episode of thrombosis are at a very high-risk of recurrence and require long-term anticoagulation. Anticoagulation is advised during pregnancy for patients who are aPL positive and have a history of repeated pregnancy loss. Corticosteroids, immunosuppressives, IVIG and plasmapheresis may be used for patients with recurrent thrombosis despite anticoagulation. More specifically targeted anti-inflammatory or immunomodulatory therapies and some newer antithrombotics are the **potential future treatments for antiphospholipid syndrome.**

KEYWORDS

Antiphospholipid, Anticardiolipin, Lupus anticoagulant, Anti-β2-GP1, CAPS

HISTORY

In 1952, a clotting inhibitor was described called lupus anticoagulant.[1] It was initially reported in association with hemorrhage but later found to be paradoxically associated with recurrent thrombosis, mainly. The presence of lupus anticoagulant was frequently associated with a biological false positive test for syphilis (BFP-STS), which was later shown to be due to a common specificity for cardiolipin- a negatively charged phospholipid antigen. Subsequently, the antiphospholipid antibodies were shown to bind diverse protein antigens, most commonly β₂ glycoprotein

(β_2 GP-1) and prothrombin[2,3] as well as negatively charged phospholipids. This whole spectrum of aPL antibodies and their clinical associations has been termed as antiphospholipid syndrome (APS).

EPIDEMIOLOGY

The prevalence of APS is unknown. In young, healthy control subjects, the prevalence for both lupus anticoagulant and anticardiolipin antibodies (aCL) is about 1 to 5%.[4] Low titre anticardiolipin antibodies occur in 10% of normal blood donors[5,6] and moderate to high titre anticardiolipin or a positive lupus anticoagulant occurs in < 1%. The prevalence increases with age, especially in elderly individuals with chronic disease. Positive tests are detected in 10-40% patients with SLE, 20% of patients with RA[7] and also in other related systemic autoimmune disorders. Various studies from India have also investigated the prevalence of aPLs in cases of suspected primary APS[8] as well as in patients with SLE.[9,10] One of the studies showed the positivity of anti-β_2GP-1 antibodies in 51%, anticardiolipin antibodies in 29% and lupus anticoagulant in 9% of SLE patients.[10] It is also detected in patients using various drugs or suffering from infectious disorders like syphilis, AIDS and other disorders.

The risk of thrombosis in patients with APS varies from 0.5% to 30%[11] depending upon the underlying disorder (far more in patients with autoimmune disorders such as SLE than in asymptomatic subjects) and the characteristics of aPL (antibody isotype, titre, etc.). A study on 25 Indian patients positive for lupus anticoagulant found that 40% developed thrombosis whereas 20% presented with bleeding manifestations. Nearly 20-25% of the female patients who conceived had recurrent first trimester fetal losses. Thus the spectrum of hemostatic disorders in patients with lupus anticoagulant can be highly variable.[12] According to analysis of 1000 patients reported by the multicenter Euro-Phospholipid Project, APS is 5 times more common in women than men.[13]

Etiology

The principal antigenic target of aPL is not phospholipids but a phospholipid binding plasma protein- β_2 GP-1 (apolipoprotein H). A common domain in the molecule is responsible for phospholipid binding as well as antigenicity. It naturally binds to phosphatidylserine on activated or apoptotic cell membranes including those of trophoblasts, platelets and endothelial cells and may be involved in physiological function of the elimination of apoptotic cells as well as natural anticoagulation.[14,15] Besides β_2 GP-1, many other antigens are targeted by aPLs. The molecules include prothrombin, annexin V, protein C, protein S, high and low molecular kininogens, tissue plasminogen activator, factor VII, factor XI, factor XII, complement component C4 and factor H.[16]

The origin of aPLs is unclear. One of the most probable mechanisms is exposure to various infectious agents including viruses like HIV, bacteria

(Treponema, Borrelia, Leptospira), parasites and drugs (chlorpromazine, procainamide, quinidine, phenytoin).[17,18] aPLs are also documented in patients with lymphoproliferative disorders. Autoimmune mechanisms play an important role in origin of aPLs as documented by their presence in SLE, RA, and other autoimmune disorders. The presence of low levels of aPLs in normal individuals may point to a physiological presence of these antibodies and a possible role in the removal of oxidized lipids.[7]

PATHOGENESIS

A. **Cellular, Subcellular and Extracellular Factors Related to Thrombosis**
   Some subsets of aPL antibodies act in concert with other factors to produce a procoagulant state. The pathogenesis of aPL-mediated thrombosis may comprise the following phases:
   a. *Activation of endothelial cells, PMNs and monocytes and production of proinflammatory and procoagulant state:* Evidence suggests that the antibody-β_2 GP-1 dimer activates the complement cascade. Through C5a and β_2 GP-1 surface receptors, aPL antibodies cause β_2 GP-1 dependent activation of intracellular signalling pathways involving p38 mitogen-activated protein kinase (MAPK) in platelets, endothelial cells and monocyte as well as NFKB in endothelial cells.[19,20] The intracellular effects lead to the following:[19-23]
      i. Upregulation and expression of adhesion molecules such as ICAM-1, VCAM-1 and P-selectin on endothelial cells.
      ii. Upregulation and expression of proinflammatory molecules as IL-1, IL-6, IL-8, TNF α, oxidants and proteases
      iii. Tissue factor synthesis by leukocytes.[24] Tissue factor activates factor VII, thus activating the extrinsic pathway of coagulation.
      All these effects ultimately create a procoagulant state and explain at least in part why aPL autoantibodies cause thrombosis.
   b. Alternatively, aPL might promote thrombosis by *platelet activation* leading to enhanced platelet adhesion and increased thromboxane synthesis.[25]
   c. *Inhibition of protein C activation system.* Activated protein C inactivates factors Va and VIIIa and thus inhibits thrombus formation. aPL can inhibit protein C activation and produce unopposed thrombin formation.[26]

   High levels of aPL may persist for years in asymptomatic persons before evidence of thrombosis appears. It appears that vascular injury and endothelial cell activation precede the occurrence of thrombosis in aPL positive people.[27,28] This 'second-hit' is important for precipitation of thrombosis.

B. **Factors Related to Pregnancy Loss**
   The role of aPL antibodies in pregnancy loss has been demonstrated in several studies. In addition to the mechanisms discussed above, other possible contributory mechanisms include:

a. *aPL displacement of annexin V proteins from trophoblast surfaces:*[29] Annexin V is a protein expressed on surface of placental trophoblast with potent anticoagulant activity and thus plays a role in maintaining an anticoagulant trophoblastic surface. Displacement of annexin V may make trophoblast surfaces procoagulant, finally leading to placental thrombosis and pregnancy loss.
b. *Downregulation of signal transducer and activator of transcription 5 (stat-5):* aPLs, through downregulation of Stat-5, inhibit the production of placental prolactin and insulin-like growth factor binding protein-1 and inhibits the normal establishment of placental function by adversely affecting the formation of trophoblast syncytium, placental apoptosis and trophoblast invasion.[30]

PATHOLOGY

Vascular Thrombosis and Vasculopathy

Various tissues show noninflammatory occlusion of all caliber arteries and veins. The most frequent site of venous thrombosis is the deep and superficial veins of leg. Other sites of venous thrombosis include pelvic, renal, mesenteric, portal, hepatic, axillary and sagittal veins and IVC.[31] The intracerebral arteries are the most frequently involved arterial bed. Other arterial sites are retinal, coronary, brachial, mesenteric, renal arterioles and peripheral arteries. Usually the vascular event occurs at single site and can recur either at the same or at different sites.

Histopathology may also show evidence of endothelial injury and its sequel. Recanalization may be seen in late stages.

Uteroplacental insufficiency is contributed by spiral artery vasculopathy characterized by atherosis, intimal thickening, fibrinoid necrosis and thrombosis.[32] Recent evidence also suggests an inflammatory contribution to placental injury.[33]

CLINICAL FEATURES OF APS

Patients with APS form a heterogeneous group with clinical manifestations ranging from asymptomatic to catastrophic APS. Recurrent vascular thrombosis, presenting with various organ dysfunctions and pregnancy losses associated with persistently positive anticardiolipin or lupus anticoagulant tests, however, constitute the clinical hallmarks of APS. Many patients also have clinical and laboratory features of other autoimmune disorders and these are known as 'Secondary APS', distinguishing them from patients with features of APS alone, who are termed as 'Primary APS'.

In patients with secondary APS or even in primary APS, careful search should be made for factors other than those related to APS, which can contribute to complications such as thrombosis or pregnancy losses, e.g.

hypercoagulable state in SLE patients with membranous lupus nephritis producing nephrotic syndrome or pregnancy loss due to complete heart block in fetus.

Though many of the clinical features of APS are related to thrombosis of vessels, there are some features such as thrombocytopenia, hemolytic anemia, abnormalities of cardiac valves, nonthrombotic skin lesions, nonthrombotic CNS abnormalities whose pathophysiological mechanisms are not known at present. The clinical features in various organs may manifest as:

Venous Thrombosis

Venous thrombosis typically presents with deep venous thrombosis (DVT) in the lower extremities.[34,35] More than half of the patients with symptomatic DVT have asymptomatic pulmonary embolism (PE). No particular clinical pattern of venous thrombosis is characteristic of APS. Unusual sites of venous thrombosis have included the upper extremities, intracranial veins, inferior and superior vena cava, hepatic veins (Budd-Chiari syndrome), portal vein, renal vein, and retinal vein.

Arterial Thrombosis

Arterial thromboses are less common than venous thromboses and occur in a variety of settings in patients with primary APS.[35] Patients with arterial thrombosis most commonly present with transient ischemic attack or stroke (50%) or myocardial infarction (23%).[13] These relatively common arterial occlusive events are suggestive of APS when they occur in individuals under age 60 without classical risk factors for atherosclerosis like family history, cigarette smoking, hyperlipidemia, hypertension and diabetes mellitus. Arterial thrombosis may also involve other large and small vessels, which is somewhat unusual for other thrombophilic disorders or atherosclerotic occlusive disease. These potential sites include thromboses of brachial and subclavian arteries, axillary artery (aortic arch syndrome), aorta, iliac, femoral, renal, mesenteric, retinal, and other peripheral arteries.

Nervous System

Stroke and TIA are the most frequent neurological complications.[36] Recurrent strokes may occasionally present with multi-infarct dementia. Central venous sinus thrombosis may be a manifestation of APS. Many neurological abnormalities are not clearly linked to thrombosis but may result from the direct effect of aPL or immune complex deposition in cerebral or spinal cord vessels. These include transverse myelopathy, chorea, GB syndrome, psychosis and migraine.[36] Seizures may also be a primary manifestation of APS. Some patients develop nonfocal neurological symptoms such as lack of consciousness, forgetfulness and dizzy spells.

Cardiac

The cardiac valves can be affected by diffuse valvular thickening, vegetations, stenosis and regurgitation. Mitral followed by aortic regurgitation is more frequent but is usually mild and does not produce symptoms or require surgical management. Myocardial infarction may develop due to involvement of larger vessels or microvascular thrombosis. Myocarditis or intracardiac thrombi can be the other features.

Pulmonary

Pulmonary hypertension, pulmonary arterial thrombosis, pulmonary emboli and rarely diffuse pulmonary hemorrhage and acute respiratory distress syndrome can be the features of APS.

Gastrointestinal and Hepatobiliary

Budd-Chiari syndrome can be a presenting complaint in these patients. Infarction of any part notably intestine, liver, spleen, gallbladder may develop. Rarely patients may present with ischemic colitis, esophageal perforation, pancreatitis or ascites.

Renal

Renal vein or renal artery thrombosis may develop which may be associated with renal infarction. Thrombotic microangiopathy is a distinctive feature. The patients may present with acute renal failure, hypertension or proteinuria, nephritic syndrome or hematuria.

Skin

Leg ulcers, livedo reticularis (Fig. 7.1), cutaneous necrosis, gangrene of digits (Fig. 7.2) or extremities, thrombophlebitis, necrotizing pupura and nailfold infarcts can all occur. Leg ulcers can be multiple, painful, have sharp margins and commonly occur in pretibial area and ankle or can occasionally occur as a single large ulcer.[37]

Ophthalmic

Retinal vein or artery thombosis, amaurosis fugax or retinitis.

Hematological

Mild thrombocytopenia (1-1.5 lakh/mm^3), seldom low enough to cause hemorrhage, is an important feature of APS.[13] Various hypotheses to explain thrombocytopenia include direct binding of aPL to platelet membrane or β_2 GP-1/phospholipids complex or coexisting antibodies to platelet membrane glycoproteins. Also, hemolytic anemia, hemolytic uremic syndrome or thrombotic thrombocytopenic purpura may occur. Rarely antiprothrombin antibodies may cause hemorrhage by depleting prothrombin (lupus anticoagulant hypothrombinemia syndrome).[38]

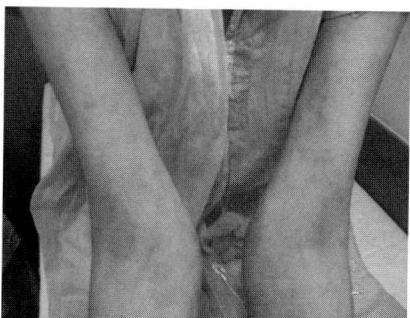

Fig. 7.1: Livedo reticularis over the forearms in a patient with APS
(For color version, see Plate 1)

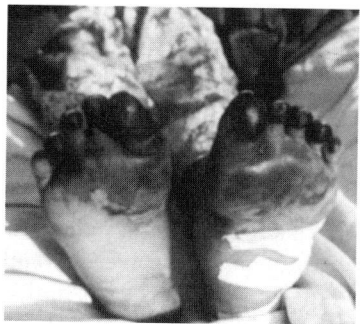

Fig. 7.2: Digital gangrene in another patient with APS secondary to SLE
(For color version, see Plate 1)

Endocrine

Infarction of major endocrine glands including adrenal, testicular and pituitary may result in failure of these glands.

Miscellaneous

Thrombosis of major vessels like aorta or vena cava may occur. Thrombosis in extremities, mesentry or splenic vein may develop. Occasionally features like perforation of nasal septum or avasular necrosis of bone may point to an underlying APS.[39]

Catastrophic Antiphospholipid Syndrome

Catastrophic APS is a rare but a life-threatening complication characterized by thrombosis of multiple medium and small arteries occurring concurrently over a short period of days. The common sites of involvement (ischemia) are renal, pulmonary, cerebral, cardiac, gastrointestinal and cutaneous vessels. Rarely, other sites like adrenal, testicular, splenic and pancreatic involvement can also occur. Thrombotic microangiopathy is a characteristic feature resulting in symptoms related to dysfunction of the affected organs especially hypertension and renal failure, ARDS, alveolar hemorrhage and capillaritis, confusion and disorientation, abdominal pain and distension or peripheral gangrene. Acute adrenal failure may be the initial clinical event.[7] Patients often have moderate thrombocytopenia. Tissue biopsy shows noninflammatory vascular occlusions.

Preliminary Criteria for the Classification of Catastrophic Antiphospholipid Syndrome (CAPS)[40]

1. Evidence of involvement of three or more organs, systems, or tissues
2. Development of manifestations simultaneously or in less than 1 week
3. Confirmation by histopathology of small vessel occlusion in at least one organ or tissue
4. Laboratory confirmation of the presence of antiphospholipid antibody (lupus anticoagulant or anticardiolipin or anti–β2-glycoprotein 1 antibodies).

Definite Catastrophic APS: All 4 criteria; else Probable Catastrophic APS.

Precipitating factors contributing to the development of CAPS most commonly include infections, oral contraceptives, surgical procedures or withdrawal of anticoagulation.

Pregnancy Morbidity

The risk for pregnancy morbidity is unknown in asymptomatic patients who are aPL-positive and in APS patients who have only vascular events but it can be as high as 90% in untreated patients who have APS and a previous history of pregnancy morbidity. Pregnancy losses are a frequent complication; reported in more than 50% of women with high or medium titres of IgG anticardiolipin. The aborted fetus is morphologically normal in most cases. HELLP syndrome, pre-eclampsia or oligohydramnios may occur.[39] Fetal distress and premature births can occur frequently. Though the fetal complications can occur at any stage of gestation, more commonly they occur in third trimester. The neonates born to mothers with APS may test positive for anticardiolipin but usually remain asymptomatic.

A study on Indian patients found primary APS as an important etiological factor in patients developing stroke at young age, premature CAD, deep vein thrombosis, primary pulmonary hypertension, peripheral arterial thrombosis and bad obstetric history. However, thrombocytopenia was rare in primary APS as compared to patients with an underlying connective tissue disease.[41]

LAB DIAGNOSIS

Lab diagnosis of APS is based on a positive lupus anticoagulant, anti-cardiolipin antibody test or anti-β_2 GP-1 antibodies.

Lupus Anticoagulant Test

It is a functional assay, which measures the ability of a subset of PL antibodies to prolong the phosholipid dependent clotting tests such as APTT or RVVT. This assay is based on the property of antibodies to inhibit clotting *in vitro,* by partially blocking the conversion of prothrombin to thrombin in the presence of phospholipids and thus finally delaying the clot formation.

The lupus anticoagulant test is performed with patient's plasma and requires following steps:
  i. Demonstration of a prolonged coagulation screening test such as APTT or dilute Russell viper venom time.
  ii. Failure to correct the prolonged screening test by mixing patient's plasma with normal plasma, thereby excluding the possibility of clotting factor deficiency and demonstrating the presence of clotting inhibitor.

iii. Normalization of the prolonged screening test by addition of excess phospholipids, thus demonstrating the 'phospholipid-dependent' character of the clotting inhibitor in patient's plasma (i.e. the aPL antibodies) and excluding other inhibitors such as anti-factor VIII or anti-factor II.

The unique and perplexing character of APS is the ability of aPL antibodies to act as clotting inhibitors *in vitro* but to promote clotting *in vivo*.

Anticardiolipin Test

It is an ELISA based test for detection of antibodies which bind cardiolipin or some combination of cardiolipin and β_2GP-1 using cardiolipin in presence of β_2GP-1 as antigen. The results are reported according to the isotype (IgG, IgM or IgA) levels and generally as semiquantitative level as normal, low positive, moderate positive or high positive. Only moderate to high levels are significant as low titres have no proven relation to APS. Moreover, a positive test should be repeated after 12 weeks to rule out a transient positivity, which again has no clinical significance.

Lupus anticoagulant is a more specific test and correlates better with aPL related clinical events. In comparison, anticardiolipin is more sensitive (positive in about 80% of patients) but less specific for the diagnosis of APS.

Other Lab Work-up

The patient with vascular occlusive disease or recurrent fetal loss should be thoroughly investigated to confirm the presence of other causes of thrombosis. Testing should be done for protein C, protein S, antithrombin III deficiency, factor V Leiden, prothrombin mutations and hyperhomocystinemia. At least 50% of APS patients with vascular events possess other acquired thrombosis risk factors at the time of event.[27,28] Thus, presence of coexisting inherited or acquired risk factors for thrombosis does not exclude the diagnosis of APS. ANA and anti-dsDNA antibodies can be positive in patients with primary APS who do not have features of SLE. Platelet count is generally modestly decreased ($\sim 50,000/mm^3$). Patients with thrombotic microangiopathy may develop proteinuria and renal insufficiency but hypocomplementemia, red blood cell casts and pyuria are not a feature.

Some patients with APS will have biological false-positive serological test for syphilis (STS) which measures the ability of aPL antibodies to precipitate VDRL antigen.

DIAGNOSIS OF APS

Diagnosis of APS requires persistently positive lupus anticoagulant test or moderate to high titre anticardiolipin anticardiolipin (IgG or IgM) or anti–β_2 GP-1 antibodies in patients with characteristic clinical features of thrombosis or pregnancy morbidity.

Revised Sapporo Criteria for Classification of Antiphospholipid Syndrome[42]

Clinical Criteria

1. Vascular thrombosis: One or more clinical episodes of arterial, venous or small vessel thrombosis in any tissue or organ.
2. Pregnancy morbidity:
    a. One or more unexplained deaths of a morphologically normal fetus at or beyond the 10th week of gestation, or
    b. One or more premature births of a morphologically normal neonate at or before 34th week of gestation because of eclampsia, severe pre-eclampsia or severe placental insufficiency, or
    c. Three or more unexplained consecutive spontaneous abortions before the 10th week of gestation in the absence of maternal anatomic or hormonal abnormalities and paternal and maternal chromosomal causes.

Laboratory Criteria

1. Lupus anticoagulant present in plasma on two or more occasions at least 12 weeks apart, detected according to the guidelines of the International Society on Thrombosis and Hemostasis (as described above).
2. Anticardiolipin antibody of IgG and or IgM isotype in serum, present in medium or high titre, on two or more occasions at least 12 weeks apart, measured by a standardized ELISA.
3. Anti-β_2 GP-1 IgG and/or IgM isotype in serum or plasma (in titer > 99th percentile), present on two or more occasions, at least 12 weeks apart, measured by a standardized ELISA, according to recommended procedures.

Definite antiphospholipid antibody syndrome is considered to be present if at least one clinical and one laboratory criterion is met.

Classification of APS should be avoided if less than 12 weeks or more than 5 years separate the positive aPL test and the clinical manifestation.

Patients with negative lupus anticoagulant and anticardiolipin tests but high suspicion of APS should be tested for IgA anticardiolipin and IgA anti β_2GP-1. Along with these, presence of certain clinical features not included in classification criteria like presence of livedo reticularis, thrombocytopenia, autoimmune hemolytic anemia, cardiac valve thickening or vegetations, early pre-eclampsia, multiple sclerosis like syndrome, chorea or myelopathy may be helpful for diagnosis in individual patients.

APS may occur as an isolated disease. At the same time positive tests may be detected in patients with SLE, RA or other related systemic autoimmune disorders. Among these, nearly 30% of patients with lupus anticoagulant and 30-50% with high or medium IgG anticardiolipin tests have clinical features of APS, known as Secondary APS. A variety of drugs, infections or other miscellaneous disorders may produce a positive test but these individuals do not have clinical features suggestive of APS.

MANAGEMENT

Patients with APS constitute a heterogenous group as far as clinical presentation is concerned and, therefore, also with regard to the treatment required.

Management of Thrombosis

Primary Thromboprophylaxis

The prophylactic treatment of patients with aPL remains controversial.[43] Present recommendations favor treatment of patients with persistently positive aPL (moderate to high titres) and/or unequivocally positive lupus anticoagulant with low dose aspirin (75-100 mg/d) for an indefinite period.[31,44] The presence of underlying CTD further supports the use of prophylactic aspirin. In addition, it is important to address factors which increase the risk of thrombosis such as smoking, estrogen containing OCPs, hypertension, hyperlipidemia or diabetes. Patients should be informed about the warning signs requiring consultation with a specialist. Any acute or high-risk situations like surgery should be managed by prophylaxis with heparin. The role of long-term anticoagulation with low intensity warfarin is being studied. In patients with SLE with aPL, hydroxychloroquine may be protective against development of both venous and arterial thrombosis.[45] Hydroxychloroquine has an immunomodulatory effect by interfering with antigen processing and inhibiting intracellular signaling pathways and activation of NF-kB. These proposed mechanisms may allow the use of hydroxychloroquine in non-SLE patients in future.

Acute Episode of Thrombosis

Parenteral anticoagulation with heparin is the treatment for acute thrombosis in APS patients. Thrombolytic agents are not generally useful because of high incidence of recurrence.

Secondary Thromboprophylaxis

The evidence suggests that APS patients who had an episode of thrombosis are at a very high-risk of recurrence which merits regular anticoagulation for secondary thromboprophylaxis.[46] Though the optimal intensity of anticoagulation is uncertain, warfarin is used to maintain an INR of 2 to 3 for both arterial and venous thrombosis patients. Patients with arterial thrombosis with high-risk for recurrence may require a more intense anticoagulation. Patients in whom INR is unreliable (due to presence of lupus anticoagulant) may be treated with unfractionated or LMW heparin and monitored by antifactor Xa activity. The duration for which the anticoagulation should be continued also remains unresolved. The present clinical data support the use of life-long anticoagulation of APS patients with an episode of vascular thrombosis. However, the patients need to be risk stratified based on clinical, thrombophilic and immunological characteristics before final decision. Recent findings of complete remission of antibody in some patients and removal of the triggers which are necessary for precipitating thrombosis in a patient may allow for discontinuing anticoagulation in selected patients. Warfarin may be used in association with low dose aspirin for secondary prophylaxis. The role of clopidogrel, pentoxyphylline, aspirin-dipyridamole, argatroban, hirudin and other newer anticoagulants is not clear.

Thromboprophylaxis in Patients with Recurrent Thrombosis

Some patients continue to experience recurrent arterial or venous thrombosis despite anticoagulation (INR 2 to 3). These patients appropriately require high-intensity warfarin (INR 3 to 4).[47] Aspirin (80-325 mg/d), hydroxychloroquine and statins can be tried along with warfarin. IVIG and plasmapheresis have also been tried with variable success. The risk-benefit ratio does not favor use of corticosteroids or immunosuppressives as prophylactic agents though they have a specific role in the management of life-threatening complications. It is important to stress here that the timely recognition of the specific triggers precipitating thrombosis and their elimination can play an important role in overall prevention of the clinical episodes.

Management of Catastrophic APS

Early recognition and timely treatment with anticoagulants and steroids can be life-saving. The clinical condition may require this treatment to be combined with repeated plasma exchange or IVIG or even fibrinolytic therapy though success is highly variable.[40] If needed, more aggressive immunosuppression with cyclophosphamide or rituximab may be tried. Despite the multi-modality treatment, the mortality is high and nearly half of the patients fail to survive.[48]

Management of Pregnancy Morbidity

Management of pregnancy in women with APS requires anticoagulation with either heparin or aspirin or both depending on the prior history of thrombosis or recurrent fetal loss.

aPL Positive Women with Prior Thrombosis

If these women are on warfarin and want to become pregnant, it is important to switch to heparin or LMWH before conception or at least at the first missed menstrual period. Patient should be fully anticoagulated receiving enoxaparin 1 mg/kg subcutaneously twice a day along with aspirin throughout pregnancy.

aPL Positive Women with Repeated Pregnancy Loss

Heparin/LMWH (30-40 mg enoxaparin/day) combined with low dose aspirin should be started after confirmation of pregnancy.[49,50] This increases fetal survival rate from 50% (untreated) to 80%. The anticoagulation should continue till 48 hours before anticipated delivery. It is resumed for 8-12 weeks postpartum because of the risk of postpartum thrombosis and then discontinued by tapering the dose. If desired, conversion from heparin to warfarin can be done as early as first or second week postpartum. Ultrasound monitoring of fetal growth and uteroplacental blood flow generally at 4 week intervals is required, allowing for timely delivery. Even with treatment, prematurity and fetal growth restriction can occur. So more frequent monitoring can be done, if required.

The role of IVIG is not clear.[43] However, it can be used in conjunction with heparin and low dose aspirin especially in patients with poor past obstetric history. Clopidogrel and newer antithrombotic agents may be tried together with IVIG and hydrocortisone for patients who are unable to use heparin or who fail heparin treatment.

Patients with *aPL and first pregnancy* or *women with very early pregnancy losses* or whose *aPL titres are low and transient* are generally not treated with heparin. However, low dose aspirin is recommended.

Management of Other Complications

Thrombocytopenia

It is generally mild but occasionally severe thrombocytopenia requiring corticosteroids may develop. Steroid resistant cases may have a trial of low dose aspirin, dapsone, danazol, hydroxychloroquine or IVIG. Anticoagulation with warfarin may also be advised though the efficacy is not clear. One study supports the efficacy of rituximab in refractory thrombocytopenia.[51] Splenectomy has also been performed successfully in some patients with APS and refractory thrombocytopenia.

Headache

Usually responds to conventional treatment. Low dose aspirin or warfarin may be required in very resistant cases.

Valvulopathy

Anticoagulation is advised for valvulopathy. In case significant hemodynamic damage occurs, surgical replacement needs to be done. All patients with APS and valve prosthesis should have full anticoagulation.

Other Issues in Management

Though the efficacy of anticoagulation is not clear, it has been used for livedo reticularis, thrombotic microangiopathy and leg ulcers. Rituximab may be tried for skin ulcers.[51] In case of SLE patients requiring renal transplant, presence of aPL antibodies is associated with poor prognosis,[52] causing thrombotic microangiopathy in the grafted tissue despite anticoagulation, thrombosis of graft's renal vein as well as increasing the risk of post-transplant thromboembolic phenomena.

Potential Current and Future Treatments for Antiphospholipid Syndrome

There are many other antithrombotic agents as well as immunomodulatory drugs which have the potential to be used for the treatment of APS but further experience and controlled studies are required to determine the exact role of these agents in the management. These may include non-aspirin antiplatelet drugs like dipyridamole, ticlopidine, or clopidogrel bisulfate; indirect and direct thrombin inhibitors; recombinant human activated protein C; prostacyclin, and anticytokine treatment. With better understanding of the intracellular mechanisms of aPL-mediated thrombosis it is likely that future therapeutic approaches to APS will include more specifically targeted anti-inflammatory or immunomodulatory therapies rather than antithrombotics. Some agents that can be considered in clinical trials in the near future include GP1b/IIIa-specific antagonists; p38MAPK inhibitors; thromboxane A2 inhibitors; tissue factor expression inhibitors; complement inhibitors and β_2GP-1 tolerogen.[53] Some newer anticoagulants in development are also potential options.

PROGNOSIS

The functional outcome of patients with isolated APS in the long-term is poor. Serious morbidity and disability occurs in patients with APS who experience major vascular events and those with delay in diagnosis and treatment. At the end of 10 years, nearly one-third of patients have permanent organ damage.[54] Also, one-third of obstetric patients experience aPL-related complications.[55] In patients with SLE, aPL positivity correlates with poor graft survival after renal transplant. Vigorous perioperative antithrombosis strategies (pharmacological as well as physical) are required in all aPL positive patients undergoing any surgical procedures as they are at high-risk of thrombosis and complications.

TAKE HOME MESSAGE

Antiphospholipid syndrome should be suspected in patients with clinical evidence of arterial or venous thrombosis in any organ of the body. It should also be suspected in patients who may not have a history of thrombosis but present with recurrent fetal loss. The availability of tests for antiphopholipid antibodies including lupus anticoagulant, anticardiolipin antibodies and anti-β_2 GP-1 antibodies helps by providing confirmatory evidence and facilitating timely intervention, which can significantly change the overall outcome.

REFERENCES

1. Conley CL, Hartmann RC. A hemorrhage disorder caused by circulating anticoagulant in patients with disseminated lupus erythematosus. J Clin Invest 1952;31:621-22.
2. Galli M, Comfurius P, Maasen C, et al. Anticardiolipin antibodies directed not to cardiolipin but to a plasma cofactor. Lancet 1990;335:1544-47.
3. Rao LVM, Hoarg AD, Rapaport SI. Differences in the interaction of lupus anticoagulant. IgG with human prothrombin and bovine prothrombin. Thromb Haemost 1995;73:668-74.
4. Petri M Epidemiology of the antiphospholipid antibody syndrome. J Autoimmun 2000;15:145-51.
5. Vila P, Hernandez MC, Lopez-Fernandez MF, et al. Prevalence, follow-up and clinical significance of the aCL in normal subjects. Thromb Haemost 1994;72: 209-13.
6. Petri M. Epidemiology of the antiphospholipid antibody syndrome. J Autoimmun 2000; 15:145-51.
7. Erkan D, Salmon JE, Lockshin MD. Antiphospholipid syndrome. In: Kelley's Textbook of Rheumatology, 8th edn, Firestein GS, Budd RC, Harris ED, McInnes IB, Ruddy S, Sergent JS (Eds), Philadelphia, Saunders 2008.
8. Shrivastava A, Dwivedi S, Aggarwal A, Misra R. Prevalence of anticardiolipin and beta-2 glycoprotein 1 antibodies in patients with suspected primary antiphospholipid syndrome: A preliminary report. JIRA 2001;9:20-22.
9. Saluja S, Kumar A, Khamastha M, Hughes GRV, Malaviya AN. Prevalence and clinical associations of anticardiolipin antibodies in patients with systemic lupus erythematosus in India. Indian J Med Res 1990;92:224-27.
10. Bhattacharya M, Kannan M, Biswas A, Kumar A, Saxena R. Beta2 glycoprotein 1 in Indian patients with SLE. Clin Appl Thromb Hemost 2005;11:223-26.
11. Gezer S. Antiphospholipid syndrome. Dis Mon 2003;49:696-741.
12. Bhattacharya M, Biswas A, Kannan M, Mishra P, Kumar A, Choudhary VP, Saxena R. Clinicohematologic spectrum in patients with lupus anticoagulant. Clin Appl Thromb Hemost 2005;11:191-95.
13. Cervera R, Piette JC, Font J, et al. Antiphospholipid syndrome: Clinical and immunologic manifestations and patterns of disease expression in a cohort of 1,000 patients. Arthritis Rheum 2002;46:1019-27.
14. Casciola-Rosen L, Rosen A, Petri M, et al. Surface blebs on apoptotic cells are sites of enhanced procoagulant activity: Implications for coagulation events and antigenic spread in systemic lupus erythematosus. Proc Natl Acad Sci USA 1996;93:1624-29.
15. Mori T, Takeya H, Nishioka J, et al. Beta 2-glycoprotein-1 modulates the anticoagulant activity of activated protein C on the phospholipid surface. Thromb Haemost 1996;75:49-55.
16. Bertolaccini ML, Hughes GR. Antiphospholipid antibody testing: Which are most useful for diagnosis?. Rheum Dis Clin North Am 2006;32:455-63.
17. Gharavi AE, Pierangeli SS, Harris EN. Origin of antiphospholipid antibodies. Rheum Dis Clin North Am 2001; 27:551-63.
18. Blank M, Krause I, Fridkin M. Bacterial induction of autoantibodies to beta 2-glycoprotein-1 accounts for the infectious etiology of antiphospholipid syndrome. J Clin Invest 2002; 109:797-804.
19. Dunoyer-Geindre S, de Moerloose P, Galve-de Rochemonteix B, et al. NF kappa B is an essential intermediate in the activation of endothelial cells by anti-beta 2-glycoprotein-1 antibodies. Thromb Haemost 2002;88:851-57.
20. Pierangeli SS, Vega-Ostertag M, Harris EN. Intracellular signaling triggered by antiphospholipid antibodies in platelets and endothelial cells: A pathway to targeted therapies. Thromb Res 2004;114:467-76.

21. Bordron A, Dueymes MY, Levy Y, et al. Anti-endothelial cell antibody binding makes negatively charged phospholipids accessible to antiphospholipid antibodies. Arthritis Rheum 1998;41:1738-47.
22. Simantov R, LaSala J, Lo SK, et al. Activation of cultured vascular endothelial cells by antiphospholipid antibodies. J Clin Invest 1996;96:2211-19.
23. Font J, Espinosa G, Tassies D, et al. Effects of β_2-glycoprotein-1 and monoclonal anticardiolipin antibodies in platelet interaction with subendothelium under flow conditions. Arthritis Rheum 2002;46:3283-89.
24. Reverter JC, Tassies D, Font J, et al. Effects of human monoclonal anticardiolipin antibodies on platelet function and on tissue factor expression on monocytes. Arthritis Rheum 1998;41:1420-27.
25. Campbell AL, Pierangeli SS, Wellhausen S, et al. Comparison of the effect of anti-cardiolipin antibodies from patients with antiphospholipid syndrome and with syphilis on platelet activation and aggregation. Thromb Haemost 1995;73:519-24.
26. Smirnov MD, Triplett DT, Comp PC, et al. On the role of phosphatidylethanolamine in the inhibition of activated protein C activity by antiphospholipid antibodies. J Clin Invest 1995;95:309-16.
27. Kaul M, Erkan D, Sammaritano L, et al. Assessment of the 2006 revised antiphospholipid syndrome (APS) classification criteria. Arthritis Rheum 2006;54:S796.
28. Erkan D, Yazici Y, Peterson MG, et al. A cross-sectional study of clinical thrombotic risk factors and preventive treatments in antiphospholipid syndrome. Rheumatology (Oxford) 2002;41:924-29.
29 Rand JH. Antiphospholipid antibody mediated disruption of the Annexin V antithrombotic shield: A thrombogenic mechanism for the antiphospholipin syndrome. J Autoimmun 2000;15:107-11.
30. Mak IYH, Brosens JJ, Christian M, et al. Regulated expression of signal transducer and activator of transcription, Stat5, and its enhancement of PRL expression in human endometrial stromal cells *in vitro*. J Clin Endocrinol Metab 2002;87: 2581-87.
31. Harris EN, Khamashta MA. Antiphospholipid syndrome: Diagnosis and management. In: Rheumatology 4th edn, Hochberg MC, Silman AJ, Smolen JS, Weinblatt ME, Weisman MW (Eds), Philadelphia, Mosby 2007;1353-60.
32. Khong TY, De Wolf F, Robertson WB, et al. Inadequate maternal vascular response to placentation in pregnancies complicated by pre-eclampsia and by small-for-gestational-age infants. Br J Obstet Gynaecol 1986;93:1049-59.
33. Stone S, Pijnenborg R, Vercruysse L, et al. The placental bed in pregnancies complicated by primary antiphospholipid syndrome. Placenta 2006;27:457-67.
34. Provenzale JM, Ortel T, Allen N. Systemic thrombosis in patients with antiphospholipid syndrome: Lesion distribution and imaging findings. Am J Roentgenol 1998;170:285-90.
35. Cervera R. Lessons from the 'Euro-Phospholipid' project. Autoimmun Rev 2008;7:174-78.
36. Brey RL. Differential diagnosis of central nervous system manifestations of the antiphospholipid antibody syndrome. J Autoimmun 2000;15:133-38.
37. Gibson GE, Su WP, Pittelkow MR. Antiphospholipid syndrome and the skin. J Am Acad Dermatol 1997;36:970-82.
38. Erkan D, Bateman H, Lockshin MD. Lupus-anticoagulant-hypoprothrombinemia syndrome associated with systemic lupus erythematosus: Report of 2 cases and review of literature. Lupus 1999;8:560-64.
39. Baker WF, Bick RL. The Clinical Spectrum of Antiphospholipid Syndrome. Hematology/Oncology Clin of North Am 2008;22:33-52.
40. Asherson RA, Cervera R, de Groot PG, et al. Catastrophic antiphospholipid syndrome: International consensus statement on classification criteria and treatment guidelines. Lupus 2003;12:530-34.

41. Malatesha G, Grover R, Kumar A, et al. Primary antiphospholipid syndrome: Clinical spectrum in Indian patients. Indian J Rheumatol 2006;14:7-15.
42. Miyakis S. International consensus statement on an update of the classification criteria for definite antiphospholipid syndrome (APS). J Thromb Haemost 2006;4:295-306.
43. Espinosa G, Cervera R. Thromboprophylaxis and obstetric management of the antiphospholipid syndrome. Expert Opin. Pharmacother 2009;10:601-14.
44. Gerosa M, Chighizola C, Meroni PL. Aspirin in asymptomatic patients with confirmed positivity of antiphospholipid antibodies. Yes (in some cases). Intern Emerg Med 2008;3:201-03.
45. Ruiz-Irastorza G, Egurbide MV, Pijoan JI, et al. Effect of antimalarials on thrombosis and survival in patients with systemic lupus erythematosus. Lupus 2006;15:577-83.
46. Ruiz-Irastorza G, Hunt BJ, Khamashta MA. A systematic review of secondary thromboprophylaxis in patients with antiphospholipid antibodies. Arthritis Rheum 2007;57:1487-95.
47. Crowther MA, Ginsberg JS, Julian J, et al. A comparison of two intensities of warfarin for the prevention of recurrent thrombosis in patients with the antiphospholipid antibody syndrome. N Engl J Med 2003;349:1133-38.
48. Vero S, Asherson RA, Erkan D. Critical care review: Catastrophic antiphospholipid syndrome. J Intensive Care Med 2006;21:144-59.
49. Kutteh WH. Antiphospholipid antibody-associated recurrent pregnancy loss: Treatment with heparin and low-dose aspirin is superior to low-dose aspirin alone. Am J Obstet Gynecol 1996;174:1584-89.
50. Rai R, Cohen H, Dave M, et al. Randomised controlled trial of aspirin and aspirin plus heparin in pregnant women with recurrent miscarriage associated with antiphospholipid antibodies. BMJ 1997;314:253-57.
51. Tenedios F, Erkan D, Lockshin MD. Rituximab in the primary antiphospholipid syndrome (PAPS). Arthritis Rheum 2005;52:4078.
52. Mc Intyre JA, Waagenknecht DR. Antiphospholipid antibodies – risk assessments for solid organ, bone marrow and tissue transplantation. Rheum Dis Clin North Am 2001;27:611-31.
53. Erkan D, Lockshin MD. New treatments for Antiphospholipid syndrome. Rheum Dis Clin North Am 2006;32:129-48.
54. Erkan D, Yazici Y, Sobel R, et al. Primary antiphospholipid syndrome: Functional outcome after 10 years. J Rheumatol 2000;27:2817-21.
55. Erkan D, Merrill JT, Yazici Y, et al. High thrombosis rate after fetal loss in antiphospholipid syndrome: Effective prophylaxis with aspirin. Arthritis Rheum 2001; 44:1466-67.

Chapter 8

Fanconi Anemia

Tulika Seth

INTRODUCTION

Fanconi anemia (FA) is a rare autosomal recessive disorder, this syndrome is characterized by pancytopenia, varied phenotypic anomalies, hyperpigmentation, developmental delay. This is associated with an increased susceptibility to leukemia, myelodysplastic syndromes and other malignancies. However, in recent studies 25 to almost 50% patients without any described phenotypic anomalies have been reported. The hallmark is chromosomal breaks and interchanges in the cells. Chromosomal breakage increases with exposure to mitomycin C (MMC), diepoxybutane (DEB) and cisplatin. Chromosomal interchanges result from double strand breaks in S phase and involve nonhomologous chromosomal regions. Fanconi anemia is associated with physical developmental anomalies. The commonly identified anomalies are absent/hypoplastic thumbs, absent radius, microcephaly, renal anomalies, short stature and abnormal skin pigmentation (i.e. café-au-lait and hyperpigmented or occasionally hypopigmented spots). However, developmental or skin manifestations are not essential for the diagnosis. Solid tumors have been reported in close to 10% of patients, often in young adults who may never have had aplastic anemia.[1]

Incidence

May be wider than originally believed, it is increasingly demonstrated that the diagnosis should be considered even in adults with bone marrow failure, myelodysplastic syndrome or early onset of an epithelial cancer. The reported incidence is 1 per 100,000 live births. The overall prevalence of Fanconi anemia is estimated at 1 case per 360,000 people, with a resulting carrier frequency of 1 per 300 individuals. A higher carrier frequency of 1 per 77 people has been reported in White Afrikaans in South African as a result of a founder effect. Indian incidence data and carrier frequency is incomplete.

Manifestations

The disorder affects all bone marrow elements and is associated with characteristic phenotypic features. Growth retardation may begin *in utero* and continue postnatally. Onset of pancytopenia and bone marrow hypoplasia can occur at any age from early childhood to patients 40 years of age. However, bone marrow failure may not occur in some patients. Risk factors for early bone marrow failure (BMF) are abnormal radii and a 5-item congenital abnormality score. The lowest risk group has an 18% risk of BMF while the highest risk group has an 83% risk. Patients who do not succumb to the pancytopenia, are at a higher risk of developing myelodysplasia (MDS), acute myeloid leukemia (AML) and solid tumors. Patients with Fanconi anemia and *BRCA2* mutations develop leukemia at a median age of 2.2 years, in contrast to 13.4 years in other patients with Fanconi anemia. These patients also develop brain tumors at a median age of 3.5 years at diagnosis. The liver is prone to peliosis hepatis, focal nodular hepatic hyperplasia, adenomas, hepatocellular carcinomas and prolonged androgen therapy have been implicated for their cause.

Sex and Age

No difference in male-female incidence has been reported in the literature. However, about 32% of males have abnormal genitalia compared to 3% of females. Short stature begins *in utero*. The average age of onset of anemia is about 8 years but tends to be highly variable with onset reported even in the third decade of life.

Screening Test

The screening test for Fanconi anemia is based on the pathognomonic hypersensitivity of Fanconi anemia cells to crosslinking agents [e.g. mitomycin C, diepoxy butane (DEB) and cisplatin]. This test is performed by exposing a culture of phytohemagglutinin (PHA) stimulated peripheral blood lymphocytes or skin fibroblasts to mitomycin C or DEB. Chromosomal breaks and radial chromosomes are increased in Fanconi cells in comparison to normal control cells. Chromosomal breaks, gaps, rearrangements, and endo-reduplication in cells grown *in vitro*.

Bone Marrow Evaluation

An aspirate and biopsy should be performed to assess the cellularity and morphology of the residual cells. To evaluate cellularity, the core biopsy specimen should be at least 1 cm long. In general, the marrow has very few hematopoietic cells which are replaced by fat cells, the stromal cells are replaced with lymphocytes. Residual erythroid cells may show evidence of dysplasia with nuclear-cytoplasmic maturation dissociation. Occasionally, localized pockets of normal marrow may be present.

Pathophysiology

Cells have deficient ability to excise UV-induced pyrimidine dimers from the cellular DNA. They are very sensitive to small concentrations of DNA crosslinking agents or oxidative stress. The defect may be in any of the proteins involved in DNA inter-strand crosslink repair; which leads to double-strand breaks in the S phase of the cell cycle and accumulation of cells in G2 stage. Occasionally patients may have 2 or more cell lines, one of which may be normal. The normal cell line is thought to arise from back mutation, gene conversion and selective loss of the abnormal cell line. If one cell type is normal, but suspicion for Fanconi anemia is high, testing should be repeated using another cell type.

Fanconi anemia (FA) is primarily an autosomal recessive disorder. There are at least mutations in 13 genes which are known to cause Fanconi Anemia—A, B, C, D1, D2, E, F, G, I, J, L, M and N. FANCB is an exception as its inheritance is X-linked recessive, as this gene resides on the X chromosome. Manifestations of the disease occur in homozygous or doubly heterozygous patients. Of 13 complementation groups identified so far, groups A and H are caused by mutations in gene – *FANCA*. The FA proteins A, B, C, E, F, G, L and M form a nuclear complex, which leads to ubiquitination of the I and D2 proteins, which are involved in DNA damage response mechanisms along with FANCD1, FANCJ, FANCN and BRCA1, RAD51 and other proteins. Although most are unique genes, several were previously known as other identified genes, e.g. *FANCD1 (BRCA2), GANCG (XRCC9), FANCI (KIAA1794), FANCJ (BRPI1/BACH1), FANCL (PHF9/POG), FANCM (Hef),* and *FANCN (PALB2)*. Heterozygotes for *BRCA2, BACH1* and *PALB2* are at increased risk for breast and other cancers.[2-4]

Some phenotype-genotype correlations occur, with some mutations causing mild disease and others severe. The wide variation in phenotype depends on whether the mutation is null or leads to a partially functional gene product rather than the specific gene affected. The specific role of FA gene mutations in the pathogenesis of birth defects, bone marrow failure, or oncogenesis has not been elucidated. However, the FA proteins help to neutralize reoxygenation-induced oxidative stress (ROS) or by undertaking DNA repair. Such mechanisms may help understand the causes behind bone marrow failure. It is known that crosslinking agents produce ROS and it is possible that FA cell hypersensitivity to crosslinkers is due to the cell's impaired ability to cope with the increased ROS.[4,5]

Common cytogenetic abnormalities found are monosomy 7, deletions of the long arms of chromosomes 5, 7, and 20 (5q–, 7q–, 20q–), trisomy 8 and translocations and rearrangements of chromosomes 1 and 3 the prognostic effect of these abnormalities needs to be evaluated.[4,5]

DNA diagnostics can be used to identify the specific mutation. It can be used to confirm the diagnosis, for carrier detection as well as for prenatal diagnosis and preimplantation diagnosis. Clinical gene mutation analysis is available for mutations in *FANCA, FANCC, FANCF,* and *FANCG*. Single-parameter flow cytometry can be used to detect a large population of cells in the G2 phase of the cell cycle, as a consequence of arrest of cells in late S phase.[4,5]

The genetic basis of Fanconi anemia needs to be evaluated to decide therapeutic options. Apparently unaffected siblings should be tested for FA homozygosity. Genetic counseling must be provided to parents, caregivers and carriers.

Management

According to the International Fanconi Anemia Registry, 73% of patients with Fanconi anemia develop overt bone marrow disease by age 10 years with median survival 7 years. Hearing and development needs to be evaluated in all children. The kidneys and urinary tract should be examined-ultrasound. Androgen therapy improves the blood count in half of Fanconi anemia patients treated.

Hematopoietic stem cell transplantation (HSCT) can be curative for the hematologic symptoms using matched related sibling bone marrow, cord blood or even unrelated donors for transplantation. According to a large International Bone Marrow Transplant Registry, 2-year survival probabilities were 66% after human leukocyte antigen (HLA)-matched sibling hematopoietic stem cell transplantation. Due to the sensitivity of patients with Fanconi anemia to chemotherapy and radiation, reduced doses are administered for conditioning.

Patients however still remain at risk for head and neck carcinomas starting 5 years after transplantation and may still develop myelodysplasia, acute myeloid leukemia, or solid tumors. Surveillance for early detection of malignancies must be started at an early stage; however, repeated radiographic tests should be avoided. Examinations should include dental and oropharyngeal check-ups, endoscopy and gynecological examination with Pap smear and rectal examination. Patients with *FANCF-* or *FANCB-* mutated tumors may treated with crosslinking chemotherapeutic agents, such as cisplatin.[1,4,5]

Indian Data

Consecutive patients of aplastic anemia, presenting to our department were evaluated in the period January 2002 to December 2007 (unpublished data). A total of 728 adult and pediatric patients presented with aplastic anemia, of these 57 patients (7%) had positive chromosomal fragility tests. FA was observed in 24.07 percent (13/54) Verma et al from India.[6]

These 57 Fanconi anemia patients underwent detailed assessment with evaluation for onset of symptoms, response to therapy, phenotypic characteristics and samples for complementation genes were taken.

The median age of onset of hematological symptoms was 15+2 years, Male : Female 4 : 1 and 3/57 developed leukemia. Patients presenting without phenotypic features of Fanconi, but with positive tests were 43%. There was no difference in severity of hematological problems in those with or without phenotypic features of Fanconi anemia. A wide spectrum of phenotypic defects were seen, the most consistent physical finding was short stature of ≥2SD, hypothenar flattening or thumb defects and hyperpigmentation. Renal anomalies were found in only 4 patients. Age of onset of symptoms or presence of phenotypic features did not predict survival. Response to androgen therapy significantly influenced survival, responders 14+2 months versus non-responders 23+8 months (p = 0.001). Complementation group A and C are being analyzed.

CONCLUSION

Gene therapy studies are underway,[7] as are clinical trials of improved treatment for malignancies associated with Fanconi anemia. Fanconi anemia should be considered in all young adults and children with hypoplastic or aplastic anemia, unexplained macrocytosis, myelodysplastic syndrome, acute myelogenous leukemia and epithelial malignancies, with or without characteristic physical anomalies

REFERENCES

1. Alter BP. Inherited bone marrow failure syndromes. In: Nathan DG, Oski SH, Ginsburg D, Look T, Hematology of Infancy and Childhood. 6th edn. Philadelphia, Pa: Harcourt Health Sciences; 2003:280-365.
2. Shimamura A. Inherited bone marrow failure syndromes: Molecular features. Hematology. Am Soc Hematol Educ Program 2006:63-71.
3. Casado JA, Callen E, Jacome A, Rio P, Castella M, Lobitz S, Ferro T, Munoz A, Sevilla J, Cantalejo A, Cela E, Cervera J, Sanchez-Calero J, Badell I, Estella J, Dasi A, Olive T, Ortega JJ, Rodriguez-Villa A, Tapia M, Molines A, Madero L, Segovia JC, Nevelling K, Kalb R, Schindler D, Hanenberg H, Surralles J, Bueren JA. A comprehensive strategy for the subtyping of patients with Fanconi anemia: Conclusions from the Spanish Fanconi Anemia Research Network. J Med Genet 2007;44(4):241-49.
4. Taniguchi T, D'Andrea, AD. The molecular pathogenesis of Fanconi anemia: Recent progress. Blood 2006;107:4223-33.
5. Rosenberg PS, Huang Y, Alter BP. Individualized risks of first adverse events in patients with Fanconi anemia. Blood 2004;104(2):350-55.
6. Varma N, Varma S, Marwaha RK, Malhotra P, Bansal D, Malik K, Kaur S, Garewal G. Multiple constitutional aetiological factors in bone marrow failure syndrome (BMFS) patients from north India. Indian J Med Res 2006;124(1):51-56.
7. Cohen-Haguenauer O, Peault B, Bauche C, Daniel MT, Casal I, Levy V, Dausset J, Boiron M, Auclair C, Gluckman E, Marty M. *In vivo* repopulation ability of genetically corrected bone marrow cells from Fanconi anemia patients. Proc Natl Acad Sci U S A 2006;103(7):2340-45.

Chapter 9
Chronic Lymphoproliferative Disorders (CLPDs)

S Varma, Neelam Varma

SUMMARY

Chronic lymphoproliferative disorders (CLPDs) show a lot of variation in the clinical presentation, natural course and require different therapeutic approaches. The definitive diagnosis of CLPDs is based on the use of multiple parameter analyses, including cell morphology, immunological markers, molecular and cytogenetic investigations.

KEYWORDS

Chronic lymphocytic leukemia, Chronic lymphoproliferative disorders, Flow cytometry, Hairy cell leukemia, Immnophenotype, Rai and Binet staging systems

Chronic lymphoproliferative disorders (CLPDs) are a heterogenous group of diseases which require targeted and specific therapeutic approaches.[1-3] CLPDs are a group of lymphoid disorders that are characterized by an indolent course, variable progression and good control but in most instances low complete cure rates. CLPDs could be both of B and T cell origin (Table 9.1), however, B cell lymphoproliferative disorders are much more frequent. Of these chronic lymphocytic leukemia (CLL) comprises 90% of CLPDs, being the commonest type worldwide.

CLL is the most common leukemia (nearly 40%) encountered in adults in the western countries. Incidence of CLL is reported to be low in Asia, specially India, China and Japan. Hairy cell leukemia (HCL) and prolymphocytic leukemia (PLL) are uncommon types of CLPDs world over.[1-7] Prognostic parameters are applicable only in the context of correct diagnosis. Therefore, it is important to make correct diagnosis of the disease under evaluation.

Table 9.1: Classification of chronic lymphoproliferative disorders (CLPD)

B Cell	T Cell	NK Cell
B-CLL, SLL, PLL	T-PLL	LGL
Hairy cell leukemia (HCL)	LGL	
Follicular lymphoma	Mycosis fungoides	
Marginal zone B cell lymphoma MALT,		
Splenic lymphoma with villous lymphocytes		
Lymphoplasmacytic lymphoma		
Mantle cell lymphoma (25% with indolent course)		

A National Cancer Institute-sponsored Working Group (NCI-WG) on chronic lymphocytic leukemia (CLL) in 1988 and 1996, published guidelines for diagnosis and treatment of CLL patients, and to establish definitions that could be used in scientific studies on the biology of this disease.[1,2]

The International Workshop on Chronic Lymphocytic Leukemia (IWCLL)-sponsored Working Group has revised the 1996 criteria, as considerable progress has been made during the last decade, in defining new prognostic markers, diagnostic parameters, and treatment options of CLL patients.[1-9]

The World Health Organization (WHO) classification of hematopoietic neoplasias describes CLL as leukemic, lymphocytic lymphoma, and is distinguished from small lymphocytic lymphoma (SLL) only by its leukemic appearance.[3] According to the WHO classification, CLL is always a disease of neoplastic B cells, whereas the entity formerly described as T-CLL is now labeled as T-cell prolymphocytic leukemia.[3,4]

CLPDs comprised of 13% of all leukemia at our institute.[10] Since CLL and HCL are encountered more frequently compared to other CLPDs, these disorders will be dealt with in greater detail.

CHRONIC LYMPHOCYTIC LEUKEMIA—DIAGNOSIS OF CLL

Other CLPDs such as small lymphocytic lymphoma (SLL), HCL, or leukemic manifestations of mantle cell lymphoma (MCL), marginal zone lymphoma (MZL), splenic marginal zone lymphoma with circulating villous lymphocytes (SLVL), or follicular lymphoma (FL) can masquerade as CLL. In order to make correct diagnosis, it is essential to evaluate the complete blood counts (CBC), blood smear, bone marrow (BM) aspiration smears, BM trephine biopsy (BMTB) and immunophenotype of the lymphoid cells in circulation and/or in BM.

Blood and Bone Marrow Features (Table 9.2)

The diagnosis of CLL requires (i) presence of $\geq 5 \times 10^9/L$ B-lymphocytes in the peripheral blood (PB) for more than 3 months duration and (ii) clonality of the circulating B lymphocytes needs to be confirmed by flow cytometry (kappa or lambda light chain restriction). Peripheral blood lymphocytosis is characteristically caused by small, mature lymphocytes with a narrow border of cytoplasm and a dense nucleus without discernible nucleoli and having partially aggregated chromatin. Gumprecht nuclear shadows, or smudge cells, found as cell debris, are other characteristic morphologic features found in PB and BM smears of CLL patients.

These typical cells may be admixed with larger or atypical cells, cleaved cells, or prolymphocytes, comprising less than 55% of the blood lymphocytes.[5] Presence of > 55% prolymphocytes would favor a diagnosis of prolymphocytic leukemia (B-cell PLL). CLL or SLL might be suspected in otherwise asymptomatic healthy adults with an absolute increase in

Chronic Lymphoproliferative Disorders (CLPDs)

Table 9.2: Characteristic morphological features of B lymphoid leukemia cells

Cell type (disease)	Size	Chromatin	Nucleolus	Cytoplasm	Other features	Trephine biopsy
CLL	< 2 RBCs	Clumped in coarse blocks	Absent	Scanty, high N/C ratio	Regular nuclear outline	Small cells, tightly packed
Large cell (CLL mixed cell)	> 2 RBCs	Clumped	Small Inconspicuous	Low N/C ratio	Variable size	Small cells, tightly packed
PLL	> 2 RBCs	Clumped	Central and prominent	Variable N/C ratio	Variable size	Medium cells, tightly packed
HCl	> 2 RBCs	Fine dispersed	Small Inconspicuous	N/C ratio low, nucleus eccenteric	Irregular fine cytoplasmic projections or villi	Cobweb appearance, Reticulin+++
SLVL	> 2 RBCs	Clumped	Small distinct	Variable	Short villi located to one pole of cell	Medium cells, tightly packed
Cleft cell	1-2 RBCs	Homogenously coarse	Absent or inconspicuous	Scanty not visible	1-2 shallow or deep narrow nuclear groove	Small cells, tightly packed

the clonal B-lymphocytes having less than 5×10^9/L B-lymphocytes in the blood. However, in the absence of lymphadenopathy or organomegaly (as defined by physical examination and CT scans), cytopenias, or disease-related symptoms, the presence of $< 5 \times 10^9$/L B-lymphocytes blood is defined as "monoclonal B-lymphocytosis.[6] The presence of a cytopenia caused by a typical marrow infiltrate defines the diagnosis of CLL regardless of the number of peripheral blood B-lymphocytes or of the lymph node involvement.

Monoclonal B-lymphocytosis is observed to progress to frank CLL at a rate of 1 to 2% per year.

The definition of SLL requires the presence of lymphadenopathy and the absence of cytopenias caused by a clonal marrow infiltrate. Moreover, the number of B-lymphocytes in the peripheral blood should not be $> 5 \times 10^9$/L. In SLL, the diagnosis should be confirmed by histopathologic evaluation of a lymph node biopsy whenever possible.

Immunophenotype

Typical immunophenotype of CLL cells is co-expression of the T-cell antigen CD5 with B-cell surface antigens CD19, CD20, and CD23. The expression levels of surface immunoglobulin, CD20, and CD79b are characteristically low compared with those found on normal B cells and many other CLPDs.[3-7] Each clone of leukemia cells has restricted expression of either kappa or lambda immunoglobulin light chains. Variations of the intensity of expression of these markers may exist and this feature does not prohibit inclusion of a patient in clinical trials for CLL.[7]

In contrast, B-cell PLL cells do not express CD5 in half of the cases, and typically express high levels of CD20 and surface Ig.[9] In addition, the leukemia cells of mantle cell lymphoma (MCL), despite also expressing B-cell surface antigens and CD5, generally do not express CD23. Flow cytometric immunophenotyping (FCM-IP) is the best modality to distinguish CLL from other CLPDs (Table 9.3).

Other Tests Performed at Diagnosis

The tests such as molecular genetics, IgV$_H$ mutation status, serum markers and BM examination, are not required to establish the diagnosis of CLL but may be useful to predict the prognosis or to assess the tumor burden. With the exception of molecular genetic analysis by fluorescence *in situ* hybridization (FISH), the application of these other tests should not be used in routine practice to influence therapy and is not generally

Table 9.3: Immunophenotypic markers in B CLPDs

Markers	CLL	PLL	HCl	HCl-V	Follicular lymphoma	MCL	SLVL	Plasma cell tumor
SmIg	Weak	Strong				Moderate	Strong	Negative
CyIg	–	–/+	–/+	–/+	–	–/+	–/+	++
M-rosette	++	–	–/+	–/+	–/+	–/+	–	–
CD5	++	–/+	–	–	–	++	–	–
CD 23	++	++	++	++	++	++	++	–
HLA-DR	++	++	++	++	++	++	++	–
FMC7/CD$_{22}$	–/+	++	++	++	++	+	++	–
CD10	–	–/+	–	–/+	+	–/+	–	–/+
CD25	–	–	++	–	–	–	–/+	–
CD38	–	–	–/+	–/+	–/+	–	–/+	++

recommended. However it is important to remember that the indication for treatment does not depend on any of these tests but only on the clinical stage and the disease activity.

Molecular Genetics

Using interphase FISH, cytogenetic lesions can be identified in more than 80% of all CLL cases.[8] The most common deletions are in the long arm of chromosome 13 [del(13q14.1)]. Additional, frequent chromosomal aberrations comprise deletions and/or trisomy of chromosome 12, deletions in the long arm of chromosomes 11 [del(11q)] and 6 [del(6q)], and in the short arm of chromosome 17 [del(17p)].[8] When stimulated *in vitro,* CLL cells can have detectable chromosomal translocations, which are of potential prognostic significance.[11] However, certain translocations can help distinguish other lymphoproliferative diseases from CLL [eg, t(11;14)], which generally is found in mantle cell lymphoma.

The results of prospective clinical trials have provided increasing evidence that detection of certain chromosomal deletions has prognostic significance (Table 9.4). CLL patients with del(17p) have an inferior prognosis and appear resistant to standard chemotherapy regimens using alkylating drugs and/or purine analogs. In a retrospective analysis on several chromosomal aberrations as detected by FISH, CLL patients with chromosomal aberrations del(11q) and del(17p) had an inferior outcome compared with patients who had a normal karyotype or del(13q) as the sole genetic abnormality. On the other hand, patients with leukemia cells having del(17p) may respond to therapy with alemtuzumab, either alone or in combination with other antileukemic agents.

Table 9.4: Correlation of specific chromosome aberrations with clinical characteristics and outcome in patient with B-CLL

Aberrations	Gene involved	Clinical characteristics and outcome	Frequency (%)
Trisomy 12	CLLU-1	Atypical morphology, intermediate outcome	16
13q aberration: del(13q)	miR15a, miR16-1	Favorable outcome if isolated aberrations	55
11q aberration: del(11q)	ATM	Extensive lymphadenopathy, short treatment free interval, shorter survival time	18
17p aberration del(17p)	p53	Shorter treatment free interval, shorter survival time, resistance of fludarabine; (may respond to therapy with alemtuzumab)	7
Normal karyotype	–	Favorable outcome	18

Detection of these cytogenetic abnormalities has obvious prognostic value and is likely to influence therapeutic decisions. It is recommended that cytogenetic analysis be performed before treating a patient on protocol under clinical trials. Additional genetic defects may be acquired during the course of the disease; therefore, FISH analyses may be justifiably repeated, before subsequent, second- and third-line treatment.

Mutational Status of IgV$_H$, VH3.21 Usage and Expression of ZAP-70 or CD38

CLL cells expressing immunoglobulin may or may not have incurred somatic mutations in the immunoglobulin heavy chain variable region genes (IgV$_H$ genes). The outcome of patients with CLL cells that use an unmutated IgV$_H$ gene is inferior to those with CLL cells that use a mutated IgV$_H$ gene. In addition, the VH3.21 gene usage is an unfavorable prognostic marker independent of the IgV$_H$ mutational status. Leukemia-cell expression of ZAP-70 and CD38 is reported to correlate with the expression of unmutated IgV$_H$ genes and to predict a poor prognosis. However, the association between expression of unmutated IgV$_H$ genes with the expression of ZAP-70 or CD38 is not absolute. It is still not certain whether leukemia-cell expression of unmutated IgV$_H$ genes or ZAP-70 predicts the response to treatment or overall survival, once therapy is required. Therefore, further clinical trials are warranted to standardize the assessment of these parameters and to determine whether they should affect the management of patients with CLL.

MicroRNAs (miRNAs) Expression

Aberrant expression of miR-29c and miR-223 was shown to be linked with outcome of CLL and could predict treatment-free survival (TFS) and overall survival (OS).[9]

Serum Markers

Several studies have found that serum markers soluble CD23 (sCD23), thymidine kinase, lactic dehydrogenase (LDH) and β_2-microglobulin may predict survival or progression-free survival. Assays for these markers need to be standardized and used in prospective clinical trials to validate their relative importance in the management of patients with CLL.

Lymphocyte Doubling Time (LDT)

One of the easiest parameters to assess, LDT of less than 6-12 months indicates a less favorable prognosis.

Staging and Prognosis

The staging systems proposed by Rai (Table 9.5) and Binet (Table 9.6) remain the gold standard for prognostication of CLL patients.

Table 9.5: Rai clinical staging system for CLL

Risk group, stage	Features at diagnosis	Median survival (months)
Low-risk		
Stage 0	Blood and marrow lymphocytosis	> 120
Intermediate risk		
Stage I	Lymphocytosis and adenopathy	108
Stage II	Lymphocytosis and splenomegaly or hepatomegaly with or without adenopathy	94
High-risk		
Stage III	Lymphocytosis and anemia (Hb < 11 g/dl)	60
Stage IV	Lymphocytosis and thrombocytopenia (platelets < 100 × 10^9/l)	60

Table 9.6: Binet clinical staging system for CLL

Risk group, stage	Features at diagnosis	Median survival (months)
Stage A	Blood and marrow lymphocytosis, < 3 areas of palpable adenopathy	>120
Stage B	Lymphocytosis, > 3 areas of palpable adenopathy	84
Stage C	Same as B, plus anemia (Hb < 11 g/dl in men, < 10 g/dl in women), or thrombocytopenia (platelets < 100 x 10^9/l)	60

Marrow Examination

The role of bone marrow aspirate and BM biopsy can not be ignored in the present scenario. Although BM aspirate and biopsy generally are not required for the diagnosis of CLL, however, these can help in evaluation of factors that might contribute to cytopenias (anemia, thrombocytopenia) that may or may not be directly related to leukemia-cell infiltration of the bone marrow. Because such factors could influence the susceptibility to drug-induced cytopenias, a marrow biopsy is recommended before starting therapy. It is recommended to repeat a marrow biopsy in patients with persisting cytopenia after treatment to detect disease-related versus therapy-related causes. Characteristically more than 30% of the nucleated cells in the aspirate are lymphoid cells, in CLL patients. Although the type of bone marrow infiltration (diffuse vs nondiffuse) reflects the tumor burden and provides prognostic information, recent studies of the German and Spanish study groups suggest that the prognostic value of BM biopsy may now be superseded by new prognostic markers.

Determinants of Prognosis in CLL

I. Patient characteristics: Age, performance status and co-morbidities.
II. Disease characteristics: Disease burden (clinical presentation, stage); cell kinetics (S-phase, LDH); biological parameters (cytogenetics, IgV_H, ZAP70, CD38).
III. Response to treatment.

Use in Clinical Practice

A number of un-answered questions remain regarding the real utility of newer disease markers (cytogenetic/FISH, IgV_H mutation status, expression of ZAP70 and CD38) vis-à-vis therapy decision-making.

There is no clear evidence to suggest that earlier initiation of therapy benefits patients with high-risk disease.

Parameters like cytogenetics/FISH, IgV_H mutation status, expression of ZAP70 and CD38 are yet not within reach of most of the hematologists and cost is a major deterrent. Methodologies are difficult to standardize and consensus regarding cut-off limits for expression of ZAP70 and CD38 is still not achieved.

The data of the newer parameters has so far mostly failed to guide treatment decisions.

More number of parameters means more variations of data, thus more discordant prognostic information is likely to emerge.

However new markers are most likely to provide useful information in future, regarding better patient management. Presently only symptoms, stage and standard indications should guide the treatment of CLL.

HAIRY CELL LEUKEMIA

HCL is an uncommon CLPD and presents usually with splenomegaly and pancytopenia. Leucocytosis (with leukemic cells $> 5 \times 10^9/l$) is seen only in 10-20% patients, however circulating hairy cells can be detected in almost all patients. Monocytopenia is consistently found. Hairy cells possess unique morphological and immunophenotypic features (Tables 9.1 and 9.2), therefore, distinction from other CLPDs is greatly facilitated. However, HCL-variant (HCL-V) and a blastic variant must always be kept in mind, in the presence of leukocytosis, larger/immature cell morphology or atypical immunophenotype (CD 25 negative).

BM aspirate is usually a dry tap, due to reticulin fibrosis. BM biopsy reveals characteristic 'fried egg' or 'honey comb' appearance of large cells with bland-looking nuclei. Pericellular reticulin fibrosis is a typical finding. Immunohistochemistry (IHC) on BM biopsy provides very useful information regarding status of residual disease.

PROLYMPHOCYTIC LEUKEMIA

PLL usually presents with splenomegaly and leucocytosis. The cell morphology is very characteristic, with very prominent nucleoli, clumped—

slightly opened chromatin, moderate amount of cytoplasm in moderately large cells (Table 9.2). FCM immunophenotyping may be completely 'CLL' like, may have a proportion of CD 19 and 5 double positive cells or may not have any CD 19 and 5 double positive cells (Table 9.3). PLL patients generally do not respond well to available therapeutic agents.

MANAGEMENT—PRINCIPLES

Management of CLPD is evolving. For the indolent forms, wait and watch is prudent for asymptomatic patients. A number of new agents have been used in this group of disorders that have increased the overall response and progression free survival. However, the management algorithm is still evolving though several areas of consensus have appeared.

CLL

It is generally agreed that most asymptomatic patients with early stage disease (Rai's 0/Binet's A) need to be monitored without any treatment. Earlier studies had shown that treating asymptomatic early stage patients by alkylating agents did not offer any survival advantage whereas the long-term treatment related risks would be unacceptable. Patients in Rai's class II or Binet's B can also be monitored unless they have features suggestive of active disease (Table 9.7). Advanced stage disease (Rai's III-IV) or Binet's C) would merit treatment. The treatment modalities include cytotoxic chemotherapeutic agents and biological agents (monoclonal antibodies) either as single agents or in combination and HSCT in selected patients.

Chlorambucil and other alkylating agents were the first agents used in the management of advanced stage CLL. These may still be used for patients who may not tolerate or afford purine analogues. Use of these agents is associated with symptomatic improvement but low complete response rates.

Table 9.7: NCI WG guidelines defining active disease in CLL (updated 2008)

- Progressive marrow failure
- Splenomegaly: Massive (> 6 cm BCM)/progressive/symptomatic
- Lymphadenopathy: Massive nodes (> 10 cm in longest diameter) or progressive or symptomatic
- Progressive lymphocytosis: > 50% in 2 months or lymphocyte doubling time (LDT) < 6 months
- Autoimmune anemia and/or thrombocytopenia poorly responsive to corticosteroids or other standard therapy
- At least one of the following disease-related symptoms:
  - Unintentional weight loss ≥ 10% within the previous 6 months.
  - Significant fatigue (i.e. ECOG PS 2 or worse; cannot work or unable to perform usual activities)
  - Fever > 38.0°C for ≥ 2 weeks without other evidence of infection
  - Night sweats for > 1 month without evidence of infection

Purine analogues: After decades of use of alkylating agents, availability of purine nucleoside analogues was the first major improvement in the management of CLL. Fludarabine and cladribine were found to be active in the management of CLL. These showed higher complete response rates and progression free survival; however initial studies did not show a clear survival advantage. Patients with adverse cytogenetic profile (del17p13.1 and del11q22.3 fare poorly with fludarabine as compared to those without these abnormalities.

Purine analogues have been subsequently used in combination with alkylating agents. Combination with chlorambucil was found to be more toxic however combining fludarabine with cyclophosphamide improved the overall response rates as well as median progression free survival though no overall survival advantage has been demonstrated. The combination is also associated with increased toxicity and its acceptability for older patients needs to be established.

Biologicals: Rituximab has been used in patients with CLL and has been shown to be effective with a good safety profile. Combination of rituximab with fludarabine and cyclophosphamide have given superior response rates with improvement in progression free survival. Alemtuzumab is the other agent that has been tried in relapsed CLL as well previously untreated CLL patients. It has shown overall response in 33-54% patients who have relapsed after previous chemotherapy. However, it has not been useful in patients with large lymph nodes (> 5 cm) and is also associated with higher incidence of infections.

Other agents that have been used are high dose dexamethasone, lenalidomide, Humanised anti-CD20 antibodies (Ofatumumab), Anti-CD23 antibodies (Lumiliximab) and flavopiridols. HSCT may be an option in younger patients with relapsed or progressive disease.

Hairy Cell Leukemia

Patients with HCl need treatment when they have symptomatic cytopenia(s) or bulky organomegaly. The treatment options are 2-chloro-deoxyadenosine as (0.1 mg/kg/day) continuous infusion for 7 days, interferon-α (2 million units/m^2) three times a week for 12-18 months or deoxycoformycin 4 mg/m^2 for 3-6 months. Five year survival with purine analogues is around 85%. Patients with variant hairy cell disease do not respond very well to the conventional treatment and treatment strategies for these patients need to be defined.

Other CLPDs

CLPDs or indolent lymphomas if asymptomatic, may not need any treatment but would need a careful monitoring. The treatment options need to be carefully weighed and need to be based upon factors such as patient's age, performance status, co-morbidities and patient preferences. The goals of therapy may vary from attempt to complete response to control of symptoms and improving the quality of life. The chemotherapeutic agents that have been used include alkylating agents like chlorambucil and cyclophosphamide, purine nucleoside analogues, combination chemotherapy such as CVP, Rituximab either alone or with combination chemotherapy, intensive chemotherapy with autologous or allogeneic stem cell transplantation.

TAKE HOME MESSAGE

In the present scenario, differential diagnosis of CLPDs can only be attempted with application of immunophenotyping of malignant cells. Cytogenetic/molecular genetic studies provide crucial information regarding the disease behavior and treatment response.

REFERENCES

1. Hallek M, Cheson BD, Catovsky Dl, Caligaris-Cappio F, Dighiero G, Döhner H, Hillmen P, Keating MJ, Montserrat E, Rai KR, Kipps TJ. Guidelines for the diagnosis and treatment of chronic lymphocytic leukemia: A report from the International Workshop on Chronic Lymphocytic Leukemia updating the National Cancer Institute Working Group 1996 guidelines. Blood 2008;111: 5446-56.
2. Cheson BD, Bennett JM, Grever M, et al. National Cancer Institute-Sponsored Working Group guidelines for chronic lymphocytic leukemia: Revised guidelines for diagnosis and treatment. Blood 1996;87:4990-97.
3. Muller-Herelink HK, Monteserrat E, Catovsky D, Harris NL. Chronic lymphocytic leukemia/small lymphocytic leukemia. In: Jaffe ES, Harris NL, Stein H, Vardiman JW (Eds). World Health Organization Classification of tumours: Pathology and genetics of tumours of Haematopoietic and lymphoid tissues. Lyon, France:IARC Press 2001:127-30.
4. Kipps TJ. Chronic lymphocytic leukemia and related diseases. In Lichtman MA, Beutler E, Kipps TJ, Seligsohn U, Kaushanky K, Prchal JT (Eds) Williams Hematology. 7th edn. New York: McGraw Hill Inc 2006;1343-84.
5. Johnston JB. Chronic lymphocytic leukemia. In Greer JP, Foerester J, Lukens JN, Rodgers GM, Paraskevas F, Glader B (Eds). Wintrobe's Clinical Hematology. 11th edn. Philadelphia: Lippincott Williams and Wilkins 2004;2429-63.
6. Johnston JB. Hairy cell leukemia. In Greer JP, Foerester J, Lukens JN, Rodgers GM, Paraskevas F, Glader B (Eds). Wintrobe's Clinical Hematology. 11th edn. Philadelphia: Lippincott Williams and Wilkins 2004;2465-84.
7. Catovsky D, Ralfkier E, Muller-Herelink HK. T cell prolymphocytic leukemia. In: Jaffe ES, Harris NL, Stein H, Vardiman JW (Eds). World Health Organization Classification of tumours: Pathology and genetics of tumours of Haematopoietic and lymphoid tissues. Lyon, France:IARC Press 2001;195-96.
8. Wierda WG, O'Brien S, Wang X, et al. Prognostic nomogram and index for overall survival in previously untreated patients with chronic lymphocytic leukemia. Blood 2007;109:4679-85.
9. Stamatopoulos B, Meuleman, et al. MicroRNA-29c and microRNA-223 down-regulation has *in vivo* significance in chronic lymphocytic leukemia and improves disease risk stratification. Blood 2009;113:5237-45.
10. Kumar N, Varma N, Varma S, Malhotra P. Study of Diagnostic and Prognostic Parameters (including Flow cytometry) in Chronic Lymphoproliferative Disorders: The Indian Perspective. Anal Quant Cytol Histol 2009 (accepted for publication).

Chapter 10

Aspirin Resistance: Expectations and Limitations

Gundu HR Rao

SUMMARY

Aspirin as a therapeutic drug has been in the use for over hundred years. Its use as an antiplatelet drug was recognized in the early 70s. For secondary prophylaxis of vascular disease, it is the most useful and cost-effective drug. Large number of clinical trials using aspirin have concluded that (low to medium dose of aspirin, 80-160 mg), at any given vascular risk, it is as effective as any other drug of choice. However, in recent years, there are several studies in which aspirin resistances in patients with various vascular diseases have been demonstrated. Furthermore, some studies have suggested worst outcome in aspirin nonresponders. Studies from our laboratory over three decades have not found any individual whose platelets are resistant to the action of aspirin. In other words, aspirin inhibited the cyclooxygenase (COX-1) of platelets of all the individuals tested. Therefore, we feel that the confusion comes from the way people test platelets for evaluating aspirin or clopidogrel resistance. In this overview we will discuss the expectations and limitations of aspirin as anti-platelet drug.

KEYWORDS

Aspirin resistance, Platelet hyperfunction, Endothelial dysfunction, Antiplatelet therapy.

INTRODUCTION

Role of platelets in the pathogenesis of atherosclerosis, thrombosis and stroke is well documented.[1] Therefore, there is a great need for developing specific and effective drugs for modulating platelet function. A thorough understanding of the signaling mechanisms involved in the regulation of platelet function will facilitate the development of better antiplatelet drugs. Agonists interact with the platelets at specific receptor sites on the plasma membrane of platelets and initiate a series of signaling events.[2-10] In spite of the fact that there are very few drugs capable of modulating platelet function, there have been extensive clinical studies to demonstrate the beneficial effects of antiplatelet drugs. Several clinical studies have established the beneficial effect of antiplatelet therapy in reducing the risk of acute vascular events. Data from large number of clinical studies done with aspirin have demonstrated that at any given risk, irrespective of the disease state, aspirin at low to medium concentration is as effective as any other drug.[2-5]

Although ability of a plant bark (bark of willow, *Salix alba*) product to reduce fever was discovered two hundred years ago, the mechanism of action of aspirin remained elusive till late 1900.[6] Nobel laureate Sir John R Vane and his associates at the Royal College of Surgeons, in London, in 1971 proposed the first satisfactory mechanism as to how it works.[7,8] Within a short period of time extensive work was done by various groups to elucidate the mechanism of action of aspirin like compounds.[8-20] At the same period, another Nobel Laureate Bengt Samuelsson of the Karolinska Institute, Stockholm, Sweden, discovered that the prostaglandin synthase produces transient bioactive prostanoids like PGG_2/PGH_2 and thromboxane from the substrate arachidonic acid.[10] These findings revolutionized the research in platelet physiology and pharmacology.[2-21]

Platelet Physiology

Blood platelets interact with a variety of soluble agonists such as epinephrine, adenosine diphosphate, thrombin and thromboxane; many cell matrix components, including collagen, laminin, fibronectin, and vonWillebrand factor and biomaterials used for construction of invasive medical devices.[21-29] These interactions stimulate specific receptors and glycoprotein-rich domains (integrin and non-integrin receptors) on the plasma membrane and lead to the activation of intracellular effector enzymes. Agonist-mediated activation of platelets stimulates phospholipase C (PLC) and it then triggers the hydrolysis of phosphatidyl inositol 4, 5-bisphosphate, the formation of second messengers such as 1, 2 diacyl glycerol and inositol 1, 4, 5-trisphosphate. Diacylglycerol activates protein kinase and inositol trisphosphate facilitates the mobilization of free calcium from the storage sites. The majority of regulatory events appear to require free calcium. Ionized calcium is the primary bioregulator, and a variety of biochemical mechanisms modulate the availability of free calcium. Elevation of cytosolic calcium stimulates phospholipase A_2 and liberates arachidonic acid (AA). Free arachidonic acid is transformed to a novel metabolite thromboxane, a potent platelet agonist. This is the major metabolite of AA metabolism and plays an important role in platelet recruitment, granule mobilization, secretion of granule contents, and expression of activated GP11b/111a ($\alpha_{11b}\beta_3$) receptors. Up regulation of activation signaling pathways, will increase the risk for clinical complications associated with thromboembolic episodes.

Arachidonic Acid Metabolism

Arachidonic acid is a 20 carbon polyunsaturated fatty acid (20:4w6) found in membrane phospholipids. Cell activation stimulates phospholipase A_2, which facilitates the release of this fatty acid from phospholipids.

AA is converted to prostaglandin (PG) endoperoxides (PGG$_2$/PGH$_2$) by cyclooxygenase (Prostaglandin G/H synthase; COX1)). These transient metabolites are converted by thromboxane synthetase to thromboxane A$_2$, which is the major metabolite of this pathway in platelets.[10] Whereas, in vascular tissues, the endoperoxides generated by COX1 are transformed by prostacyclin synthetase to prostacyclin. Thromboxane is a potent platelet agonist and a vasoconstrictor. Prostacyclin is an antiplatelet compound and exerts vasodilatory effects on vascular tissues. Thus from a single substrate two pharmacologically opposing vasoactive prostanoids are generated by platelets and vascular tissues.[3] Aspirin selectively acetylates the hydroxyl groups of a single serine residue (position 529) in the prostaglandin G/H synthase and causes irreversible inhibition of the activity of this enzyme.[12,13] Inhibition of PG synthase results in the decreased conversion of AA to PG endoperoxides, PGG$_2$/PGH$_2$. Molecular mechanisms involved in aspirin-mediated inhibition of prostaglandin G/H synthase are well documented.

However, little is known about how other nonsteroidal anti-inflammatory drugs inhibit this enzyme. To elucidate the mechanism by which this enzyme oxidizes arachidonic acid, we developed a cell free assay system. This system used ferrous iron induced oxidation of AA. Oxidation of the fatty acids by iron was followed by nitroblue tetrazolium.[31] Several drugs known to be inhibitors of this enzyme were used in this system to evaluate the affinity of these compounds to ferrous iron. Results demonstrated these compounds could form a complex with ferrous iron and inhibit arachidonic acid metabolism.[32,33] Using a ferrous iron chelator, bypirydil, we demonstrated the ability of this compound to inhibit platelet prostaglandin synthesis and function.[34] In a separate study, we showed ibuprofen, a short acting drug, interacted with the active site of PG synthase and blocked the ability of aspirin to acetylate the enzyme.[35] Based on these results and other studies, we concluded aspirin like compounds devoid of acetyl group interact with the heme part of the PG synthase and block arachidonic acid oxidation. In platelets AA is converted by lipoxygenase to 12-hydroxyeicosatetraenoic acid. This pathway is not inhibited by aspirin.

Clinical Use of Aspirin

Single oral doses of 10-100 mg of aspirin can significantly inhibit the platelet PG synthase activity.[36] The inhibitory effect is fast and probably occurs in the portal circulation. The half-life of aspirin is very short (15-20 minutes) but sufficient to inhibit PG synthase of circulating platelets. Since these cells lack DNA and the ability to resynthesize the enzyme, the dysfunction caused by aspirin cannot be overcome. Therefore, platelets exposed to aspirin loose the ability to make the prostanoids completely. However, one should keep in mind that once the aspirin is hydrolyzed to salicylic acid, ability to inhibit prostaglandin synthase is lost. Hence, the platelets produced from the marrow after the aspirin is hydrolyzed, will have active prostaglandin synthase. Approximately 10% of fresh platelets are added on to the circulating blood every day. Although aspirin treated blood do not make prostaglandins, they respond with aggregation to the stimulation by prostaglandin endoperoxides and thromboxane. Fresh platelets formed after the hydrolysis of aspirin, can synthesize prostanoids and these newly formed metabolites of AA can cause aggregation of aspirin exposed platelets. In view of the fact that aspirin irreversibly inhibits prostaglandin synthase, it is possible to take advantage of daily low-dose aspirin to achieve a cumulative effect. Even doses as low as 30-50 mg aspirin taken daily will suppress platelet thromboxane synthesis significantly in 5 to 10 days.

Vascular tissues on the other hand have the ability to resynthesize prostaglandin G/H synthase.[36] Therefore, these cells can recover the enzyme activity following aspirin exposure. It is therefore, possible to develop a strategy to promote the biochemical selectivity of aspirin in terms of inhibition of platelet prostaglandin synthase. This is done by modification of the drug delivery, so the amount of drug delivered is just enough to inhibit platelet enzymes in the peripheral circulation and spare the systemic effect on vascular endothelium.[37,38] Several studies have demonstrated the feasibility of this approach and various control release or timed release formulations have been developed for this novel therapy.[37-39]

As mentioned earlier, aspirin is metabolized rapidly and the major metabolite, salicylic acid is a poor inhibitor of platelet prostaglandin synthase. Therefore, it is essential to develop appropriate strategies to maximize the beneficial effect of this novel drug. As low dose as 20 mg taken daily, reduces the platelet thromboxane formation by more than 90 percent. However, it is generally believed that higher doses are essential for preventing thromboxane dependent platelet activation. Studies by Wilson et al demonstrated that maximal plasma concentration of 12 umol/L could be achieved by a single oral 50 mg dose of enteric-coated aspirin.[17] This dose was found sufficient to cause significant inhibition of platelet function and daily ingestion of low-dose aspirin demonstrated a cumulative effect. In a separate study, McLeod et al used doses ranging from 50-3900 mg of aspirin and monitored platelet function, bleeding time and concluded maximum dysfunction was obtained with daily doses of about 100 mg and no further changes were observed in these studies with higher doses.[18] Several workers have demonstrated the efficacy of low-dose oral aspirin in preventing platelet thromboxane production.[2-4,18,44] Indeed one of these studies has demonstrated beneficial effect of a dermal aspirin preparation on selective inhibition of platelet prostaglandin synthase, sparing the prostacyclin biosynthesis.[38] Studies done with low-dose aspirin and the data generated by the two major clinical studies support the use of 80-160 mg aspirin per day as a prophylactic drug for the primary prevention of clinical complications associated with platelet hyperfunction.[19,20]

The two major clinical trials on aspirin concluded that ingestion of 160 mg per day or 325 mg alternative day provided significant benefit in preventing fatal events associated with CAD.[20,21] It is very well established that 100 mg of aspirin per day is sufficient to significantly reduce the platelet thromboxane production.[2-4,20,21,40-42] Furthermore, studies by McLeod et al have shown that dosages higher than 100 mg per day do not produce any greater inhibition of platelet function or enhance bleeding times.[18] Therefore, it is reasonable to conclude that 80-160 mg aspirin per day should be the choice for an ideal preventive protocol.[41] However, there is considerable room for improvement to maximize the benefits by better understanding the pharmacology of aspirin and platelet physiology.[2-4] It is possible to customize the aspirin treatment based on the individual patient needs. One can monitor the platelet prostaglandin synthase activity following aspirin ingestion and recommend a dose that is appropriate.[34,41] It is possible to monitor the platelet response to agonists such as ADP or arachidonate and determine the degree of inhibition by aspirin like compounds.[18] In order to get maximum inhibition of platelet enzymes, continuous release aspirin formulations can be developed and tested against currently available aspirin formulations. Platelets are produced and released constantly to the circulation. Therefore, a time release aspirin which would make available small amounts of aspirin into the circulation may be effective. For instance, a 100 mg formulation capable of releasing 10 mg acetyl salicylic acid per hour may be better than a preparation which releases all of its active principle in a short span of time. Using the strategy of slowing down the release of active principle newer formulations could be used effectively to provide needed amounts of the drug into circulating blood at regular intervals. These novel formulations may also provide selectivity of aspirin action by preventing platelet thromboxane production and sparing the endothelial prostacylcin synthesis. McLeod et al studied the effect of various doses of aspirin (50, 100, 325, 1000 mg) on platelets and vascular tissues.[44] They did not observe inhibition of urinary 6-keto-PGF1 alpha production at low doses of 50 and 100 mg. They attributed these findings to the differential and selective inhibition of platelet function and the sparing effect on vascular COX enzymes. Sullivan and associates studied the effect of two different doses of aspirin on platelet function and TXA2 production.[45] Platelet function in healthy volunteers was inhibited by both the doses (75 and 300 mg). Low dose failed to inhibit completely TXB2 production 24 hours later, whereas 300 mg aspirin did. Even alternate day regimen of these doses prevented platelet function and significantly inhibited the urinary levels of the 11-keto-TXB2. In a separate study, in healthy volunteers, formation of thrombin (Fibrinopeptide A; FPA), alpha granule release (beta-thromboglobulin; beta TG), and thromboxane (TXB) were monitored *in vivo*, in blood emerging from a template bleeding incision.[47] At the site of plug formation significant platelet activation and thrombin generation was observed as indicated by 110 fold, 50 fold, and 30 fold increase in FPA, beta TG, and TXB2, within the first minute. A low dose regimen (0.42 m/kg/day for 7 days) caused greater than 90% inhibition of TXB2 formation in both bleeding time and clotted blood in these studies, suggesting critical role of platelet activation at the site of hemostatic plug formation. In a study to evaluate the effect of low dose aspirin (0.5 and 15 mg/kg/day) on platelet and renal prostanoids, Wilson et al monitored serum TXB2 and urinary 6-keto PGF1 alpha.[47] Serum TXB2 level was reduced to 3% of control by low dose and to 0.1% by the higher dose. Urinary TXB$_2$ was reduced only to 68% by low dose aspirin, and to 51% by high dose. Urinary 6-keto-PGF1 alpha was not reduced by either dose. Based on their observation, they concluded low dose aspirin could significantly affect platelet PG production without affecting stimulated release of PGI2 production.

Several earlier studies evaluated the effect of low dose aspirin on normal healthy volunteers as well as patients with various vascular diseases. However, earlier studies did not report prevalence of any aspirin resistance. Zucker et al evaluated the effect of low dose aspirin (0.45 mg/kg/day) and a high dose (900 mg/day) in type 11 hyperlipoproteinemic subjects.[48] They found that low dose aspirin effectively inhibited platelet function in these patients. Increased platelet thromboxane production has been described in several disorders including type-2 diabetes and type 11a hypercholesterolemia. This increased production of TXB2 in hypercholesterolemic patients is attributed to abnormal cholesterol levels in these patients. Even a low dose such as 50 mg for 7 days significantly reduced 11 dehydro-TXB2, in these patients.[49] The effect of low dose aspirin has been evaluated in patients with diabetes, coronary heart disease, myocardial infarction (MI), cerebrovascular disease, peripheral artery disease and a variety of surgical procedures. Diminno et al studied the effect of single doses of 100 and 1000 mg aspirin for 1 month in normal volunteers and patients with diabetic angiopathy.[50] They found a dose schedule of aspirin, which may suffice in normal volunteers, was not effective in patients with diabetic angiopathy. Contrary to this observation, Terres et al found a low dose of aspirin (100 mg) caused significant inhibition of platelet function in both healthy subjects and patients with coronary heart disease.[51] Similarly, a low dose (0.45 mg/kg/day) was found adequate for selective inhibition of TXA2-related platelet function, in patients recovering from MI.[52] Looks like the results vary considerably, depending upon the type and stage of disease, dose of aspirin, and severity of procedure. In a study evaluating the effect of low dose aspirin (100 mg) on hematological activity of left ventricular (LV) thrombus in anterior wall acute MI (AMI), Kupper et al found that low dose had no effect on the incidence of hematologic activity and embolic potential of LV thrombosis in anterior wall AMI.[53] On the other hand, a low dose aspirin (40 mg/day) daily was found to be as effective as higher doses in preventing platelet responses in patients who had recent cerebral ischemia.[54] Uchiyama et al evaluated the effect of low dose aspirin, ticlopidine, and a combination of both these drugs in patients with cerebral ischemia.[55] Aspirin alone markedly inhibited platelet aggregation induced by AA, partially inhibited aggregation induced by ADP and did not inhibit aggregation by platelet activating factor. Combination of these drugs inhibited aggregation by all agonists. Rao et al demonstrated, in healthy volunteers, low doses of aspirin (40-80 mg) had no inhibitory effect on the response of platelets to ADP, epinephrine and thrombin, but effectively inhibited the platelet response to threshold concentrations of arachidonic acid. Epinephrine at concentrations too low to cause aggregation restored the sensitivity of aspirin-treated platelets to AA. This phenomenon, in which weak agonists restore the sensitivity of drug-induced refractory platelets to the action of other agonists, was described from our laboratory as "mechanism of membrane modulation".[57-64]

Aspirin Resistance

Studies from our laboratory for the first time demonstrated that one could induce drug mediated resistance in platelets to the action of aspirin.[65] In this study, the subjects were given a short acting inhibitor of COX1, Ibuprofen. This was followed by administration of a full strength (325 mg) aspirin. Ibuprofen-mediated inhibition of COX1 enzyme lasts for a short time, whereas, aspirin induced inhibition is irreversible. Ibuprofen treated platelets recovered their sensitivity to the action of AA by 24 hours. Whereas, aspirin treated platelets failed to respond to the action of AA even after 24 hours. In those subjects who had ingested aspirin after taking Ibuprofen first, aspirin failed to inhibit irreversibly the COX1, suggesting Ibuprofen molecules effectively prevented the acetylation of COX1. One of the earliest work describing "nonresponders" and "responders" evaluated the effect of low dose aspirin and a thromboxane synthetase inhibitor dazoxiben (UK3724B) in healthy subjects.[56] These studies demonstrated low dose aspirin and ingestion of two dazoxiben tablets prevented the release of granules from platelets in response to AA in some individuals (responders) and not in others (nonresponders). These subtle differences in response of platelets to various drugs as well as differences in response to various agonists may be critical when considering the outcome of acute vascular events. For instance, collagen seems to exert its effect by multiple mechanisms. In a study, using aspirin, monoclonal antibodies to 11b-111a receptor and fibrinogen, it was demonstrated that there exists at least three mechanisms by which collagen activates platelets; (1) GP11b-111a associated activation, (2) prostaglandin dependent pathway, (3) alternate pathway responsible for 20-30% platelet aggregation.[66]

Although, it is well known there are individual differences in response to drugs as well as agonists, this subject has not been studied thoroughly. Therefore, the time has come for an in depth study. There is a need to explain why the protection offered to the subjects is not complete although many antiplatelet drugs are used. Furthermore, several recent studies have demonstrated variable degree of aspirin resistance exists in patients with a variety of vascular diseases. This subject currently is a very hot topic and has made national headlines. Andrew Pollack published an article in July of 2004 in New York Times, on this subject titled, "For Some, Aspirin May Not Help Hearts".[67] According to this article, 5-40% of aspirin users are "nonresponders" or "resistant" to the medicine. In the same article, he cites the opinion of Dr Daniel I Simon, which reads as follows: "They are taking it for stroke and heart attack prevention and it not going to work". He also reports the opinion of Dr Michael J Domanski; Head of Clinical Trials Unit at the NIH, in his opinion, the nonresponders may represent a huge number of patients. According to Dr Deepak L Bhatt, Director of Interventional Cardiology Cleveland Clinic, aspirin resistance is associated with worst outcome. Professor Eric Topol, Chairman, Cardiovascular Medicine Cleveland Clinic, USA states, "Aspirin resistance carries high-risk, with over 20 million Americans taking aspirin to prevent heart attacks or strokes, it is important that further work to be done to confirm our findings and develop a rapid detection method. He also assures that for individuals with aspirin resistance, there are excellent alternatives".

These observances from health care providers and researchers raise number of issues. Do we know enough about aspirin resistance? What causes this resistance to develop in patient populations? Are there specific, rapid cost-effective tests available? What alternative long-term treatments are available, if patients are resistant to common antiplatelet drugs such as aspirin and Clopidogrel? Should the doses of these drugs used for therapy be increased? Should we drop the use of these drugs in nonresponders? We need to find answers to these and other emerging questions soon. In the next few paragraphs a brief overview of what is known about the prevalence of aspirin resistance, clinical findings, and methodologies available, will be provided.

The first and foremost need at this time is to standardize a definition of aspirin resistance. The mechanism of action of aspirin is very well documented.[7-13] The drug acetylates the platelet COX1 enzyme and irreversibly inhibits its ability to convert AA to PG endoperoxides.[12,13] In the absence of this step, platelets do not respond to AA stimulation with aggregation. Weak agonists such as ADP, Epinephrine depend on the formation of PG endoperoxides to initiate secondary wave of aggregation and promote release of platelet granule contents. Therefore, weak agonists fail to induce platelet aggregation and release of granules from aspirin-treated platelets. Failure of AA, ADP and Epinephrine to cause aggregation of platelets more or less establishes drug-induced platelet dysfunction. If platelets obtained from individuals who have ingested a full strength aspirin, respond with aggregation to the action AA, ADP and Epinephrine, and release their granule contents, then one can safely conclude these platelets are resistant to aspirin action. Further proof for aspirin resistance of platelets can be provided by studying AA metabolism by such platelets, monitoring serum TXB2 levels, or urinary levels of TXB2 or its metabolite, 11-dehydro-TXB2. Methods are available to monitor all these parameters.

Prevalence of Aspirin Resistance

Aspirin resistance has been poorly defined, variety of nonspecific methods have been employed to monitor the "aspirin resistance" and conflicting reports have been published on the rates of prevalence and outcome of continuing this therapeutic modality.[68-70] Aspirin resistance has been reported in patients with cardiovascular, cerebrovascular, and peripheral vascular disease.[71] Because of the differences in methodologies used to monitor this phenomenon and lack of a specific assay to determine the true aspirin resistance there is considerable confusion and the true significance of this observation remains obscure.[70,71] It also raises the question as to how we missed this phenomenon all these years. Large numbers of clinical trials have demonstrated the beneficial effects of aspirin therapy irrespective of the disease state.[40] Is it possible that these earlier trials missed nonresponders? Is it possible that only responders got the benefit of this therapy?

Studies in our laboratory over three decades, have failed to show any aspirin resistance in normal healthy subjects. The only subject whose platelets failed to aggregate in response to arachidonate was found to be deficient in platelet COX1.[59] Platelets obtained from this subject responded with aggregation when stirred with epinephrine and arachidonate, suggesting PG endoperoxides and TAX2 are not essential to cause irreversible aggregation of platelets. There is not much data on the prevalence of aspirin resistance in general healthy subjects. In patients with various vascular diseases, the rate of nonresponders reported varies between less than 2% to over 60%. Since the methods used to monitor aspirin resistance in these reports are not specific, the prevalence rate published is debatable.

Hurlen et al used the method of Wu and Hoak to determine the platelet aggregation ratio as a marker for assessing platelet function and evaluated the effect of aspirin (160 mg/day) in 143 patients who had survived myocardial infarction.[72,73] Based on their definition, they could only identify two subjects as primary nonresponders. Gum et al from Cleveland Clinic studied 326 stable cardiovascular subjects on aspirin (325 mg/day) and tested aspirin sensitivity by platelet response to aggregating agents such as ADP and AA. They found 5.5% as nonresponders to aspirin and 24% as semiresponders.[74] Gum and associates used the PFA 100, a method that is supposed to measure platelet function, to determine aspirin resistance in their patient population.[75] Based on their studies with this methodology they found 9.5% to be nonresponders to aspirin action.

Some studies have reported as high as 30-40% nonresponders of stroke or vascular disease patients and predicted > 80% increase risk for a repeat event during a 2 years follow-up period.[76-79] Eikelboom et al analyzed base line urinary levels of TXB2 metabolites 11-dehydro thromboxane B2 in 5529 patients enrolled in the Heart Outcomes Prevention Evaluation (HOPE) Study.[80] Of these subjects 488 were on aspirin regimen. On the basis of their findings they concluded that in aspirin-treated patients, increased levels of urinary metabolite of TXB2 predict future risk of myocardial infarction or cardiovascular death. The patients with the highest levels of TXB2 metabolite had 3-5 fold higher risk of cardiovascular death compared to those in the lowest quartile. Another study reporting clinical outcomes of aspirin resistance is from Austria.[79,81,82] In this study patients undergoing arterial angioplasty were on 100 mg aspirin per day. Platelet function was assessed by whole blood aggregometry. This study demonstrated that reocculsion at the sites of angioplasty occurred only in men for whom platelet dysfunction was evident by aggregometry.[79] Zimmerman et al identified aspirin nonresponders as those who had > 90% inhibition of TXB2 formation in presence of 100 umol/L aspirin and 1 mmol/L arachidonate.[83] In patients who had undergone coronary bypass surgery (CABG), AA and Collagen stimulated formation of TXB2 was same before and after CABG, indicating oral aspirin did not significantly inhibit platelet COX1. However, the *in vitro* studies with 100 umol/L aspirin on blood obtained from these subjects showed decreased TXB2 (> 10%) in most samples studied. They concluded that platelet inhibition by aspirin is compromised for several days after CABG, probably due to an impaired interaction between aspirin and platelet COX1. This observation indicates how complex the issues are when evaluating the effect of antiplatelet drugs during and after interventional procedures. Sane et al evaluated the effect of aspirin (325 mg/day/month) in patients suffering from congestive heart failure (left ventricular ejection fraction <40%).[84] They used whole blood aggregometry (Chronolog, Chronolog Corp, PA, USA), Platelet receptor expression by flow cytometry and PFA 100. Patients were considered nonresponders when 4 of the 5 parameters assayed were observed. Using this complex rating, persistent platelet activation was observed in 50 of the 88 patients (56.8%). These observations remind us of the inadequacy of the existing methods to detect what truly represents "aspirin resistance".

Methodologies

Researchers have used a variety of methods to assess the aspirin and Clopidogrel resistance.[90-97] In spite of the inherent problems associated with platelet aggregometry, it still is the gold standard to detect aspirin sensitivity of platelets. Studies from our laboratory and that of others have shown even low doses (40-80 mg) of aspirin effectively inhibit arachidonate-mediated platelet aggregation. In the absence of any other specific rapid point-of-care assay system for detecting the sensitivity of platelets to aspirin or lack of aspirin sensitivity, it is preferable to use optical aggregometry to validate the results obtained by other methods. Hurlen et al used platelet aggregate ratio (PAR) to evaluate the effect of aspirin in post-MI patients. Basically the method developed by Wu and Hoak uses a ratio of platelets obtained with EDTA/formalin as anticoagulants and comparing the counts of platelets obtained with EDTA.

In the presence of platelet aggregates the ratio is <1.0. Using this method they found two individuals as primary nonresponders and 14 patients as secondary nonresponders.

Several researchers have used Platelet Function Analyzer PFA 100 (Dade International Inc, Miami USA), to evaluate aspirin resistance in patients with various vascular diseases. This analyzer measures platelet function as their ability to occlude a membrane coated with collagen and epinephrine (EPI) or collagen and ADP under high shear stress. Sambola et al evaluated the effect of low dose aspirin (100 mg/day/1 month, 6 months) in 100 patients with acute coronary syndrome. At one-month post-aspirin therapy, they found 49 patients to have suboptimal response to aspirin (SASAR), whereas only 25 of them showed SASAR by conventional aggregometry. Anderson et al evaluated the effect of 75 mg aspirin in patients (n = 202) with MI. In patients on aspirin alone they found 25/71 as nonresponders with the epinephrine cartridge. They did not find a significant difference between EPI cartridge and ADP cartridge. Gum et al evaluated the phenomenon of aspirin resistance in 325 stable cardiac patients. They found 5 percent were nonresponders and 23 percent semiresponders by optical aggregometry. Whereas, using PFA 100 they found 9.5% as aspirin resistant. This detection system does not seem to detect difference between the effects of low and high-dose aspirin on platelet function. Since, it evaluates the synergistic effect of a combination of two agonists on platelet function, the results obtained or similar to that obtained in our aggregation studies. In a series of studies we have demonstrated a combination of two agonists overcomes the inhibition by aspirin and other drugs. Studies by Kawasaki et al have demonstrated increased sensitivity to collagen in individuals resistant to low-dose aspirin.

Malinin et al used the Ultegra RPFA-ASA (VerifyNow; Accumetrics, Inc., San Diego, California, USA) to monitor the effect of a single dose of aspirin (325 mg) in subjects with multiple risk factors.[92] This system uses turbidimetric optical detection system. It uses a test cartridge that contains lyophilized preparation of human fibrinogen-coated beads, platelet agonist, and buffer. Fibrinogen-coated beads bind available receptor on platelet membrane. A cationic agonist, propyl gallate, is used to obtain complete activation of platelets. It uses citrated whole blood for assays. The results are expressed in aspirin response units (ARU). Of the 14 subjects studied, only one was found to be nonresponsive by aggregometry, whereas they found 10 subjects as nonresponders by RPFA-ASA. They concluded this system was a sensitive device for measuring antiplatelet responsiveness. Newly introduced "VerifyNow" kit includes arachidonic acid as an agonist for activating platelets. Inclusion of this agonist instead of propyl gallate has considerably improved the performance of this system. In our hands, this system is as good as whole blood aggregometry in identifying aspirin nonresponders.

Aspirin resistance could be monitored by a variety of assays, including platelet aggregometry, PAR, PFA100, RPFA-ASA; plasma, serum, urinary

TXB2 and urinary 11-dehryothromboxane-2. We use majority of these methods to validate data in our efforts to develop a rapid, specific point-of-care assay system, for monitoring platelet function. Majority of these methods are labor intensive, time consuming and expensive. Technologies are available to develop a rapid and specific assay system, which can monitor platelet function. Specific fluorescent antibodies can be used to detect platelet bound fibrinogen, P-selectin or released granule products such as beta-thromboglobulin, platelet factor 4, soluble P-selectin. Furthermore, ATP release or thromboxane generated also could be easily monitored. All the available methods use large quantities of blood and take considerable amount of time. It is possible to device methods that use only small quantities of blood obtained from a finger stick. By using state-of-the-art detectors one could detect the luminescence (ATP) or fluorescence (specific antibodies) in minutes and develop needed software to standardize the results. If the assay uses AA as standard platelet agonist then specificity could be built into this system for monitoring aspirin sensitivity. Similarly by using ADP as agonist one can build the needed specificity to monitor nonresponders to Clopidogrel. The limiting factors for nonavailability of such a system are lack of funds and the assumption, that currently available methods detect platelet sensitivity or otherwise to antiplatelet drugs effectively.

Discussion

Aspirin is the mosteffective, widely used, relatively inexpensive antiplatelet drug currently available. In the developing world, aspirin is the most cost-effective drug for primary as well as secondary prophylaxis for platelet-mediated vascular complications.[3-5] The mechanism by which it inhibits platelet function is well documented.[7-14] Many large clinical trials have established beyond any doubt that aspirin therapy significantly reduces the incidence of acute events in a variety of vascular diseases.[40] Recent studies have provided evidence to suggest that some subpopulation of patients on aspirin therapy may have developed resistance to the action of aspirin.[67-90] These observations have raised alarm in the public as to who is getting benefited and who is not? Since there is no simple test that can be performed at the doctor's office to detect such a condition there is some panic in the patient population. Furthermore, there is still lack of awareness of this problem in the medical community at the time of this writing. There are only two major studies which have described adverse outcome in those patients who are defined as nonresponders to the action of aspirin.[75,79]

Based on methods, which still are not very specific, researchers have identified a subpopulation of patients who are considered nonresponders and another group as semiresponders to the action of aspirin.[74-90] Although the majority of methods used for monitoring this phenomenon lack specificity, it is important to recognize the problem exists. If these patients, for whatever reason are not getting appropriate protection there is an immediate need to identify them and change their therapeutic regimen. It is equally important to recognize even those who are considered responders, may need additional protection to prevent adverse outcomes if they have hyper-responsive platelets or hyper-responsive coagulation pathways.

Subject of aspirin resistance has received lot of attention in the press and scientific publications.[67-90] However, the practicing physicians and the public are fully not aware of the problem. Therefore, there is an immediate need for the development of awareness programs to educate the health care providers as well as the public who receive health care. Since, there is considerable interest in this subject in the research community a number of reviews have been published on this subject.[67-90] No attempt has been made in this article to extensively review this subject. Focus of this article has been to bring into discussion three specific areas of concern. First and foremost is the molecular mechanism involved in the initiation of thrombosis and stroke. Basically, two major pathways play a role in the pathophysiology of this process. Therefore, there is a need to identify the hyper-responsiveness of individuals to both these pathways and develop appropriate combination therapy. Secondly, arachidonic acid pathway blocks only one of the many mechanisms modulating platelet activation. Therefore, there is an immediate need to develop appropriate drugs or drug combinations to prevent the common pathway of platelet activation. Since fibrinogen binding to activated GP 11b/111a receptor promotes thrombus formation and growth, drugs should be designed and developed to modulate these mechanisms. Third, there is a need for better point-of-care assays which can profile the coagulation pathway as well as platelet activation mechanisms. Such an assay system could be effective in identifying nonresponders to commonly used antiplatelet drugs, semiresponders or hyper-responsive individuals and those with hypercoagulable states. Since, there is no such detection system a lot of individuals at risk are not getting appropriate treatment for prophylaxis against acute vascular events.

In the early 80s, based on our extensive studies, we concluded that aspirin and other antiplatelet drugs do not prevent platelet activation under a variety of experimental conditions.[57-65] Aspirin only inhibits one of the many platelet activation mechanisms. Furthermore, it does not prevent platelet interaction with vessel wall. However, in large number of clinical studies, it has been shown to offer significant beneficial effect to patients with various vascular diseases. Several recent studies have demonstrated there exists some degree of nonresponders to the action of aspirin. [67-90] Therefore, it is of great importance to thoroughly examine this issue and determine the prevalence of true "aspirin resistance" among the patients and provide them alternate therapies. Since, our studies have clearly demonstrated epinephrine, nor-epinephrine, and ADP can potentiate the action of other agonists on platelets we may as well screen those who are hyper-responsive to various agonists so these individuals also could be provided appropriate therapeutic regimen. There are reports suggesting, those who are nonresponders to the action of aspirin may be more responsive to the action of agonists such as ADP or collagen. Studies should take into consideration platelets can be stimulated by a variety of soluble agonists as well as cell matrix components and increased shear stress.

In spite of the fact that several attempts have been made to explain the mechanisms involved in aspirin resistance, there exists no clear explanation. Serious attempts have to be made to understand the mechanism by which an individual develops resistance to these drugs. Since, platelets lack DNA it is highly unlikely that they re-synthesize COX1 enzyme. Since many of these patients are on long-term aspirin therapy the effect of aspirin on megakaryocytes is poorly understood. Platelets are formed from megakaryocytes and these cells do have DNA, hence, studies are warranted to explore the effect of aspirin on bone marrow megakaryocytes. Majority of patients with vascular disease also will be taking many other drugs. As such, some amount of drug-drug interaction cannot be ruled out. Whatever may be the mechanism by which individuals with vascular disease develop resistance to aspirin, a better understanding of the molecular mechanisms involved will facilitate the development of appropriate therapeutic regimen.

CONCLUSION

Platelets play a very important role in the pathogenesis of atherosclerosis, thrombosis and stroke. Aspirin, even at a low to medium dose (80-120 mg day) has been shown to offer significant protection to individuals from developing acute vascular events. Aspirin is the most cost-effective drug available for the secondary prophylaxis of cardiovascular diseases. In view of these earlier observations, expectations of clinicians on the beneficial effect of aspirin therapy was very high. However, from the available evidence both experimental and clinical, it is reasonable to conclude, that significant number of patients are not getting full protection from the use of aspirin. Even those who are considered responders to aspirin therapy may need additional protection, if their platelets are hypersensitive or have a hyper-responsive coagulation pathway. Therefore, there are some limitations in the benefit derived from currently available antiplatelet therapy. Since, currently available methods to assess aspirin sensitivity are not specific, labor intensive and time consuming; efforts should be made to develop specific rapid detection methods. Serious attempts should be made to develop state-of-the-art, Point-of-Care assay systems which are capable of detecting hyper-responsiveness to both platelet and coagulation activation mechanisms. In addition efforts should be made to develop better and effective antiplatelet drugs.

TAKE HOME MESSAGE

Aspirin resistance is a rare phenomenon in healthy individuals. Observed aspirin resistance in clinical situations may be the result of altered sensitivity of platelets to the action of other stimulants. Furthermore, as demonstrated by Rao et al in their studies, endogenous agonists such as epinephrine, and ADP potentiate the action of other platelet stimulants. There is a great need for the development of Point-of-Care devices for monitoring antiplatelet therapy. Antiplatelet and antithrombotic therapy should be monitored in clinical situations and appropriate customized treatment plans should be developed to suit the needs of individual patients. The development of newer antiplatelet agents and antithrombotic agents should be prioritized. This strategy will provide safer and effective drugs and will be the choice of the future antiplatelet regimens, for the better management of individuals with thrombotic tendency.

REFERENCES

1. Sherry S, Scriabine A. Platelets and Thrombosis. University Press, USA 1999;309.
2. Suldow C, Baigent C. Randomized Trials of Antiplatelet Therapy. Handbook of Platelet Physiology and Pharmacology. Rao GHR, (Eds) Kluwer Academic Publishers, USA 1999;526-49.
3. Rao GHR, Rao AT. Pharmacology of Platelet Inhibitory Drugs. Ind. J. Physiol 1994;38:69-84.
4. Rao GHR, Rao ASC, White JG. Aspirin in Ischemic Heart Disease—an overview. Ind Heart J 1993;45:73-79.
5. Rao GHR. Aspirin and Coronary Artery Disease: Coronary Artery Disease in South Asians: Epidemiology, Risk Factors and Prevention. Rao GHR, Kakkar VV (Eds), Jaypee Brothers Medical Publishers, India 2001;263-78.
6. Weisman G. Aspirin. Sci Am 1991;264:84-91.
7. Vane JR. Inhibition of prostaglandin synthesis as a mechanism of action of aspirin-like drugs. Nature 1971;231:232-35.
8. Vane JR, Flower RJ, Botting RM. History of aspirin and its mechanism of action. Stroke 1990;21:IV-12.
9. Ferreira SH, Vane JR. Newer aspects of the mode of action of non-steroidal anti-inflammatory drugs. Ann Rev Pharmacol 1974;14:57-73.
10. Hamberg M, Svensson J Samuelsson B. Thromboxanes: A new group of biologically active compounds derived from prostaglandin endoperoxides. Proc Natl Acad Sci 1975;72:2994-98.
11. Marcus AJ. Aspirin as an anti-thrombotic medication. N Engl J Med 1983;309: 1515-17.
12. Roth JG, Caverley DC. Aspirin, Platelets and Thrombosis: Theory and Practice. Blood 1994;83:885-98.
13. Roth JG, Stanford N, Majerus PW. Acetylation of prostaglandin synthetase by aspirin Proc Natl Acad Sci 1975;72:3073-76.
14. Meade EA, Smith WL, Dewitt DL. Differential inhibition of prostaglandin endoperoxide syhthase (cyclooxygenase) isoenzymes by aspirin and other non-steroidal anti-inflammatory drugs. J Biol Chem 1993;268:6610-14.
15. Burch JW, Stanford N, Majerus PW. Inhibition of platelets prostaglandin synthetase by oral aspirin. J Clin Invest 1978;61:314-19.
16. Reilly IA, FitzGerald GA. Aspirin in Cardiovascular Disease. Drugs 1988;35: 154-76.

17. Wilson KM, Siebert DM, Duncan EM, et al. Effect of aspirin infusions on platelet function in humans. Clin Sci 1990;79:37-42.
18. McLeod LJ, Roberts MS, Cossum PA, et al. The effects of different doses of some acetyl salicylic acid formulations on platelet function and bleeding times in healthy subjects. J Haematol 1986;36:379-84.
19. Masptti G, Galanti G, Pogessi L. Differential inhibition of prostacyclin production and platelet aggregation by aspirin. Lancet 1972;2:11213-16.
20. Steering Committee of the Physicians Health Study Research Group. Preliminary Report: Findings from the aspirin component of the ongoing physicians' health study. N Engl J Med 1988;318:262-64.
21. Steering Committee of the Physicians Health Study Research Group. Final Report. N Engl J Med 1989;321:129-35.
22. Hallam TJ, Sanchez A, Rink TJ. Stimulus response coupling in Platelets. Biocem J 1984;218:819-27.
23. Zucker MB Nachmias VT. Platelet Activation. Arteriosclerosis 1985;5:2-18.
24. Edridge MJ. The molecular basis of communication within the cells. Sci Am 1985; 253:142-52.
25. Holmsen H. Platelet metabolism and activation. Semin Hematol 1985;22:219-40.
26. Seiss W. Molecular mechanism of platelet activation. Physiol Rev 1990;70:115-64.
27. Rao, GHR. Physiology of blood platelet activation. Ind J Physiol Pharmacol 1993; 37:263-75.
28. Rao, GHR. Signal transduction, second messengers and platelet function. J Lab Clin Med 1993;121:18-21.
29. Rao, GHR. Signal transduction, second messengers and platelet pharmacology. Pharmacol 1994;13:39-44.
30. Packham MA. Role of platelets in thrombosis and hemostasis. Can J Physiol Pharmacol 1993;72:278-84.
31. Rao GHR, Gerrard JM, Eaton JW, White JG. The role of iron in prostaglandin synthesis: Ferrous iron mediated oxidation of arachidonic acid. Prost and Med 1978;1:55-70.
32. Peterson DA, Gerrard JM, Rao GHR, Mills EL, White JG. Interaction of arachidonic acid and heme iron in the synthesis of prostaglandins. Adv Prost and Thromb Res 1980;6:157-61.
33. Peterson DA, Gerrard JM, Rao GHR, White JG. Inhibition of ferrous iron induced oxidation of arachidonic acid by indomethacin. Prost and Med 1979;2:97-108.
34. Rao GHR, Cox AC, Gerrard JM, White JG. Effects of 2,2' dipyrydil and related compounds on platelet prostaglandin synthesis and platelet function. Biochem Biphys Acta 1980;628:468-79.
35. Rao GHR, Johnson GJ, Reddy KR. Ibuprofen protects cyclooxygenase from irreversible inhibition by aspirin. Arteriosclerosis 1983;3:384-88.
36. Patrono C. Aspirin as an antiplatelet drug. N Engl J Med 1994;330:1287-94.
37. Hanley SP, Cockbill SR, Bevan J, et al. Differential inhibition by low-dose aspirin of human venous prostacyclin synthesis and platelet thromboxane synthesis. Lancet 1981;2:969-71.
38. Keimowitz RM, Pulvermacher G, Mayo G, et al. Transdermal modification of platelet function: A dermal aspirin preparation selectively inhibits platelet cyclooxygenase and preserves prostacyclin biosynthesis. Circ 1993;88:556-61.
39. Clarke RJ, Mayo G, Price P, et al. Suppression of thromboxane A_2 but not systemic prostacyclin by controlled release aspirin. N Engl J Med 1991;325:1137-41.
40. Antiplatelet Trialists' Collaboration. The Aspirin Papers. Brit J Med 1994;308:71-72;81-106.
41. Fuster V Dyken ML, Vokomas PS. Aspirin as a therapeutic agent in cardiovascular disease. Circ 1993;87:659-75.

42. Rao GHR, Reddy KR, White JG. Low-dose aspirin, platelet function and prostaglandin synthesis: Influence of epinephrine and alpha-adrenergic receptor blockade. Prost and Med 1981;6:485-94.
43. McLeod LJ, Roberts MS, Seville PR. Selective inhibition of platelet cyclooxygenase with controlled release low dose aspirin. Aust N Z J Med 1990;20:652-56.
44. Rao GHR, Radha E Johnson GJ, et al. Enteric coated aspirin, platelet cyclooxygenase activity and platelet function. Prost Leukot Med 1984;13:3-12.
45. Sullivan MH, Zosmer A, Gleeson RP, et al. Equivalent inhibition of *in vivo* platelet function by low dose and high dose aspirin. Prost Leukot Fatty Acids 1990;39: 319-21.
46. Kyrle PA, Eichler HG, Jager U, et al. Inhibition of prostacyclin and thromboxane A2 generation by low dose aspirin at the site of plug formation in man *in vivo*. Circ 1987;75:1025-29.
47. Wilson TW, McCauley FA, Wells HD. Effects of low dose aspirin on responses to Furosemide. J Clin Pharmacol 1986;26:100-05.
48. Zucker Ml, Trowbridge C, Woodroof J, et al. Low- vs high-dose aspirin. Effects on platelet function in hyperlipoproteinemic and normal subjects. Archintern Med 1986;146:921-25.
49. Davi G, Averna M, Catalano I, et al. Increased thromboxane biosynthesis in type 11a hypercholesterolemia. Circ 1992;85:1792-98.
50. Diminno G, Silver MJ, Cerbone AM, et al. Trial of repeated low-dose aspirin in diabetic angiopathy. Blood 1986;68:886-91.
51. Terres W, Schuster O, Kupper W, et al. Effects of low-dose acetylsalicylic acid on thrombocytes in healthy subjects and in patients with coronary heart disease. Dtsh Med Wochenschr 1989;18:1231-36.
52. De Caterina R, Giannessi D Bernini W, et al. Low-dose aspirin in patients recovering from myocardial infarction. Evidence for a selective inhibition of thromboxane-related platelet function. Eur Heart J 1985;6:409-17.
53. Kupper AJ, Verheugt FW, Peels CH, et al. Effect of low-dose acetylsalicylic acid on the frequency and heamtologic activity of left ventricular thrombus in anterior wall acute myocardial infarction. Am J Cardiol 1989;63:917-20.
54. Weksler BB, Kent JL, Rudolph D, et al. Effects of low-dose aspirin on platelet function in patients with recent cerebral ischemia. Stroke 1985;16:5-9.
55. Uchiyama S, Sone R, Nagayama T, et al. Combination therapy with low-dose aspirin and ticlopidine in cerebral ischemia. Stroke 1989;20:1643-47.
56. Jones EW, Cockbill SR, Cowley AJ, et al. Effects od dazoxiben and low-dose aspirin on platelet behavior in man. Brit J Pharmacol 1983;15:395-445.
57. Rao GHR, White JG. Epinephrine-induced Platelet Membrane Modulation. The Platelet Amine Storage. Myers KM, Barnes CD (Eds) CRC Press, Roca Baton, USA 1992;117-49.
58. Rao GHR, Johnson GJ, White JG. Influence of epinephrine on the aggregation response of aspirin-treated platelets. Prost Med 1980;5:45-58.
59. Rao GHR, White JG. Epinephrine potentiation of arachidonate-induced aggregation of cyclooxygenase deficient platelets. Am J Hematol 1981;11:355-66.
60. Rao GHR, White JG. Role of arachidonic acid in human platelet activation and irreversible aggregation. Am J Hematol 1985;19:339-47.
61. Rao GHR, White JG. Aspirin, PGE1 and Quin-2 AM induced platelet dysfunction. Restoration of function by norepinephrine. Prost Leukot Essen Fatty Acids 1990;39:141-46.
62. Rao GHR, Escolar G, White JG. Epinephrine reverses the inhibitory influence of aspirin on platelet vessel wall interaction. Thromb Res 1986;44:65-74.
63. Rao GHR, Escolar G, Zavrol J. Influence of adrenergic receptor blockade on aspirin-induced inhibition of platelet function. Platelets 1990;1:145-50.

64. Rao GHR, Reddy KR, White JG. Modification of human platelet response to sodium arachidonate by membrane modulation. Prost Med 1981;6:75-90.
65. Rao GHR, Johnson GJ, Reddy KR. Ibuprofen Protects Platelet Cyclooxygenase from Irreversible Inhibition by Aspirin. Arteriosclerosis 1983;3:383-88.
66. Connelan JM, Thurlow PJ, Barlow B, et al. Investigation of alternative mechanisms of collagen-induced platelet activation using monoclonal antibodies to glycoprotein 11b-111a and fibrinogen. Thromb. Haemost 1986;55:153-57.
67. Pollack A. For Some, Aspirin May Not Help Hearts. New York Times. 2004.
68. Weber AA, Przytuski B, Schanz A, et al. Platelets 2002;13:37-40.
69. Yilmaz MB, Balbay Y, Korkmaz S. Aspirin resistance. Anadolu Kardiyol Derg 2004;4:59-62.
70. Patrono C, Coller B, FitzGerald GA, et al. Platelet-Active Drugs: The Relationships Among Dose, Effectiveness, and Side Effects. Chest 2004;126:2348-2645.
71. Howard PA. Aspirin resistance. Ann Pharmacother 2002;36:1620-24.
72. Hurlen M, Seijeflot I, Arnesen. The Effect of Different Regimens on Platelet Aggregation After Myocardial Infarction. Scand. Cardiovasc. J 1998;32:233-37.
73. Wu KK, Hoak JC. A new method for the quantitative detection of platelet aggregation in patients with arterial insufficiency. Lancet 1974;11:924-26.
74. Gum PA, Kottke-Marchant K, Poggio ED, et al. Profile and prevalence of aspirin resistance inpatients with cardiovascular disease. Am J Cardiol 2001;88:230-35.
75. Gum PA, Kottke-Marchant K, Welsh PA, et al. A prospective, blinded determination of the natural history of aspirin resistance among stable patients with cardiovascular disease. J Am Coll Cardiol 2003;41:961-67.
76. Deliargyris E, Boudoulas H. Aspirin Resistance. Hellenic J. Cardiol 2004;45:1-5.
77. Grotemeyer KH. Effects of acetylsalicyclic acid in stroke patients; evidence of non-responders in a subpopulation of treated platelets. Thromb Res 1991;63: 587-93.
78. Grotemeyer KH. Two-year follow-up of aspirin responder and aspirin non-responder. A pilot-study including 180 post-stroke patients. Thromb Res 1993; 71:397-403.
79. Mueller MR, Salat A, Stangi P, et al. Variable platelet response to low-dose ASA and the risk of limb deterioration in patients submitted to peripheral arterial angioplasty. Thromb Haemost 1997;78:1003-07.
80. Eikelboom JW, Hirsh J, Weitz JI, et al. Aspirin-resistant thromboxane biosynthesis and the risk of myocardial infarction, stroke, or cardiovascular death in patients at high-risk for cardiovascular events. Circ 2002;105:1650-55.
81. Smout J, Stansby G. Aspirin resistance. Brit J Surgery 2002;89:4-5.
82. Helgason CM, Bolin KM, Hoff JA, et al. Development of aspirin resistance in persons with previous ischemic stroke. Stroke 1994;25:2331-36.
83. Zimmerman N, Wenk A, Kim U, et al. Functional and biochemical evaluation of platelet aspirin resistance after coronary artery bypass surgery. Circ 2003;108: 542-47.
84. Sane DC, McKee SA, Malinin AI. Frequency of aspirin resistance in patients with congestive heart failure treated with antecedent aspirin. Am J Cardiol 2002;90: 893-95.
85. Muller I, Besta F, Schulz C, et al. Prevalence of Clopidogrel non-responders among patients with stable angina pectoris scheduled for elective coronary stenting. Thromb Heamost 2003;89:783-87.
86. Lau WC, Gubrel PA, Watkins PB, et al. Contribution of hepatic cytochrome P450 3A4 metabolic activity to the phenomenon of Clopidogrel resistance. Circ 2004; 109:166-71.

87. Angiolilo DJ, Fernandez-Ortiz A, Bernardo E, et al. High Clopidogrel loading dose during coronary stenting: Effect on drug response and interindividual variability. Eur Heart J 2004;25:1903-10.
88. Serebruany VL, Steinhubl SR, Berger PB, et al. Variability in platelet responsiveness to Clopidogrel among 544 individuals. J Am Coll Cardiol 2005;45:246-51.
89. Dziewierz A, Dubek D, Heba G, et al. Inter-individual variability in responses to Clopidogrel with cardiac diseases. Polis Heart J 2005;62:1-6.
90. Altman R, Luciardi HL Muntaner J, et al. The antothrombotic profile of aspirin, aspirin resistance or simply failure? Thromb J 2004;2:1-8.
91. De Gaetano G, Cerletti C. Aspirin resistance: A revival of platelet aggregation tests. J Thromb Haemost 2004;1:2048-61.
92. Malinin A, Spergling M, Muhlestein B, et al. Assessing aspirin responsiveness in subjects with mutiple risk factors for vascular disease with a rapid platelet function analyzer. Blood Coag Fibrinol 2004;1%:295-301.
93. Sambola A. Heras M, Escolar G, et al. The PFA-100 detcts suboptimal antiplatelet responses in patients on aspirin. Platelets 2004;1-8.
94. Coleman JL, Wang JC, Simon DI. Determination of individual responses to Aspirin therapy using the Accumetric Ultegra. The J. Near-Patient Testing and Technol 2004;3:77-82.
95. Feuring M, Hasseroth K, Janson CP, et al. Inhibition of platelet aggregation after intake of acetylsalicylic acid detected by a platelet function analyzer (PFA 100). Int J Clin Pharmacol Ther 1999;37:584-648.
96. Andersen K, Hurlen M, Arnesen H, et al. Aspirin-responsiveness as measured by a PFA 100 in patients with coronary artery disease. Thromb Res 2002;108:37-42.
97. Christiaens L, Allal J, Corbi C, et al. Impact of ABO blood group on the detection of aspirin resistance with the Platelet Function Analyzer PFA-100. Thromb Res 2003;108:115-19.

Chapter 11

Hemovigilance

Neelam Marwaha

SUMMARY

Hemovigilance is a surveillance system to detect, report and analyze untoward effects of blood collection and transfusion in order to prevent their occurrence and recurrence. It can be organized in a country either through voluntary reporting or legislation. However, for logistic reasons, hemovigilance is organized based on the existing network for collection of data related to blood transfusion services in various countries. Near Miss events are errors which are detected before the transfusion of incorrect blood and help to identify hot spots for transfusion errors. Rapid alert system within hemovigilance assists in taking corrective measures within shortest possible time. Recipient hemovigilance data has lead to numerous blood safety initiatives. Donor hemovigilance is essential as the blood supply is dependent on safe blood donors. Thus, hemovigilance data can provide a powerful input into decision-making in transfusion safety.

KEYWORDS

Hemovigilance, Transfusion hazards, Adverse donor events

INTRODUCTION

Transfusion of blood and its components is an inherent modality of treatment for a large number of hereditary and acquired disorders. It is prescribed by almost all medical and surgical specialists, but like any other form of therapy has its unique adverse effects. A gradual awareness of the risks was becoming increasingly apparent particularly with respect to transmission of viral diseases and immunological problem between allogeneic blood and its recipients. However, there was scant information on the safety of the whole transfusion process from blood collection to component preparation and its final administration at the bedside. Another significant factor is the fact that in the developed countries almost the entire blood collection is from voluntary nonremunerated blood donors. Even in the developing countries there is a gradual but continuous rise in voluntary blood donations. This imposes a great responsibility on all the health care professionals who collect, prescribe and transfuse blood and its components. The safety of the entire transfusion chain, i.e. from the donor to the recipient needs monitoring. This can only be achieved by vigilance of adverse events, hence, hemovigilance, it is best defined as "a set of surveillance procedures, from the collection of blood and its components to the follow-up of recipients to collect and assess information on unexpected or undesirable effects resulting from the therapeutic use of labile blood products and to prevent their occurrence or recurrence".[1]

EVOLUTION OF HEMOVIGILANCE

The concept of hemovigilance emerged from an already existing system of pharmacovigilance which is a system of surveillance of medicinal products with particular reference to adverse reactions as well as serious misuse and abuse of these drugs. In 1974 European Council adopted a directive that required member states to establish national pharmacological systems to collect the above information on drugs.[2] In the early nineties when blood transfusion appeared to be one of the major routes of transmission of hepatitis C virus, the French health authorities took initiative and introduced the concept of hemovigilance in their Blood Transfusion Safety Act of 1993. In 1995, the European Council passed a resolution on blood safety that identified development of a hemovigilance system to improve public confidence in the safety of the blood system. Details of historical aspects are shown in Table 11.1.

The scope of vigilance of health products has widened considerably and presently there are multiple vigilance systems (Table 11.2). The plasma derivatives like albumin, factor concentrates and immunoglobulin preparations which are prepared through plasma fractionation are covered under pharmacovigilance, in most of the countries.

The main objectives of hemovigilance can be listed as follows:
- To make transfusion of blood and blood products safer (recipient safety).
- To make donation safe and comfortable (donor safety).

Table 11.1: Evolution of hemovigilance

Year	Development
1974	European council directed member states to develop pharmacovigilance
1993	French Blood Transfusion Safety Act introduced the concept of hemovigilance
1995	European council passed a resolution identifying the need for hemovigilance
1996	Serious Hazards of Transfusion (SHOT) project was started in UK
1997	Quality Plan was swung into action in USA by the FDA (Food and Drug Administration) and AABB (American Association of Blood Banks)
1998	Initiation of the European Hemovigilance Network
1998	Establishment of a working party on hemovigilance by the International Society of Blood Transfusion.
2002	European Union Blood Directive for legal notification of serious adverse events in member countries.

Hemovigilance

Table 11.2: Health care related vigilance systems

System	Product under surveillance
Pharmacovigilance	Drugs
Hemovigilance	Labile blood components
Biovigilance	Cellular and organ transplants
Materiovigilance	Medical devices
Infectiovigilance	Emerging infectious agents
Reactiovigilance	Reagents, equipments, sample containers

- To restore public confidence in the blood transfusion services by presenting risks and benefits in a balanced perspective.
- To recognize serious adverse events.
- To analyze factors leading to such adverse events.
- To implement preventive strategies to minimize adverse events.
- To assess the outcome of preventive strategies.

HEMOVIGILANCE SYSTEMS

Hemovigilance may be performed at an institutional level to improve existing transfusion practices, but this does not constitute a system. A hemovigilance system comes into existence only when adverse event data is collected through an organized network, reported finally to a central agency where it is analyzed and recommendations made at the national level. Wherever, it started, the system has been organized within the existing network for collection of data related to blood transfusion, for obvious logistic reasons. There are at least three district patterns of hemovigilance.

Through Legislation

Prototype of such a system started in France as a component of the Blood Transfusion Safety Act in 1993. As per the Act, notification of transfusion incidents is mandatory.[3] At least one medical personnel in blood centers and the hospital are designated as hemovigilance correspondents. Any transfusion incident report is sent to the local health authorities for onward transmission to regional hemovigilance coordinators and finally to a centralized hemovigilance cell (Fig. 11.1). The data is analyzed here by a group of experts comprising of transfusion medicine specialists, public health physician, epidemiologists and statistician. Within four years of its inception 2000 hemovigilance correspondents were linked to 24 regional coordinators.

Voluntary Reporting of Adverse Events of Transfusion

An alternative approach initiated in 1996 in the United Kingdom was to create a system of voluntary reporting.[4] The strategic direction of SHOT comes from a steering group represented by medical, nursing and laboratory staff. SHOT was affiliated to the Royal College of Pathologists

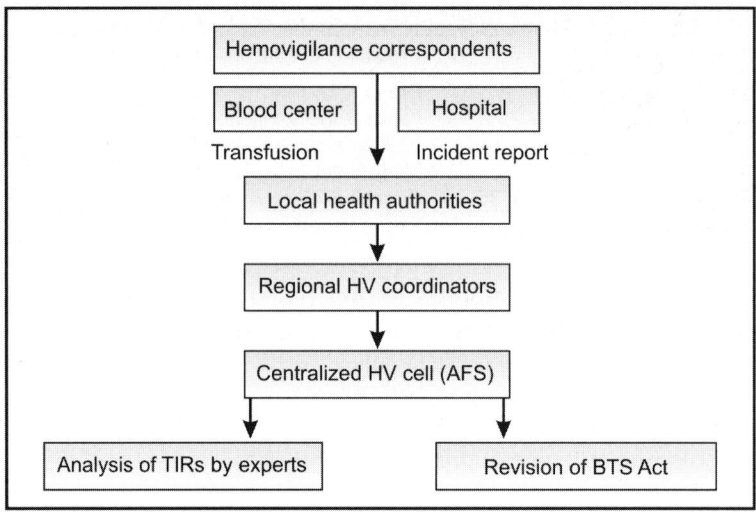

Fig. 11.1: French hemovigilance system

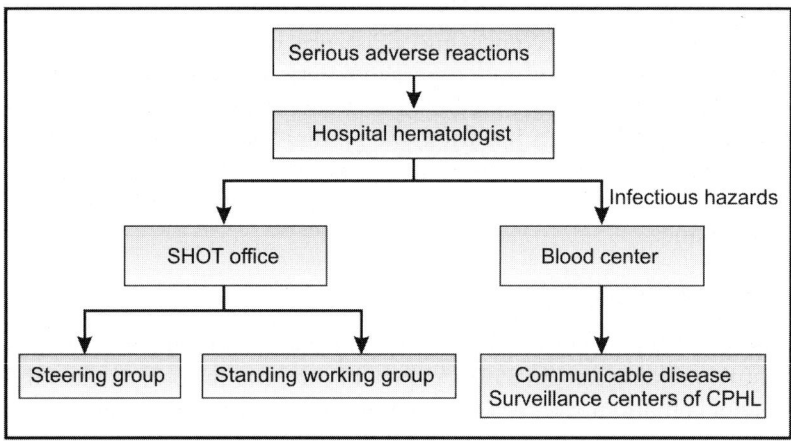

Fig. 11.2: Serious hazards of transfusion (SHOT) initiative, UK

in 1997. The operational aspects are organized by a standing working group which is accountable to the streering group (Fig. 11.2). In general the hospital hematologist is entrusted the responsibility of reporting transfusion related events. The noninfectious adverse event is reported to the SHOT office where confidentiality of the reporting personnel is maintained. The infectious complications are notified to the blood center, so that any components still in inventory can be removed to prevent transmission to other recipients. The blood center then notifies to the Communicable Disease Surveillance Center.

Multidisciplinary Approach

In USA, blood banking and transfusion medicine quality programs fall into two distinct disciplines.[5] Blood collection, component preparation and testing constitute the manufacturing side. Quality measures were strengthened in 1991 by the US Food and Drug administration and blood centers were directed to comply with current Good Manufacturing Practices.[6] Subsequently the American Association of Blood Banks (AABB) the main professional and standards determining organization introduced a Quality Plan. The transfusion medicine practices which include blood component requisitioning, compatibility testing and bedside transfusion, the standard setting organizations are National Institutes of Health (NIH) which develop guidelines based on Consensus Development Conference statements. Besides these, there are many professional organizations which provide expert opinions about appropriate use of blood. The standard setting organizations conduct periodic inspections to ensure compliance, identify adverse events and recommend corrective action.

OBSERVATIONS THROUGH HEMOVIGILANCE

Initially when hemovigilance systems were established emphasis was laid on adverse effects of transfusion, i.e. recipient safety. In France, since reporting was bound by legislation all transfusion incident reports (TIRs) were sent to health authorities. The TIRs were graded according to severity as Grade 1 (minor reactions) Grade 2 (Incidence with long term consequences) Grade 3 (Life-threatening) and Grade 4 (leading to mortality).[7] TIRs were also categorized according to time of occurrence, i.e. acute or delayed and also depending upon the pathogenesis. Acute reactions were mostly febrile nonhemolytic transfusion reactions (41%) and allergic reactions (31%). Hemolytic transfusion reactions (HTRs) were observed due to ABO mismatch resulting in death of 4 out of 58 cases (risk approximately 1 per 2 million units). Non-ABO HTRs involved antibodies against antigens of Rh, Kidd, Duffy, Kell and MNS systems. Bacteria associated transfusion reactions appeared to be the leading cause of mortality.

Delayed TIRs were primarily due to alloimmunization to red cell antigens. 23.3% were due to lack of antibody screeing and identification. 51.4%, i.e. majority were due to incomplete transfusion history provided by the clinicians.[3] 2 cases of HIV transmission were reported and in both the cases the blood units were negative by antibody and P24 antigen screening, but PCR positive on testing stored donor samples. One HBV and one HCV transmission was reported since 1994. Surprisingly even predeposit autologous blood donation was not entirely risk free. Bacterial contamination and one ABO mismatch due to clerical error was noted.

The UK SHOT project identified only serious reactions for reporting.[4] These included:
1. Incorrect blood/component transfused
2. Major acute or delayed reaction

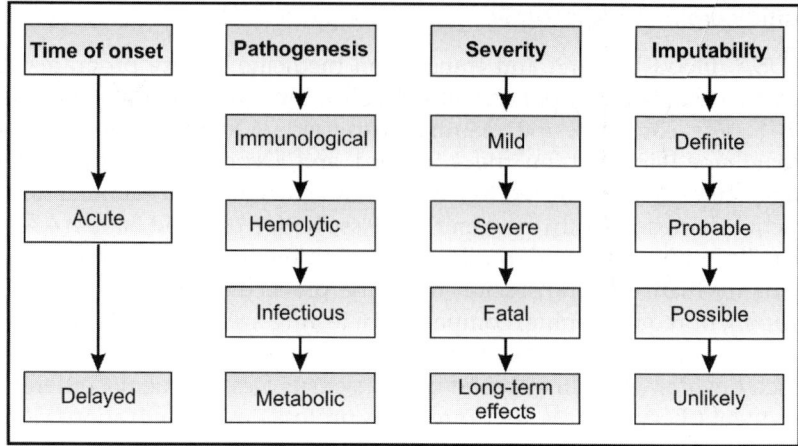

Fig. 11.3: Analysis of adverse reactions

3. Transfusion related GVHD (graft vs host disease)
4. Transfusion related acute lung injury (TRALI)
5. Post-transfusion purpura (PTP)
6. Transfusion transmitted infections.

The data was analyzed as per the format shown in Figure 11.3. It was observed over the years that incorrect blood/component transfused constituted almost 50% of the adverse events. Majority of the errors occurred at the bedside either due to incorrect sampling, misidentification of blood/component with the intended recipient or wrong prescriptions. Several other studies have also highlighted the element of human error leading to incorrect blood/component transfused.[8-12] In a study reported from our center 123 errors were detected out of 60,500 blood/components transfused, 107 out of 123 errors occurred outside the blood bank, majority (73/107) were labeling errors. Out of 16 errors in the blood bank 12 were clerical and only 4 technical.[12] As a result of these errors there was delay in issue, incorrect blood/component issued and acute HTR occurred in 3 patients.

Of the immunological complications of blood transfusion TRALI, PTP and TA-GVHD were reported. In cases of TA-GVHD, the blood components issued were not irradiated. As far as transfusion transmissible infections were concerned, bacterial sepsis predominated over viral infections. One case of transfusion transmitted falciparum malaria leading to fatal outcome was also reported. The donor had lived in a malarious area as a child and had visited a different geographical but malaria endemic area within the previous 4 years. This rapidly resulted in amendment to selection criteria for donors. Continuous reporting to the SHOT office have added two more categories of serious adverse events and these include transfusion associated circulatory overload (TACO) and events related to administration of anti-D immunoglobulin.[13] In the latter category the events include omission or late administration, anti-D given to a D positive patient or an alloimmunized patient, anti-D given to mother of a D negative newborn/wrong patient or incorrect dose/outdated anti-D.

NEAR MISS EVENTS

"Near Miss" events are errors which are detected before the transfusion of incorrect blood/component, and hence a major transfusion error can be avoided.[14] Reporting of "Near Miss" events helps in identifying "hot spots" for transfusion errors and is of immense value for hemovigilance purposes. "Near Miss" reporting has revealed that blood sampling is a common site of error, although in some cases this can be detected in the laboratory due to history of previous transfusion records. Another important fact observed is that generally excess of errors occur during emergency hours especially night shifts. Hence, clinical staff should, as far as possible, avoid requisitioning blood and transfusing it overnight, unless absolutely essential.

RAPID ALERT SYSTEM

The objective of a rapid alert system is to take corrective measures in the shortest possible time.[1] It has been used to alert the appropriate authorities to take note of appearance of clusters of transfusion reactions, defects in disposable materials in the transfusion chain or defective equipments, etc. To cite an example in most of the tertiary care hospitals in our country, blood components are transfused in preference to whole blood. The shelf-life of each component is different, hence the time of actual transfusion of each component from the same donor may be different. Platelets have a short shelf-life (3 to 5 days) while red cells have shelf-life of 35 days and fresh frozen plasma and cryoprecipitate for one year. In case platelets have been detected to have bacterial contamination, a rapid alert to the blood center will lead to immediate removal of other components from that donor unit from the inventory. A platelet rich plasma (PRP) unit showed a puffy appearance on Day 1 of preparation which was noticed prior to release by our staff. The puffy appearance was suggestive of gas formation and hence bacterial contamination. The red cell unit from this donor was immediately quarantined and samples from both grew *klebsiella pneumoniae*. Thus timely detection and alert prevented acute bacterial sepsis.[15]

OUTCOME OF HEMOVIGILANCE

As a result of increasing implementation of hemovigilance in various countries the following observations are being summarized.
1. Bacterial contamination of blood and components constituted a more frequent infectious hazard of blood transfusion rather than viral diseases.
2. The risk of transmitting viral infection by use of screened blood is almost negligible and is mainly linked to donations occurring in the window period, when sensitive testing technologies are applied.

3. Administration of ABO incompatible blood was invariably due to failure to detect incorrect identity of patient or the blood unit. Errors occurred both in the blood center and at the patient bedside, the latter being more common.
4. Administration of ABO compatible but noncompatibility due to other alloantibodies occurred on two accounts (a) failure of clinicians to provide information regarding prior transfusions and (b) technical limitations of alloantibody detection technology.
5. Immune nonhemolytic complications of transfusion like TRALI, PTP and TA-GVHD were unpredictable and presumably under reported.
6. The causes of transfusion related mortality were TA-GVHD, TRALI, bacterial sepsis of contaminated blood components and incorrect blood/component transfused.
7. Pre deposit autologous transfusion could also not guarantee 100% safety as there was occurrence of clerical errors leading to ABO mismatched blood issue and bacterial contamination on storage.
8. Continued surveillance has shown TACO a significant transfusion related acute event especially in the elderly patients.[16]
9. Awareness has been generated regarding anti-D related administration events.

RECOMMENDATIONS AND INITIATIVES FOR BLOOD SAFETY

Based on analysis of hemovigilance data various countries where such a system has been established have developed transfusion guidelines to minimize serious adverse events.

1. **Transfusion Errors:** "Getting the right blood/component to the right patient at the right place at the right time" involves patient's bedside sampling through laboratory testing, issuing and finally transfusion to the patient. Errors as noticed may occur at any stage of the process. Each hospital needs to formulate and adopt guidelines when patient identification and blood/component intended for transfusion are made in accordance with strict procedures. The guidelines need to be circulated to all user departments periodically. Use of computerization in transfusion services with barcode identities of patients and blood units and introduction of an IT "block" to the administration of blood without confirming the identity of the patient and blood have been implemented in many hospitals. Post-computerization there has definitely been a reduction in such errors.[17]

2. **Bacterial Contamination:** Careful donor screening and proper phlebotomy site with two antiseptic solutions are the initial essential steps to reduce bacterial contamination. Visual inspection of blood/component prior to issue decreases the chances of a grossly contaminated unit to be issued. Automated rapid bacterial detection systems have been developed and are being used to screen platelet

concentrates, since these are stored at temperature of 22 ± 2°C, hence most likely for bacterial contamination.[18]

3. **Immune Complications:** Irradiation of blood components in patients susceptible to TA-GVHD has markedly reduced the incidence of this fatal complication. TRALI, an adverse event mediated by plasma containing components generally from female multiparous donors sensitized by HLA antigens, is being prevented by using male donor derived fresh frozen plasma. The incidence of TRALI has significantly declined as per data from UK SHOT project,[13] American Red Cross[19] and other centers.[20] HTRs due to non-ABO clinically significant alloantibodies can be avoided by type and antibody screen policy in blood centers rather than type and cross-match as is being practiced in most developing countries.

4. **Viral Disease Transmission:** Despite screening for antibodies for viral antigens and testing for the antigen too, window period transmission can occur due to circulating viral nucleic acids. Implementation of nucleic acid amplification technology (NAT) has reduced the risk of HIV and HCV to almost neglible level (1 in 4.5 million and 1 in 4.36 million respectively).[21] The risk of HBV still remains 1 in 63000. Automated platform for rapid screening by NAT where results are available within few hours are available.

5. **Leukodepletion of Cellular Blood Components:** Universal leukodepletion of packed red cells and platelet concentrates to leukocyte levels of $< 5 \times 10^6$ per unit have reduced the incidence of febrile non-hemolytic transfusion reactions, HLA alloimmunization and CMV transmission.[22]

6. **New Technologies for Alloantibody Screening and Identification:** The conventional tube technique may miss some of the clinically significant alloantibodies. Sensitive column agglutination technology (CAT), solid phase red cell adherence (SPRCA) and erythrocyte magnetized (EMA) methods have made compatibility testing safer.[23]

7. **Development of prior filters to intercept transmission of new variant Creutzfeld Jakob disease.**

8. **Pathogen inactivation of fresh frozen plasma and platelet concentrates.**

9. **Formation of hospital transfusion committees for appropriate use of blood/components and transfusion audits.**

10. **Regular training on blood safety for blood bank staff and sensitization programs for clinicians.**

DONOR HEMOVIGILANCE

Initial surveillance was largely restricted to adverse events of transfusion in the recipient. However, it is equally important to recognize adverse events in donors, since the blood supply is entirely dependent on donors. Donor reactions have a negative impact on voluntary blood donation program. In a recent study by the American Red Cross on more than 6 million blood donors it was observed that systemic reactions (Vasovagal reactions) were observed more frequently in whole blood donors, double unit red cell donors and in younger age donors.[24] Phlebotomy related complications were more common in plateletpheresis donors and in those beyond 60 years of age.[24] In two institutional studies from India[25-27] vasovagal reactions were seen most frequently in donors of younger age, lower weight, female gender and first time donation status. Such information is relevant for formulating appropriate donor motivational strategies and postdonation care of donors.

ROLE OF INTERNATIONAL SOCIETY OF BLOOD TRANSFUSION (ISBT) IN HEMOVIGILANCE

The Working Party of the ISBT includes members from 26 countries from all over the world. The terms of reference were as follows:
- To develop the different elements to be included in hemovigilance (donor, recipient, process)
- To help standardize surveillance data elements (definitions, diagnostic criteria, flow charts, forms)
- To exchange information between countries on the operation of hemovigilance systems and to exchange data on the results
- To be a source of information and guidance for countries setting up new hemovigilance systems.

Two subgroups were designated—one for adverse donor events and the other for adverse transfusion events. The second group worked closely with the European Hemovigilance Network (EHN) which is a well organized and coordinated network. Definition of various adverse events have been agreed upon and there is also provision for including previously unknown complication of transfusion (PUCT).[28]

HEMOVIGILANCE IN INDIA

The government of India has taken initiative in this regard.[29] Objective 5.7 of the National Blood Policy States:

"NBTC (National Blood Transfusion Council) will develop a program of national hemovigilance with the help of the technical resource group and a monitoring committee. This should be implemented by all SBTCs (State Blood Tranfusion Councils)."

Perhaps, the hospital transfusion committees, which have already started functioning in some of the hospitals, should take initiative in this regard and coordinate with the SBTCs whenever the hemovigilance strategy is finalized. However, great care is needed that this program remains descriptive and constructive with the overall objective of improving transfusion practice.

CONCLUSION

In the developed countries, the blood services have established such system for collecting, testing, and labeling of blood/blood components, which have an extremely high degree of accuracy and low incidence of errors. The clinical environment is still error-prone for which corrective measures at the bedside have been initiated. The bedside errors can ultimately be reduced by education of nursing and medical staff, circulation of guidelines for appropriate transfusion practices and continued reporting and analysis of adverse events of transfusion. In developing countries, there is a need to improve laboratory and clinical aspects of blood transfusion. Implementation of accreditation for transfusion laboratories and hemovigilance for clinical practices of transfusion can meet the international standards for blood safety.

TAKE HOME MESSAGE

Blood and blood component therapy is life-saving but has serious potential hazards. The only source of safe blood are voluntary blood donors. Hemovigilance is a system of recognizing and reporting the adverse events of blood collection (donor hemovigilance), blood processing (process hemovigilance) and transfusion (recipient hemovigilance) with the objective of preventing their occurrence and/or recurrence. Hemovigilance systems may be put in place through legislation or on a voluntary basis by technical experts and thus varies in different countries. For meaningful analysis uniform formats need to be established for classification of transfusion reactions and donor events as has been done by the ISBT. Hemovigilance data helps in redefining transfusion policies and priority setting of healthcare resources. Numerous blood safety initiatives have resulted from such data analysis. "Near Miss" events are errors detected prior to transfusion of incorrect blood/component. Although transfusion error is prevented, but reporting of such events identifies error-prone areas. "Rapid Alert" is an early warning system for corrective measures in the shortest possible time when clusters of transfusion reactions are anticipated. The National Blood Policy of the Govt of India aims at establishing a hemovigilance system in the country through networking of the National Blood Tansfusion Council, State Blood Transfusion Councils and Hospital Transfusion Committees.

REFERENCES

1. http://www.ehn-org.net.
2. McClelland B, UK SHOT project, Love E, Scott S and Williamson LM. Hemovigilance: Concept, Europe and UK initiatives Vox Sang 1998:74 (Suppl 2):431-39.
3. Rouger Ph, Nozart-Pirenne F, LePennec P.Y. Hemovigilance and Transfusion Safety in France Vox Sang 2000;78 (Suppl2):287-89.
4. Williamson LM, Cohen H, Love E, Jones H, Todd A and Soldan K. The Serious Hazards of Transfusion initiative: The UK approach to Hemovigilance Vox Sang 2000;78 (Suppl 2):291-95.
5. Menitove JE. Hemovigilance in the United States of America Vox Sang 1998;74 (Suppl 2) 447-55.
6. Food and Drug Administration: Guidelines for Quality Assurance in Blood Establishments 1995.

7. Noel L, Debeir J, Cosson A. The French Hemovigilance system. Vox Sang 1998; 74 (Suppl 2):441-45.
8. Sazama K. Reports of 355 transfusion associated deaths: 1976 through 1985. Transfusion 1990;30:583-90.
9. Baele PL, De Bruyere M, Deneys Y, Dupont E, Flament L, Lambermont M, et al. Bedside Transfusion Errors. Vox Sang 1994;66:117-21.
10. Mercuriali F, Inghilleri G, Colotti MT, Fare M, Biffi E, Vinci A, et al. Bedside Transfusion Errors: Analysis of 2 years use of a system to monitor and prevent transfusion errors. Vox Sang 1996;70:16-20.
11. Linden JV, Wagner K, Voytovich AE and Sheehan J. Transfusion errors in New York State: An analysis of 10 years' experience. Transfusion 2000;40:1207-13.
12. Sharma RR, Kumar S, Agnihotri SK. Preventable errors related to transfusion. Vox Sang 2002; 82:37-41.
13. www.shot-uk.org.
14. Audrey T. Hemovigilance—closing the loop. Vox Sang 2002;83 (Suppl 1) 13-16.
15. Thakral B, Dhawan HK, Das A, Saluja K, Sharama RR, Marwaha N, et al. Bacterial contamination of platelets: Abnormal appearance prevents catastrophic events. Transfusion 2007;47:1961-62.
16. Popovsky MA. Transfusion-related acute lung injury and transfusion-associated circulatory overload. ISBT Science series 2006;1:107-11.
17. Sawfenberg J, Hogman CF, Cassemar B. Computerized delivery control: A useful and safe complement to the type and screen compatibility testing. Vox Sang 1997; 72:162-68.
18. Brecher ME, Hay SN, Rothenberg SJ. Evaluation of a new generation of plastic culture bottles with an automated bacterial detection system for nine contaminating organisms found in PLT components. Transfusion 2004;44:359-63.
19. Eder AF, Herron R, Strupp A, Edward BD, Notari P, Chambers LA, et al. Transfusion related acute lung injury surveillance (2003-2005) and the potential impact of the selective use of plasma from male donors in the American Red Cross. Transfusion 2007;47:599-607.
20. Insunza A, Romon I, Gonzalez Ponte ML, Hoyos A, Pastor JM, et al. Implementation of a strategy to prevent TRALI in a regional blood centre. Transf Med 2004; 14:157-64.
21. Stramer SL. US NAT yield: Where are we after 2 years? Transf Med 2002;12:243-53.
22. Dzik WH. Leukoreduced blood components. Laboratory and clinical aspects. In Simon TL, Dzik WH, Stowell CP (Eds) Principles of transfusion medicine. 3rd edn. Baltimore, MD: William and Wilkins 2002;270-87.
23. Weisbach V. Comparison of testing with Tube LISS-IAT, CAT, SPRCA for clinically significant antibodies (cs-ab) and antibodies of minor clinical significance (ms-ab). Tranf Med 2006;16:276-82.
24. Eder AF, Dy BA, Kennedy JM, Notari VI EP, Strupp ME, Wissel R, et al. The American Red Cross donor hemovigilance programme : Complications of blood donation reported in 2006. Transfusion 2008;48:1809-19.
25. Agnihotri N, Sharma RR, Rao UV, Marwaha N. Comparison of adverse reactions in voluntary and replacement whole blood donors and its impact on donor retention. Transfusion 2005;45 (Suppl) 172A.
26. Sharma RR, Saluja K, Thakral B, Marwaha N. Frequency of adverse events in plateletpheresis donors. J Clin Apheresis 2007;22:72.
27. www.isbt-web.org.
28. Tondon R, Pandey P, Chaudhary R. Vasovagal reactions in 'at risk' donors: A univariate analysis of effect of age and weight on the grade of donor reactions. Tranf Apheresis Science 2008;39:95-99.
29. An Action Plan for Blood Safety. National Aids Control Organization, Ministry of Health and Family Welfare Govt. of India, 2003.

Chapter 12

Allogeneic Hematopoietic Stem Cell Transplantation in Hematologic Disorders

Rajat Kumar

SUMMARY

Allogeneic hematopoietic stem cell transplantation (SCT) is curative in many potentially fatal conditions. The procedure is expensive as a lot of resources in the form of supportive therapy are required. Early complications of infections and conditioning toxicity, and late complications of graft versus host disease (GVHD) remain obstacles in progress. Worldwide, unrelated transplants, including cord blood transplants are being increasingly used. Unrelated transplants need a far greater precision in HLA matching as well as facilities for management of more severe GVHD and complications due to the greater immunosuppression which is required. In India very few centers are performing allogeneic SCTs and these are predominantly related SCTs. The indications for allogeneic SCTs are based on the relative risks and benefits of transplant versus nontransplant therapy. These indications are constantly changing, as improvements take place in both types of therapies. An overview of the indications for the more common hematological disorders is provided in this chapter. Due to differences in resources and patient population, indications and practices for allogeneic SCT in developing countries may vary from those practiced in the more advanced countries. An informed consent and patient preference are extremely important in any decision-making.

KEYWORDS

Bone marrow transplantation, Stem cell transplantation, Leukemia, Aplastic anemia, Graft versus host disease

INTRODUCTION

Bone marrow transplantation (BMT) or hematopoietic stem cell transplantation (SCT) is a life saving procedure for a number of malignant and nonmalignant life threatening diseases.[1,2] The procedure itself has many technical variations according to the primary disease, age of the patient, facilities available and experience of the center. Allogeneic bone marrow transplantation involves the transplantation of hematopoietic stem cells derived from the bone marrow of a matched donor, ideally an HLA identical sibling, into the patient. Hematopoietic stem cells can also be collected from the peripheral blood or cord blood.[3,4]

Table 12.1: Indications for allogeneic stem cell transplantation

Malignant disorders	Nonmalignant disorders
Acute myeloid leukemia	Thalassemia major
Acute lymphoblastic leukemia	Aplastic anemia
Chronic myeloid leukemia	Fanconi's anemia
Multiple myeloma (mainly autologous)	Myeloproliferative disorders
Chronic lymphocytic leukemia	Sickle cell anemia
Myelodysplastic syndromes	Paroxysmal nocturnal hemoglobinuria
Hodgkin's disease	Severe combined immune deficiency
Non-Hodgkin's lymphoma	Inborn errors of metabolism

INDICATIONS FOR SCT

The indications for allogeneic (allo) hematopoietic stem cell transplantation in hematological disorders can be conveniently divided into two groups (Table 12.1): (a) Malignant disorders—like leukemias, lymphomas and multiple myeloma. In all these indications, the cure or palliation is by the high doses of chemotherapy or radiation therapy, while the transfused stem cells serve to rescue the patient from the myelotoxic effects of the anticancer therapy. In allogeneic type of transplants, there is an additional immunological advantage of graft versus cancer effect, which contributes to the cure (b) Nonmalignant diseases—like aplastic anemia, thalassemia, Gaucher's disease, etc. In these conditions the abnormal marrow is replaced by the healthy donor marrow.

ALLOGENEIC SCT

Stem Cell Source

The three sources of stem cells used in hematopoietic SCT are the bone marrow, peripheral blood and cord blood. The three sources differ in the stem cell content, composition and state of activation of immune cells. Quantitatively, peripheral blood represents the richest and cord blood the poorest stem cell source. Peripheral blood contains more lymphocytes than the other two sources. The most rapid engraftment is observed with peripheral blood transplants and the slowest with cord blood transplants. The risk of developing graft versus host disease (GVHD) also varies with the source of stem cells. Peripheral blood stem cells, which contain more T cells than marrow does, increase the incidence and severity of chronic GVHD compared with bone marrow, while cord blood transplants have a lower risk of GVHD.[4,5] The trends in stem cell source for transplantation are changing. A report from the European Group for Blood and Bone Marrow Transplantation (EBMT) published in 2009 highlights these changes. In 2007, there were 25,563 first HSCTs, 10,072 allogeneic (39%), 15,491 autologous (61%) and 3606 additional transplants reported from 613 centers in 42 countries. The main indications were leukemias (8061 (32%; 89% allogeneic)); lymphomas [14 627 (57%; 89% autologous)], solid tumors [1488 (6%; 96% autologous)] and nonmalignant disorders [1302 (5%; 91% allogeneic)].

Peripheral blood was the main source of stem cells for autologous SCT (98%) and the predominant source for allogeneic SCT (71%).[6]

Donor Requirement

For an allogeneic BMT, an HLA identical sibling is the ideal donor. A sibling who is identical in the HLA-A, B, DR loci is considered HLA identical implying a 6/6 match. In spite of HLA identity, there are always variations in the minor histocompatibility loci. These antigenic differences lead to graft rejection or graft versus host disease unless immunosuppression is used. It is also possible to have a successful transplant using a partially matched sibling as a donor, or an unrelated HLA identical donor, but the complications of graft versus host disease (GVHD) and graft rejection increase. For unrelated transplants, the HLA-C and HLA-DQ loci are also tested and a 10/10 match is ideal. For unrelated cord blood transplants, a 6/6 or even a 4/6 match is acceptable as the cord blood cells are immunologically naïve and the risk of GVHD is less. With improvements in HLA typing at the molecular level, results of unrelated transplants are often equivalent to matched sibling transplants and at times may be preferred. The EBMT 2007 data shows, for the first time since the activity survey began the numbers of unrelated HSCT equal the number of HLA-identical sibling transplants. There are several reasons behind this development. The massive increase of unrelated donor registries has increased the likelihood of finding a well-matched unrelated donor (www.wmda.org). In addition, there is increasing evidence that the well-matched donor in certain situations might be preferable to a sibling donor, for example, in the situation of an older male patient with the choice between an older female sibling donor and a young well-matched unrelated male donor.[6] There are currently more than 13 million unrelated bone marrow voluntary donors registered and more than 350,000 unrelated cord blood units cryopreserved worldwide (www.bmdw.org). Most of those represented in these are Caucasians and other races like the Asians and Africans are underrepresented.[7]

Most centers in India are not conducting any unrelated SCTs.

Conditioning Procedure

Myeloablative Conditioning

The standard preparatory regimens given prior to SCT are myeloablative. Patients receive extremely high doses of chemotherapy or radiotherapy or both. The aim is three-fold: (a) Eradication of malignant cells or, in cases of genetic disorders it is eradication of the abnormal clone of cells, (b) Suppression of the immune system of the host (recipient) so that the allograft is not rejected, and (c) Clearing a "physical space" to allow adequate growth of the donor stem cells. The conditioning, which is myeloablative, is also toxic to various organs like the liver, lungs, kidneys, gastrointestinal tract and reproductive system.

Nonmyeloablative Conditioning

The association of graft-versus-host disease with diminished relapse rates following allogeneic hematopoietic SCT, together with the dramatic responses sometimes seen following donor lymphocyte infusions demonstrates the potential of the human immune system to eradicate hematological malignancies. The curative potential of allogeneic BMT is mediated in part by an immune mediated graft-versus-tumor effect. This has prompted some workers to focus on the use of donor T cells to eradicate both nonmalignant and malignant cells of host origin, without the use of myeloablative conditioning regimens. This reduced-intensity conditioning (RIC), aims to suppress the immunity of the recipient sufficiently to allow allogeneic engraftment, without destroying the recipient's marrow, with lower regimen related toxicity. This represents an important step in capitalizing on the allogeneic graft-versus-tumor effect.[8] Allogeneic transplantation after RIC is most effective in treating slow-growing cancers like chronic lymphocytic leukemia and low-grade non-Hodgkin's lymphoma while this approach is under evaluation for acute leukemia in remission and myelodysplasia.[2]

Technical Aspects of Allogeneic Transplantation

The actual SCT is not complicated. The donor's marrow is harvested by repeated aspiration from the posterior iliac crests, under general or spinal anesthesia. The marrow is collected in a bag with anticoagulant. The number of marrow cells or total nucleated cells (TNC) required for successful engraftment is estimated to be at least 1 to 3×10^8 per kg of recipient's body weight. Bone marrow is transfused through the veins and the donor marrow cells home into the recipient's marrow space and start engrafting. Engraftment is considered established when the peripheral neutrophil count reaches 500/cu mm on 3 successive days.

Supportive Care of the Patient

Protective Isolation

After transplantation of the marrow, it takes about two to three weeks before engraftment occurs, that is the time when the stem cells start producing adequate number of neutrophils, platelets and erythrocytes. During this period very intensive support is required. Some centers have reported carrying out stem cell transplants without protective isolation, or even in outpatient setting, without increase in morbidity or mortality.[9] This is only feasible if the home offers a clean environment, the patient can be monitored closely and admitted immediately, if required. At the All India Institute of Medical Sciences, the Department of Hematology recently published its experience of performing 40 consecutive allogeneic transplants from July 2004 to November 2007 in single non-HEPA filter rooms for a variety of indications. Source of stem cells was peripheral blood in 33, bone marrow in six and combined in one. The indications were severe aplastic anemia-18, CML-7, AML-7, ALL-2, myelodysplastic syndrome-2 and thalassemia major-4. The median age was 19 years (range 2.2-46) with 29 male and 11 female participants. The 30-day mortality was nil, and 100-day mortality was 1 (2.5%). This experience suggests that allogeneic SCT can be safely performed in non-HEPA filter rooms in India.[10]

Venous Access

The transplant process typically involves the use of a long-term, silastic, multilumen, flexible catheter for chemotherapy administration, infusion of stem cells and supportive care management including frequent blood sampling, intravenous antibiotics, blood components and parentral nutrition.[11]

Infections

Infection remains an important cause of morbidity and mortality after bone marrow or stem cell transplantation, with bacterial, fungal infections and viral infections being the predominant cause.[12] The EBMT analyzed a large homogeneous group of 14,403 patients transplanted for early leukemia from an HLA-identical sibling and reported to the EBMT from 1980 to 2001. Of the 597 deaths with infection as the primary cause of death, 217 (36%), were attributed to bacteria, 183 (31%) to viruses, 166 (28%) to fungi and 31 (5%) to parasites. The cumulative incidence of deaths with infection at 5 years was 5% with a cumulative incidence of 1.8% attributed to bacteria, 1.6% to viruses, 1.4% to fungi and 0.3% to parasites.[12] During the early neutropenic period, bacterial and fungal infections predominate while viral infections are frequent after engraftment when the cell mediated immunity is impaired, the most important viruses being CMV, HSV, and VZ. Bacterial infections with encapsulated organisms again predominate after three to six months of engraftment, akin to the condition in post-splenectomized patients. Antimicrobials should be administered after establishing the cause of infection, but in practice an etiological agent is often not identified. During the neutropenic phase, early institution of empirical antibiotics to cover gram-negative and gram-positive bacteria, with addition of antifungal drugs like amphotericin or voriconazole if fever persists, is practiced in most centers in India.[10]

Blood Component Support

After conditioning therapy, patients require multiple red cell and platelet transfusions during the 2-4 week period of pancytopenia, till engraftment occurs. Patients are profoundly immunosuppressed and at risk of developing transfusion associated - graft versus host disease (TA-GVHD) after receiving cellular blood products. To prevent this, all cellular blood products should be irradiated prior to transfusion, to inactivate the donor lymphocytes.

Hematopoietic Growth Factors

Hematopoietic colony stimulating factors (CSF) like G-CSF and GM-CSF are often administered to patients after infusion of stem cells in order to reduce the duration of neutropenia. More recently, studies have shown that even without use of these factors there is no adverse impact on outcome, and many centers use them only in cases with delayed engraftment.

Toxicity Related to Conditioning

The conventional myeloablative therapy given before infusion of bone marrow causes organ toxicity, in addition to myelotoxicity. These are: (a) Veno-occlusive disease (VOD) of the liver, more accurately termed as "sinusoidal obstruction syndrome". It is characterized by (i) jaundice, (ii) hepatomegaly and right upper quadrant pain, (iii) ascites, or (iv) unexplained weight gain (b) Hemorrhagic cystitis characterized by the presence of hematuria, dysuria, and urinary frequency in a patient with sterile urine; (c) Seizures, usually drug induced; (d) Pulmonary complications which can be infectious or noninfectious; (e) Skin and mucosal changes like alopecia, nail changes and oral mucositis.

Failure of Engraftment

Failure to engraft after hematopoietic stem cell transplantation (graft dysfunction) or to sustain engraftment (graft rejection) is a formidable complication due to many possible factors. These include inadequate stem cell numbers, infections, graft-versus-host disease and immunological mediated processes. Bone marrow graft may get rejected by functional host lymphocytes which survive the conditioning regimen. Fortunately, this complication is uncommon. Multiple treatment alternatives have been explored including hematopoietic growth factors, additional infusions of stem cells alone, with augmented immunosuppression or with additional cytotoxic therapy. The incidence is higher in unrelated donor BMT and whenever there is presence of any HLA mismatch. Depleting the marrow of T cells also increases graft rejection.

Graft Versus Host Disease

In allogeneic SCT patients, a unique complication occurs: Graft versus Host disease (GVHD). There are two types of GVHD, acute and chronic.[2]

Acute GVHD: This occurs within the first 100 days after transplant. It classically affects three tissues, namely the skin, gut and liver and may be accompanied by fever. The severity can be graded according to the extent of skin involvement, degree of hyperbilirubinemia and severity of diarrhea.[2]

Chronic GVHD: This usually develops later than 100 days after transplant and often follows acute GVHD but may also develop de novo. It is classified as limited or extensive chronic GVHD. Clinically it resembles autoimmune disorders like scleroderma with skin rash, sicca complex, sclerosing bronchioloitis and hepatic dysfunction. The mortality varies from 20 to 40%. Management is with immunosuppressive agents like cyclosporine, prednisolone, tacrolimus, mycophenolate, methotrexate and cyclophosphamide in various combinations. After a year or more, many patients develop self-tolerance, and these drugs can be tapered off. GVHD is more common in older patients and those with one or more HLA mismatches or unrelated HLA identical transplants. It is mainly for this reason that elderly patients do not do well with allogeneic BMT due to severe GVHD. With the use of PBSC, the time limits are not so well defined and acute GVHD may occur later while classical chronic GVHD may occur earlier.

Tumor Relapse

A successful BMT does not always mean that the primary disease is cured. A certain number of patients will relapse from the original malignancy, as the tumor cells survive the chemo/radiotherapy and graft versus tumor effect. Relapses are higher if the SCT is performed when the disease is not in remission, or at an advanced stage, or is aggressive.

Patients with hematologic malignancies in relapse after allogeneic bone marrow transplantation can be treated by infusing lymphocytes from the original stem cell donor. Donor lymphocyte infusion (DLI) induces complete remissions in the majority of patients with chronic myeloid leukemia (CML) in early-stage relapse and in less than 30% of patients with relapsed acute leukemia, myelodysplasia, and multiple myeloma.

Peripheral Blood Stem Cell Transplantation

It is well known that the peripheral blood contains a small percent of circulating stem cells, approximately 0.1%. This number can be increased by administration of colony stimulating factors, like G-CSF and GM-CSF, which mobilize stem cells form the bone marrow. For allogeneic donors, administration of colony stimulating factors, like G-CSF and GM-CSF for 4 to 5 days results in a high circulating stem cells which can be collected by a cell separator. The procedure requires venous access and takes about four hours. The donor need not be admitted, does not require anesthesia and is spared the pain of marrow aspiration. Hematopoietic reconstitution is more rapid and predictable when peripheral stem cells are used for transplantation. This translates in reduced duration of neutropenia, fewer platelet transfusions, and shorter hospital stay. Immune reconstitution may be better with PBSCT as there are more lymphocytes in the graft as compared to marrow.

Cord Blood Stem Cell Transplantation

Placental blood, which is routinely discarded in clinical practice, is potentially a vast supply of allogeneic fetal hematopoietic stem cells. Cord blood (CB) stem cells have distinctive proliferative advantages which include an (a) enriched proportion of immature stem cells, (b) higher clonogenic growth advantage, (c) increased cell cycle rate, (d) autocrine growth factors production and (e) increased telomere length.

The main limitation of cord blood transplants (CBT) is the limited number of nucleated cells available in a unit. As compared to bone marrow transplantation, the time for engraftment in cord blood transplantation is much longer, taking a month for neutrophilic engraftment and more than fifty days for platelet engraftment. There is also a higher incidence of nonengraftment. The nucleated cell dose available in a cord blood unit is critical, being 1 log less than in a bone marrow transplant (BMT). The minimum recommended dose for CBT is 2.0 to 2.5 × 10^7 nucleated cells/kg for a successful outcome and at least a 4/6 HLA match. The main advantage of CBT is a lower incidence and severity of graft versus host disease. This allows a 1 to 2 HLA antigen mismatch even in unrelated CBT. More than 6000 CBTs have been performed, mainly in the unrelated setting.

The main problem in doing CBT in adults is the limited number of nucleated cells/CD34+ cells in a cord blood collection relative to the weight of an adult. Different strategies are being investigated for this; these include (a) multiunit cord blood transplantation, (b) *ex vivo* expansion of CB hematopoietic stem cells, (c) nonmyeloablative preparative regimen to reduce the conditioning toxicity.[4] Data from the Center for International Blood and Marrow Transplant Research (CIBMTR) indicates that 5% of transplants from unrelated donors into adult recipients consist of cord blood.[2]

INDIAN EXPERIENCE

In India the first BMT was performed in Tata Memorial Hospital (TMH), Mumbai in March 1983. The next center to start BMT/SCT was Christian Medical College, Vellore where the first allogeneic BMT was done in 1986. AIIMS, New Delhi is the third largest center in the country. In the next few years the number of transplants performed in India are expected to increase sharply.[13]

INDICATIONS FOR ALLOGENEIC TRANSPLANTS

In recent years, evidence based guidelines have been formulated for indications in hematologic disorders. These may change with improvements in nontransplant therapy. Some years ago, allo-SCT was the first line treatment for patients of CML who were eligible and had a donor, but with the availability of tyrosine kinase inhibitors, the indications of transplant have reduced radically.

Table 12.2: Indications for allogeneic transplantation in AML (excluding acute promyelocytic leukemia)

Indication	Treatment recommendation	Comments
Myeloablative allo-SCT vs chemotherapy in CR1	Allo-SCT recommended in high-risk cytogenetics, age < 55; Reasonable for intermediate risk, Not recommended for low-risk	Insufficient evidence for intermediate risk. For patients with normal cytogenetics, molecular markers may serve as a guide.
RIC Allo-SCT vs chemotherapy	No recommendation	Insufficient evidence, but RIC is offered to those who would not tolerate myeloablative conditioning.
Allo- SCT vs chemotherapy in CR2	Allo-SCT recommended if donor available	
Related vs unrelated SCT	Related if available, otherwise unrelated	Unrelated may provide equivalent outcomes
BMT vs PBSCT	For high-risk: PBSCT. For low-risk both equivalent.	Insufficient data for unrelated SCT
Conditioning regimen	No recommendation	Insufficient evidence. If TBI used, fractionated rather than single dose
RIC	No recommendation	This is based on age, co-morbidities

RIC = reduced intensity conditioning, Allo = allogeneic, TBI = total body irradiation

Acute Myeloid Leukemia (AML) (Excluding Acute Promyelocytic Leukemia)

The recommendations for allogeneic SCT have been recently revised.[14] A summary is given in Table 12.2. Cytogenetic data plays a very important role in choosing who should be offered transplantation upfront in 1st CR.[15] The outcome is superior if allo-SCT is performed in first CR, but as SCT itself is complicated by morbidity and transplant related mortality, SCT is not indicated in good-risk AML who are likely to be cured with chemotherapy alone. If a relapse occurs, allogeneic transplantation offers the best chance of long-term cure.

Acute Lymphoblastic Leukemia (ALL)

There are controversies regarding the timing and indications for allogeneic transplant in ALL.[16-19] An international collaboration was set-up to prospectively evaluate the role of allogeneic transplantation for adults with ALL and compare with autologous transplantation and standard chemotherapy. Patients received 2 phases of induction and, if in remission, were assigned to allogeneic transplantation if they had a compatible sibling donor. Other patients were randomized to chemotherapy for 2.5 years versus an autologous transplantation. A donor versus no-donor analysis showed that Philadelphia chromosome–negative patients with a donor had a 5-year improved overall survival (OS), 53% versus 45% ($P = .01$), and the relapse rate was significantly lower ($P \leq .001$). The survival difference was significant in standard-risk patients, but not in high-risk patients with a high nonrelapse mortality rate in the high-risk donor group. Patients randomized to chemotherapy had a higher 5-year OS (46%) than those randomized to autologous transplantation (37%; $P = .03$). The study concluded that matched related allogeneic transplantations for ALL in first complete remission provide the most potent antileukemic therapy and considerable survival benefit for standard-risk patients. However, the transplantation-related mortality for high-risk older patients was unacceptably high and abrogated the reduction in relapse risk.[18] A contrary view is held on reviewing other studies, suggesting that there is no clear consensus as to whether there is an advantage to allogeneic HCT over chemotherapy for adults with ALL with standard-risk features while in the first complete remission (CR1). However, allogeneic HCT is recommended in CR1 for patients with high-risk ALL and for those in a second CR.[19] A summary is given in Table 12.3.

Chronic Myeloid Leukemia (CML)

The first SCTs for CML in chronic phase (CP) were performed in Seattle in the late 1970s. The stem cells were obtained from the BMs of their respective genetically identical (syngeneic) twins. The four original patients achieved

Table 12.3: Allogeneic transplantation in ALL

Indication	Treatment recommendation	Comments
Allo-SCT vs chemotherapy in first CR	Allo-SCT recommended but controversial	European data suggests first line in standard risk ALL but other data recommends in high-risk only
Allo-SCT vs chemo in 2nd CR	Allo-SCT preferred	
Related Allo-SCT vs unrelated SCT	Long-term leukemia free survival with related SCT, unrelated SCT of possible benefit in high-risk ALL	Unrelated: Greater toxicity may compromise benefit of graft vs leukemia effect
Conditioning regimen	TBI containing regimens appear better. No specific regimen is superior	
Children		
Allo-SCT in first CR	In Ph+ and other high-risk ALL (induction failure, hypodiploidy)	Not indicated in standard risk
Conditioning regimen	TBI containing regimens appear better. No specific regimen is superior	

TBI = total body irradiation

Ph negativity and remained in good health for the duration of subsequent follow-up. In 1980, transplants using HLA-identical siblings for patients with CML in CP began to be undertaken at specialist centers. Twenty years later, the standard recommendation for newly diagnosed patients with CML in CP was to offer allo-SCT as early as possible after diagnosis if the patient was relatively young (for example, less than 50 years of age) and had a suitable donor who would ideally be an HLA-identical sibling but might be a phenotypically HLA-matched family member or a voluntary unrelated donor.[20]

The indications for transplantation in CML have changed drastically with the availability of tyrosine kinase inhibitors (TKI) like imatinib, dasatinib and nilotinib. Most patients are started on imatinib 400 mg daily. In general, transplantation is no longer a first line option and is reserved for those who show suboptimal response to TKIs or those who relapse. These are the principles adopted in most countries where patients would get TKIs indefinitely. Despite these good results, allogeneic transplantation is the only curative therapy in contrast to TKIs which have to be taken life-long and have a substantial cost.

Thus, the clinician and the patient have to balance the notion that a transplant, although associated with appreciable risks, can, if successful, cure the leukemia against the knowledge that early results show that TKIs can clearly prolong life without any definite prospect of 'cure', and that possible late toxicity cannot yet be reliably predicted. A case can be made for offering an up-front transplant to the new patient who is at poor risk according to Sokal's criteria and also at good risk for surviving a transplant by European Group for Blood and Marrow Transplantation criteria.[21]

There are three possible exceptions to these rules (a) Some pediatricians believe that initial treatment by allo-SCT may be the preferred approach for children who have HLA-identical sibling donors, (b) In a situation where the cost of continuing treatment with TKIs for some considerable number of years is prohibitive, then up-front allografting should be considered, especially if this procedure can be carried out more cheaply than is usual in the western world, (c) Allo-SCT should still be considered as part of the therapeutic strategy for a patient who presents *de novo* in accelerated phase or blastic transformation. For such patients, treatment should begin either with imatinib alone at 600 or 800 mg/day, followed by an appropriate combination of cytotoxic drugs, or alternatively, imatinib may be given simultaneously with cytotoxic drugs. Once Ph-negative status is achieved, a patient should, if possible, proceed to allo-SCT with minimum delay.[20]

Patient preference and counseling is extremely important. There is consensus that if a patient does not show adequate response to TKIs or shows a relapse, Allo-SCT should be offered.[20,22,23] A summary is given in Table 12.4.

Table 12.4: Allogeneic transplantation in chronic myeloid leukemia (CML)

Indication	Treatment recommendation	Comments
Timing at presentation	Upfront Transplant: Patient preference, cost of transplant less than overall cost of TKI, in pediatric patients, patient with high-risk disease (Sokal's score) but low-risk of TRM (EBMT score)	Most centers in the Western world offer TKI in preference to transplant.
Timing in course of therapy	(a) No cytogenetic response at 6 months, (b) have cytogenetic relapse after 12 or 18 months after achieving initial hematological remission, (c) partial cytogenetic response at 18 months, (d) patients with T315I mutations unresponsive to TKIs, (e) progress to accelerated or blastic phase, (f) intolerant to TKI	

Table 12.5: Allogeneic transplantation in chronic lymphocytic leukemia (CLL)

Indication	Treatment recommendation	Comments
Timing	(a) Non-response or early relapse (within 12 months) after purine analogues, (b) relapse within 24 months after having achieved a response with purine-analogue-based combination therapy, (c) Patients with p53 abnormalities (del17p)	Both BM and PBSCT can be done
Conditioning regimen	RIC	High TRM with myeloablative transplant

Chronic Lymphocytic Leukemia (CLL)

The majority of patients with CLL are elderly and are not candidates for transplantation. Moreover, the disease is heterogeneous in its course and many patients would live for many years without the need for therapy, or be controlled very easily with short courses of chemotherapy. The indications for allo-SCT in CLL are ill-defined. An EBMT consensus meeting has identified indications where allo-SCT may be a preferred treatment modality in CLL.[24] The panel suggested that allo-SCT is a procedure with evidence-based efficacy in poor-risk CLL. A summary is given in Table 12.5.

Myelodysplastic Syndrome (MDS)

The only curable treatment for MDS is allogeneic SCT. As the patients suffering from MDS are often elderly and transplant is toxic, allo-SCT is often not a valid option. The indications, timing, conditioning regimen and need for pretransplant chemotherapy are all controversial.[25] A study from the EBMT recommended early transplant as front line therapy in patients younger than 40 years in early disease for the best outcome.[26] In contrast, another study made the opposite recommendations, suggesting

Table 12.6: Allogeneic transplantation in myelodysplastic syndrome (MDS)

Indication	Treatment recommendation	Comments
Timing	Early SCT for IPSS score Int-2 or high-risk at diagnosis and selected patients of low-risk and int-1 who have refractory cytopenias	The IPSS score did not include some high-risk features
Pre-SCT induction chemotherapy	No recommendation	Insufficient data to recommend for or against pre-SCT induction
Related vs unrelated	No recommendation	No evidence of survival advantage based on donor selection. In practice, if a related donor is available, it is preferred
BM vs PBSC	No recommendation	In related donors, high-risk patients may benefit from PBSCT. For unrelated donors, insufficient evidence
Myeloablative vs RIC	No recommendation	Insufficient evidence. The choice is based on age, co-morbidities

that delaying transplant in young patients with early disease was the best course, while monitoring for disease progression.[27] Evidence based guidelines have been formulated and recently published.[28] These are given in Table 12.6.

Lymphomas

In lymphomas, autologous SCT is recommended in case of relapse. Allo-SCT has a role when autologous stem cells cannot be collected, due to bone marrow involvement.[29] Allo-SCT is generally offered to younger patients with a suitable donor. Table 12.7 highlights some of these recommendations.

Aplastic Anemia

Severe aplastic anemia (SAA) is potentially curable with allo-SCT, the only limiting factor being, the transplant related morbidity and mortality. Guidelines suggest that in young patients with an HLA matched sibling donor, allo-SCT should be first line therapy, as the complications are much less. In those who are older than 40 years, immunosuppression should be tried first[30,31] (Table 12.8). The source of stem cells is also controversial. A recent study showed better outcome with bone marrow versus peripheral blood. This was mainly due to a higher GVHD in the PBSC group.[32] This study analyzed the outcome of 692 patients with severe aplastic anemia receiving transplants from HLA-matched siblings. A total of 134 grafts were PBSC grafts, and 558

Table 12.7: Allogeneic transplantation in NHL

Indication	Treatment recommendation	Comments
High grade		
Timing	Autologous SCT is first choice (see comments). Allo-SCT when (a) failure to enter first complete remission, (b) first relapse or second remission, (c) first remission if high IPI.	Allo-SCT indicated in chemotherapy sensitive disease and (a) Unacceptable autologous hematopoietic stem cell graft or (b) Progression after autologous transplant, inability to harvest an engrafting dose of autologous hematopoietic progenitors or (c) Bone marrow or peripheral blood involvement
Follicular		
Timing	Autologous SCT is first choice (see comments). Allo-SCT when (a) first relapse or (b) failure to enter first remission	Age <70 years age with (a) chemosensitive disease, (b) inability to harvest an engrafting dose of autologous hematopoietic progenitors, (c) bone marrow or peripheral blood involvement

Table 12.8: Aplastic anemia

Indication	Treatment recommendation	Comments
Severe aplastic anemia	If HLA Identical Sibling Available. (a) Age < 40 yr : BMT 1st line treatment. (b) Age > 40 yr: BMT as 2nd line treatment if immunosuppression fails in 3-4 months, (one or two cycles may be tried). If only HLA Identical Unrelated Donor available. Age < 40 years: BMT if immunosuppression fails.	The indications of age may be relaxed for: (a) Patients who are infected and would not tolerate immunosuppression or (b) Very severe aplastic anemia

were bone marrow grafts. Rates of hematopoietic recovery and grades 2 to 4 chronic graft-versus-host disease (GVHD) were similar after PBSC and BM transplantations regardless of age at transplantation. In patients older than 20 years, chronic GVHD and overall mortality rates were similar after PBSC and BM transplantations. In patients younger than 20 years, rates of chronic GVHD (relative risk [RR] 2.82; $P = .002$) and overall mortality (RR 2.04; $P = .024$) were higher after transplantation of PBSCs than after transplantation of BM. These authors concluded that bone marrow grafts are preferred to PBSC grafts in young patients undergoing HLA-matched sibling donor transplantation for SAA.[32]

This view is not accepted by many transplanters in the developing world. Patients with aplastic anemia who come for transplantation in developing countries are often multi-transfused and the blood products they receive are usually not leucodepleted. They are, therefore, alloimmunized and have a high-risk of graft rejection. PBSC transplant reduces the chances of graft rejection due to a higher stem cell dose and the higher T cell content. Moreover, many patients are infected prior to coming for transplant and a PBSC has the advantage of an earlier engraftment as well as immune reconstitution. The transplant centers at AIIMS, New Delhi and CMC, Vellore routinely use PBSC as a preferred source for allo-SCT in aplastic anemia.[33,34] The success rates of 70-80% survival suggest that in the Indian context, PBSC may be a preferred source of stem cells in the kind of patients seen in India.

Thalassemia Major

A major indication for Allo-SCT in India is thalassemia major. This disease is potentially curable with an allogeneic transplantation. The results are excellent if the transplantation is done prior to the complications of iron overload, transfusion complications and alloimmunization. Results from Pesaro, Italy, suggest more than 85% disease free survival for patients transplanted early, in Pesaro Class 1.[35] In India, similar results have been attained at CMC, Vellore.[13] When a child is diagnosed with thalassemia major, treatment should be started with optimal blood transfusion and iron chelation instituted before there is a significant rise in ferritin levels. All siblings should be typed for an HLA identical match. If a match is available, the child should be referred to a transplant center. An allo-SCT should be performed as soon as feasible. For convenience of nursing and post-transplant care, allo-SCT in India is generally performed after the child is more than 3 years of age.

Paroxysmal Nocturnal Hemoglobinuria (PNH)

BMT is still the only curative therapy for PNH, but is associated with significant morbidity and mortality. The International Bone Marrow Transplant Registry (IBMTR) reported a two-year survival probability of 56% in 48 recipients of HLA-identical sibling transplants between 1978 and 1995. Their median age was 28 years. The majority of the deaths in this study occurred within one year of transplantation. The European Blood and Marrow Transplant group reported a 5-year survival rate of 70% following allogeneic BMT for PNH; however, only 54% met criteria for classical PNH.[36] The course of PNH is unpredictable and indications for transplant are bone marrow failure, recurrent thrombosis or single severe thrombosis and severe hemolysis.

Acute Promyelocytic Leukemia (AML-M3)

The treatment and outcome for APL has improved dramatically after the introduction of ATRA and Arsenic therapy. In case of a relapse, salvage therapy is advised. For patients with a molecular remission, autologous transplant is preferred. Allogeneic SCT is only indicated for those who do not achieve molecular remission and have a donor.

Other Indications

Allogeneic hematopoietic SCT is also offered to a number of other hematologic conditions. As these are rare, there is insufficient evidence to provide definite guidelines regarding the indications, types of transplant conditioning and the outcome. These conditions include Fanconi's anemia, sickle cell anemia, severe ITP, myelofibrosis, inherited disorders of metabolism. Usually these are done in selected cases where the disease is progressive, a donor is available and sufficient expertise is available with the center.

TAKE HOME MESSAGE

Allogeneic SCT should be offered to patients where the benefits outweigh the risks. Non-transplant therapy should be compared to SCT, before making any recommendations. Counseling of the patient and patient preference is extremely important, as SCT involves considerable expense, often prolonged morbidity and even fatality. In India, where the cost is usually borne by the patient and family, economic factors need consideration. In general, early transplant offers better results than SCT performed in advanced disease, but in those disorders where nontransplant therapy offers similar outcomes, SCT is offered when there is failure of alternative therapy. In hematological malignancies, cytogenetic and molecular prognostic markers usually guide the timing of transplantation. Potential transplant candidates should be referred early to a transplant center where facilities for assessment are available. For more detailed disease specific analysis, the original articles should be reviewed.

REFERENCES

1. Armitage JO. Bone marrow transplantation. N Engl J Med 1994; 330(12): 827-38.
2. Copelan EA. Hematopoietic stem-cell transplantation. N Engl J Med 2006; 354(17):1813-26.
3. Schmitz N, Barrett J. Optimizing engraftment—source and dose of stem cells. Semin Hematol 2002;39(1):3-14.
4. Ballen KK. New trends in umbilical cord blood transplantation. Blood 2005; 105(10):3786-92.
5. Couban S, Simpson DR, Barnett MJ, Bredeson C, Hubesch L, Howson-Jan K, et al. A randomized multicenter comparison of bone marrow and peripheral blood in recipients of matched sibling allogeneic transplants for myeloid malignancies. Blood 2002;100(5):1525-31.
6. Gratwohl A, Baldomero H, Schwendener A, Rocha V, Apperley J, Frauendorfer K, et al. The EBMT activity survey 2007 with focus on allogeneic HSCT for AML and novel cellular therapies. Bone Marrow Transplant 2009;43(4):275-91.
7. Johansen KA, Schneider JF, McCaffree MA, Woods GL. Council on Science and Public Health, American Medical Association. Efforts of the United States' National Marrow Donor Program and Registry to improve utilization and representation of minority donors. Transfus Med 2008;18(4):250-59.
8. Slavin S, Nagler A, Naparstek E, Kapelushnik Y, Aker M, Cividalli G, et al. Nonmyeloablative stem cell transplantation and cell therapy as an alternative

to conventional bone marrow transplantation with lethal cytoreduction for the treatment of malignant and nonmalignant hematologic diseases. Blood 1998; 91(3):756-63.
9. Russell JA, Chaudhry A, Booth K, Brown C, Woodman RC, Valentine K, et al. Early outcomes after allogeneic stem cell transplantation for leukemia and myelodysplasia without protective isolation: A 10-year experience. Biol Blood Marrow Transplant 2000; 6(2):109-14.
10. Kumar R, Naithani R, Mishra P, Mahapatra M, Seth T, Dolai TK, et al. Allogeneic hematopoietic SCT performed in non-HEPA filter rooms: Initial experience from a single center in India. Bone Marrow Transplant 2009;43(2):115-19.
11. Lazarus HM, Trehan S, Miller R, Fox RM, Creger RJ, Raaf JH. Multi-purpose silastic dual-lumen central venous catheters for both collection and transplantation of hematopoietic progenitor cells. Bone Marrow Transplant 2000;25(7):779-85.
12. Gratwohl A, Brand R, Frassoni F, Rocha V, Niederwieser D, Reusser P, et al. Cause of death after allogeneic haematopoietic stem cell transplantation (HSCT) in early leukaemias: An EBMT analysis of lethal infectious complications and changes over calendar time. Bone Marrow Transplant 2005;36(9):757-69.
13. Chandy M. Stem cell transplantation in India. Bone Marrow Transplant 2008; 42 Suppl 1S81-S84.
14. Oliansky DM, Appelbaum F, Cassileth PA, Keating A, Kerr J, Nieto Y, et al. The role of cytotoxic therapy with hematopoietic stem cell transplantation in the therapy of acute myelogenous leukemia in adults: An evidence-based review. Biol Blood Marrow Transplant 2008;14(2):137-80.
15. British Committee for Standards in Haematology, Milligan DW, Grimwade D, Cullis JO, Bond L, Swirsky D, et al. Guidelines on the management of acute myeloid leukaemia in adults. Br J Haematol 2006;135(4):450-74.
16. Hahn T, Wall D, Camitta B, Davies S, Dillon H, Gaynon P, et al. The role of cytotoxic therapy with hematopoietic stem cell transplantation in the therapy of acute lymphoblastic leukemia in adults: An evidence-based review. Biol Blood Marrow Transplant 2006;12(1):1-30.
17. Hahn T, Wall D, Camitta B, Davies S, Dillon H, Gaynon P, et al. The role of cytotoxic therapy with hematopoietic stem cell transplantation in the therapy of acute lymphoblastic leukemia in children: An evidence-based review. Biol Blood Marrow Transplant 2005;11(11):823-61.
18. Goldstone AH, Richards SM, Lazarus HM, Tallman MS, Buck G, Fielding AK, et al. In adults with standard-risk acute lymphoblastic leukemia, the greatest benefit is achieved from a matched sibling allogeneic transplantation in first complete remission, and an autologous transplantation is less effective than conventional consolidation/maintenance chemotherapy in all patients: Final results of the International ALL Trial (MRC UKALL XII/ECOG E2993). Blood 2008;111(4): 1827-33.
19. Larson RA. Allogeneic hematopoietic cell transplantation is not recommended for all adults with standard-risk acute lymphoblastic leukemia in first complete remission. Biol Blood Marrow Transplant 2008;15(1 Suppl):11-16.
20. Goldman J. Allogeneic stem cell transplantation for chronic myeloid leukemia-status in 2007. Bone Marrow Transplant 2008; 42 Suppl 1S11-S13.
21. Passweg JR, Walker I, Sobocinski KA, Klein JP, Horowitz MM, Giralt SA, et al. Validation and extension of the EBMT Risk Score for patients with chronic myeloid leukaemia (CML) receiving allogeneic haematopoietic stem cell transplants. Br J Haematol 2004;125(5):613-20.
22. Goldman J. Recommendations for the Management of *BCR-ABL*-positive Chronic Myeloid Leukaemia. British Committee for Standards in Haematology 2007.

23. Hochhaus A, Dreyling M, ESMO Guidelines Working Group. Chronic myelogenous leukemia: ESMO clinical recommendations for the diagnosis, treatment and follow-up. Ann Oncol 2008;19 Suppl 2ii63-4.
24. Dreger P, Corradini P, Kimby E, Michallet M, Milligan D, Schetelig J, et al. Indications for allogeneic stem cell transplantation in chronic lymphocytic leukemia: the EBMT transplant consensus. Leukemia 2007;21(1):12-17.
25. Marcondes M, Deeg HJ. Hematopoietic cell transplantation for patients with myelodysplastic syndromes (MDS): When, how and for whom? Best Pract Res Clin Haematol 2008;21(1):67-77.
26. Runde V, de Witte T, Arnold R, Gratwohl A, Hermans J, van Biezen A, et al. Bone marrow transplantation from HLA-identical siblings as first-line treatment in patients with myelodysplastic syndromes: Early transplantation is associated with improved outcome. Chronic Leukemia Working Party of the European Group for Blood and Marrow Transplantation. Bone Marrow Transplant 1998; 21(3):255-61.
27. Cutler CS, Lee SJ, Greenberg P, Deeg HJ, Perez WS, Anasetti C, et al. A decision analysis of allogeneic bone marrow transplantation for the myelodysplastic syndromes: Delayed transplantation for low-risk myelodysplasia is associated with improved outcome. Blood 2004;104(2):579-85.
28. Oliansky DM, Antin JH, Bennett JM, Deeg HJ, Engelhardt C, Heptinstall KV, et al. The role of cytotoxic therapy with hematopoietic stem cell transplantation in the therapy of myelodysplastic syndromes: An evidence-based review. Biol Blood Marrow Transplant 2009;15(2):137-72.
29. Hahn T, Wolff SN, Czuczman M, Fisher RI, Lazarus HM, Vose J, et al. The role of cytotoxic therapy with hematopoietic stem cell transplantation in the therapy of diffuse large cell B-cell non-Hodgkin's lymphoma: An evidence-based review. Biol Blood Marrow Transplant 2001;7(6):308-31.
30. Marsh JCW, Ball SE, Cavenagh J, Darbyshire P, Dokal I, Gordon-Smith EC, et al. Guidelines for the diagnosis and management of aplastic anaemia. British Committee for Standards in Haematology 2009.
31. Marsh JC, Ball SE, Darbyshire P, Gordon-Smith EC, Keidan AJ, Martin A, et al. Guidelines for the diagnosis and management of acquired aplastic anaemia. Br J Haematol 2003;123(5):782-801.
32. Schrezenmeier H, Passweg JR, Marsh JC, Bacigalupo A, Bredeson CN, Bullorsky E, et al. Worse outcome and more chronic GVHD with peripheral blood progenitor cells than bone marrow in HLA-matched sibling donor transplants for young patients with severe acquired aplastic anemia. Blood 2007;110(4):1397-1400.
33. Kumar R, Prem S, Mahapatra M, Seth T, Chowdhary DR, Mishra P, et al. Fludarabine, cyclophosphamide and horse antithymocyte globulin conditioning regimen for allogeneic peripheral blood stem cell transplantation performed in non-HEPA filter rooms for multiply transfused patients with severe aplastic anemia. Bone Marrow Transplant 2006;37(8):745-49.
34. George B, Mathews V, Viswabandya A, Kavitha ML, Srivastava A, Chandy M. Fludarabine and cyclophosphamide based reduced intensity conditioning (RIC) regimens reduce rejection and improve outcome in Indian patients undergoing allogeneic stem cell transplantation for severe aplastic anemia. Bone Marrow Transplant 2007;40(1):13-18.
35. Lucarelli G, Galimberti M, Polchi P, Angelucci E, Baronciani D, Giardini C, et al. Marrow transplantation in patients with thalassemia responsive to iron chelation therapy. N Engl J Med 1993;329(12):840-44.
36. Brodsky RA. How I treat paroxysmal nocturnal hemoglobinuria. Blood 2009; (online Prepublication).

Chapter

13 The Battle of Cancer is to be Won by Targeted Therapy

MB Agarwal

INTRODUCTION

The Egyptian papyri, which are thought to have been written between 3000 and 1500 BC, are considered as the earliest descriptions of human cancer. The Edwin Smith papyrus describes several cases of tumors. Egyptian physicians used surgery and cauterization as important palliative measures. After surgery and radiotherapy, which began in early 20th century, the use of chemical gases during the second world war paved the way to develop chemotherapy for treating cancer with mustered gas leading to the development of alkylating agents in 1950s. This became a major milestone in the field of cancer-therapy during the second half of the 20th century.

The cytotoxic properties of nitrogen mustards were investigated by Gilman in 1942. The dramatic therapeutic success of nitrogen mustard in patients of Hodgkin lymphoma and lymphosarcoma were described by Goodman et al in 1946. Subsequently, anti-folate drugs were used in children with acute lymphoblastic leukemia (ALL) and choriocarcinoma. Gradually, combination chemotherapy became curative in ALL and certain lymphomas. In late 1970s, cisplastin was synthesized and found to be effective for treating ovarian and testicular cancer. Development of carboplatin quickly followed. Simultaneously, there was intensive search for anti-cancer drug development from planned sources resulting into discovery of vinca-alkaloids and taxanes.

This traditional medical treatment of cancer (chemotherapy) worked by interfering with rapidly dividing cells (anti-mitotic). It has been effective and even curative for certain cancers such as gestational choriocarcinoma, childhood acute lymphoblastic leukemia (ALL), Hodgkin lymphoma and a subgroup of non-Hodgkin lymphoma. In addition, adjuvant chemotherapy for breast, colon and lung cancer can augment the survival benefit afforded by surgical therapy. Even in patients with advanced solid tumor or recurrences despite surgery, chemotherapy can offer lengthened survival of worthwhile quality. Unfortunately, with chemotherapeutic agents, the therapeutic index is narrow, responses are partial, disappointingly brief and unpredictable. These issues highlight the limitations of traditional cytotoxic chemotherapy which fail to distinguish cancer cell from normal cell.

Against this background, the advent of therapies based on mechanisms that target critical molecular pathways in the growth and development of tumors, has evoked considerable interest. During last two decades, there has been increased scientific understanding of the biology of cancer. This has changed cancer pharmacotherapy. The targeted therapies (also known as molecularly targeted therapies) block or target cancer growth by interfering with specific molecules needed for carcinogenesis and tumor growth. They hold the promise of being more selective and less harmful to the normal cells as they are focused on molecular changes specific to cancer. These agents alter the cell growth without necessarily killing them and hence can be considered as subtle but specific bullets.

The 21st century is the era of molecularly targeted anti-cancer therapy. Paul Ehrlich's concept of developing "magic bullet" for treating cancer resulted in concept of "selective toxicity" by Albert. The therapeutic armamentarium of 21st century oncologists has a greater number of complex drugs and drug-combinations which continues to expand. At the moment, over 400 small molecules and biological modifiers are undergoing clinical developments. Most of these targeted therapies are still at the level of preclinical testing or various phases of clinical trials. However, whenever, there is a clear cut known "molecular driver", one or more targeted therapies have been developed and some of these have already received US-FDA approval for treating cancers, either alone or in combination with each other or even in combination with chemotherapy.

The classical example is Philadelphia chromosome – positive chronic myeloid leukemia (CML) (Fig. 13.1). In early 1980s, it was clear that

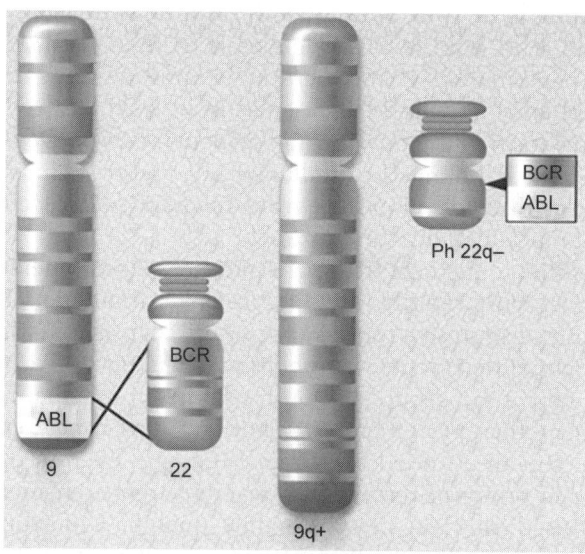

Fig. 13.1: Philadelphia chromosome
(With permission from Editor, Blood 2008;112:4808-17).

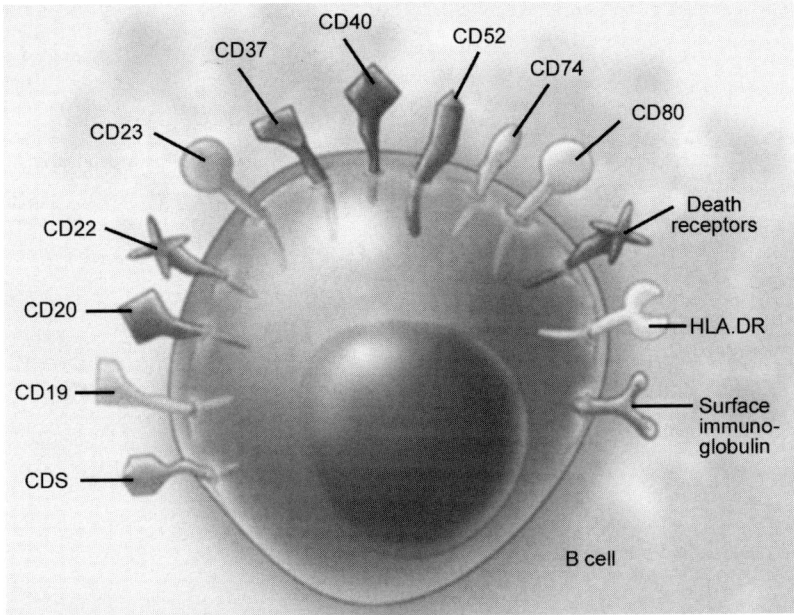

Fig. 13.4: Cell-surface antigens on B-lymphocyte
(With permission, Editor, N Engl J Med 2008; 359:613-26)

Table 13.1: Monoclonal antibodies for B-cell cancers

Antibody	Target
Rituximab (Rituxan, MabThera, Reditux)	CD20
Humanized anti-CD20 antibodies	CD20
Epratuzumab	CD22
Lumiliximab	CD23
SGN-40	CD40
Alemtuzumab (Campath)	CD52
Galiximab	CD80

this inhibitor protein, making NFκB active. It then travels to the nucleus and starts a chain of events promoting tumor growth and spread. Bortezomib blocks the activation of NFκB and thus paralyses the growth of tumor.

5. Immunotherapy: In addition, cancer vaccines and gene therapy are also considered by some to be targeted therapies as they interfere with the growth of cancer cell.

Signal-transduction research has shown the importance of members of the human epidermal growth factor receptor (HER) family of transmembrane tyrosine kinases in many solid tumors. One member of this family is HER2 (ErbB2). The gene for this receptor is modified in up to 30% of breast cancers, leading to aggressive

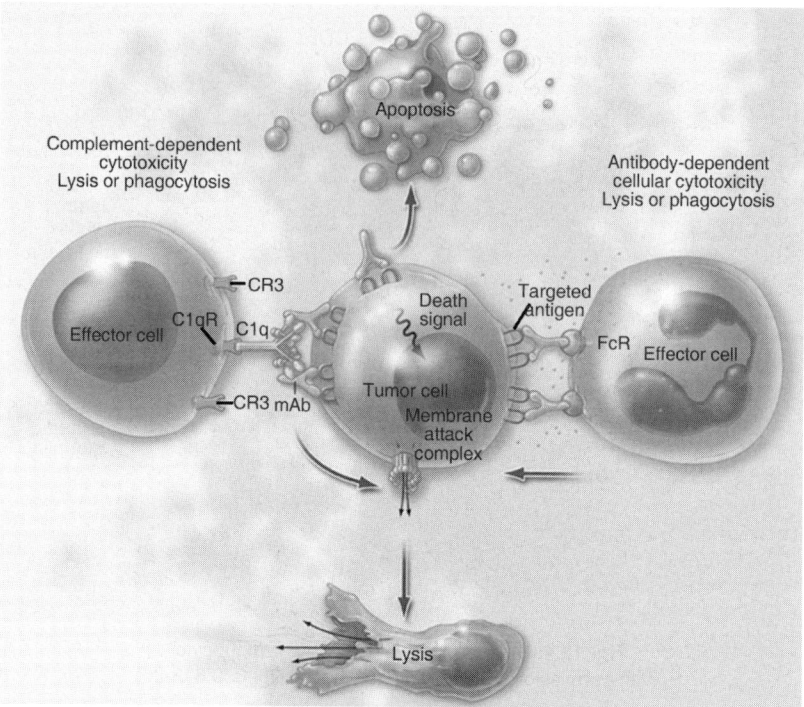

Fig. 13.5: Potential mechanisms of action of monoclonal antibodies
(With permission, Editor, N Engl J Med 2008; 359:613-26)

behavior and unfavorable prognosis. However, the overexpressed HER to receptor protein also serves as a target for anti-HER2 antibody (Trastuzumab) therapy. The presence or absence of amplification can be used to differentiate patients who may have a response to the antibody from those who will not have a response. The addition of chemotherapy further enhances the responses to antibody.

The epidermal growth factor receptor (EGFR, also known as ErbB1 or HER1), another transmembrane receptor tyrosine kinase of the HER family, has important role in the proliferation and metastasis of tumor cells. It is frequently overexpressed in common solid tumors and has become a favored target for orally administered small-molecule and antibody-based therapy. Gefitinib was approved by US-FDA as third-line therapy for non-small-cell lung cancer in May 2003.

FUTURE CHALLENGES

It is believed that target therapies, in future, are likely to replace existing chemotherapies in the treatment of cancer. Today, many cancers have become chronic lifelong disorders and no more the deadly killers. As they need lifelong treatment, any drug which is more tolerable and has less side-effects, is likely to be thoroughly investigated and clinically used.

The future of targeted therapy will focus on finding patient-specific targeted therapy (subpopulations). The route to identify these subpopulations is through biomarkers and surrogate endpoints. Unfortunately, one is forced to predict, based on the present successes and failures, that the road to further development of molecularly targeted anti-cancer drugs may not be an easy one. Firstly, the animal models are poor predictive of therapeutic efficacy against human cancer. The data generated from such studies should be viewed with caution. Secondly, human tumors that respond to drugs, still contain subclones which, become drug resistant by a broad array of mechanisms. Hence, molecular profiling of a patient's cancer before choosing therapy and as a means to define treatment modifications, is likely to become the standard of care.

Still, the knowledge-base generated over last two decades has provided us with several principles that will be applicable to develop in molecularly targeted therapies further. As stated earlier, with the availability of present molecularly targeted therapies, many human cancers which were fatal, have now become chronic conditions. Maintenance therapy, hence, is a new concept in cancer. This has become a reality because targeted therapies are relatively nontoxic and effective in maintaining minimal residual disease (MRD) as MRD.

CONCLUSION

Cancer remains the second leading cause of death in United States. All the three existing modalities, i.e. surgery, radiotherapy and drug therapy have narrow therapeutic index. Vigorous research continues to improve the efficacy of these treatment modalities, e.g. refined surgical techniques, improved radiation delivery methods (IMRT) and developing molecularly targeted therapies.

With the advent of molecularly targeted therapies, it appears that Paul Ehrlich's romantic concept of the "magic bullet" against tumor cells, which is more than a century old, has been achieved most effectively in patients with chronic myeloid leukemia with the use of Imatinib. With the current large oncology drug pipeline, we are at the dawn of an era during which "magic bullets" will be developed more and more and will be used to treat a wider spectrum of cancers more extensively and effectively. Only by undertaking thoughtfully planned studies, the future molecularly targeted therapies will change the cancer scenario.

SUGGESTED READING

1. Cheson BD, Leonard JP. Monoclonal antibody therapy for B-cell non-Hodgkin's lymphoma. N Engl J Med 2008;359:613-26.
2. DeVita VT Jr, Chu E. A history of cancer chemotherapy. Cancer Res. (American Association for Cancer Research Centennial Series) 2008;68:8643-53.

3. Druker BJ. Translation of the Philadelphia chromosome into therapy for CML (ASH 50th Anniversary Review). Blood 2008;112:4808-17.
4. Duenas-Gonzalez A, Garcia-Lopez P, et al. The prince and the pauper. A tale of anti-cancer targeted agents. Molecular Cancer 2008;7:82-115.
5. Joske DJ. CML : The evolution of gene-targeted therapy. Med J Australia (Clinical Update) 2008;189:277-82.
6. Lichtman MA. Battling the haematological malignancies : The 200 years' war. The Oncologist 2008;13:126-38.

Chapter 14

Thalassemia Screening and Control Program

VP Choudhry, Amit Upadhyay

SUMMARY

Thalassemia is the commonest hemolytic anemia in the world. In India it has been estimated that there are five crore thalassemia carriers and over twelve thousands children with thalassemia major are born in India. The cost of therapy for management of these children is beyond the reach of the families and the government. Various studies all over the World have shown that it is cost effective to control the birth of thalassemic babies. Several countries have successfully controlled the birth of thalassemia in their countries. Various strategies along with modalities for control of thalassemia program utilizing the present primary health care system or medical college system have been reviewed along with their pros and cons. There is an urgent need to initiate the thalassemia screening and control program and government of India needs to take necessary steps in that direction on top priority.

KEYWORDS

Thalassemia, Screening and coltrol.

Hemoglobinopathies is most frequent inherited disorder in the world, primarily because of high prevalence of thalassemia in the world (WHO). It is much more so in the South East Asia and in the Meditarrean region. It was in 1925 when Thomas B Cooley gave the first description of thalassemia in the Transactions of American Pediatric Society. He described children with anemia, hepatosplenomegaly, discoloration of skin and sclera and no bile in the urine. Whipple and Bradford first used the term thalassemia in 1932. Thalassemia word was taken from Greek meaning the sea, as it was more common in meditarrean area. It is widely prevalent along the meditarrean affecting Italy, Spain, Portugal, East and Central Europe, Greece, Meditarrean islands, republic of Soviet Union, Cyprus, Africa, South East Asia, North and South America, etc.[1,2]

In India there are several studies from different part of regions showing high prevalence of thalassemia carriers in different population. It varied between 0-17 percent of population with mean of nearly 4%.[3] Under the ages of ICMR, three large multicentric studies have been conducted which have revealed the mean prevalence of beta thalassemia varying between 2.9 to 4.6%[4] (Table 14.1).

Table 14.1: Multicentric studies—ICMR

Period	Group	No. screened	% beta thalassemia
1984-87	High school children 3 centers	12000	4.6%
1996-98	Pregnant women 5 centers	7000	3.8%
2000-05	Jai Vigyan program College students, pregnant women	60000	2.9%

Table 14.2: Thalassemia control program—why prevention

- High prevalence
- Traits are normal and healthy
- Marriages within the same community
- Death certain if no treatment
- Survival based on repeated blood transfusion
- Blood is a scarcity and carries risk of TTI
- Treatment costly, painful and has complications
- Permanent cure BMT-HLA match not easily available, enormous cost, high-risk

Why Thalassemia Control (Table 14.2)

With the present birth rate in our country, it has been estimated that over twelve thousand children with thalassemia major are born every year. Presently there is no national data that how many thalassemics are in our country. However there are over fifty-five thalassemia societies who are working for the noble cause of thalassemia in our country. It has been estimated that there are over one lac thalassemic children. Even if very we take very conservative estimates, around fifty thousand thalassemic are on regular transfusion and taking some form of chelation. Availability of blood is a scarcity even though we are over 100 crore in population as our youth does not come forward to donate blood. Under present scenario, 15,00,000 units of blood are required every year for thalassemic children. Cost of therapy for management of thalassemia including the need for regular blood transfusions and iron chelation therapy is quite high and is beyond the reach of majority. It was estimated that if all these children are given proper care, the cost of therapy for these children alone will be nearly 650 crore. Other reasons why it is essential to control thalassemia are summarized in Table 14.2. Thus it is essential to initiate the screening and control program.[5,6] Many countries in the world have already initiated the screening and control program (Table 14.3). Countries such as Cyprus, Greece, etc. have already brought birth of thalassemia to zero (Fig. 14.1).[7]

Target population: It is essential to define the target population for screening program for control of thalassemia. School children can be screened easily under school health program or along with any other program under government of India. The success of this program will be delayed. A study conducted at Mumbai revealed that it was not a satisfactory method as a baby with thalassemia was born among those who were screened during

Thalassemia Screening and Control Program

Table 14.3: Thalassemia control program

Thalassemia prevention scenario worldwide		
Italy	:	Mandatory antenatal screening
Iran	:	Premarital thalassemia screening
Palastine	:	Free health insurance
		Premarital test is necessary
Pakistan	:	Shows documentary in all its international flights
Taiwan	:	National screening program
Maldives	:	National screening program
UK, US	:	Newborn screening program

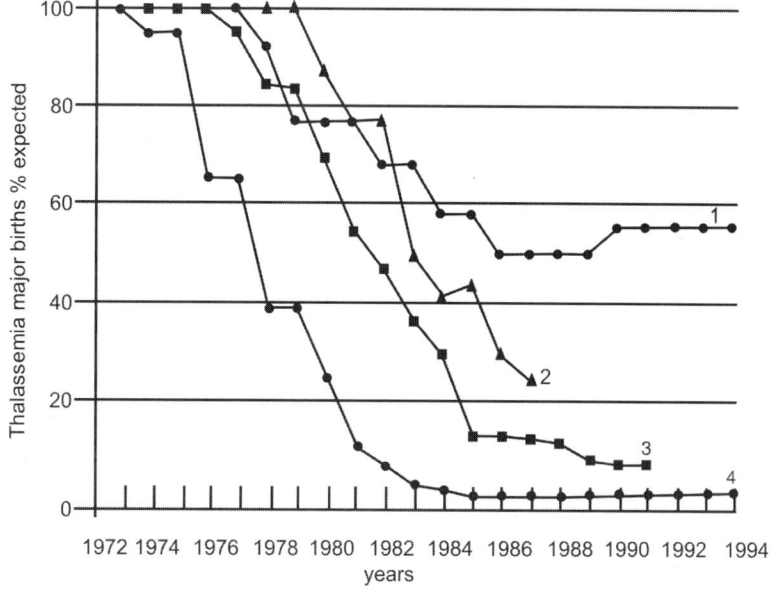

1=UK, 2=Italy, 3=Greece, 4=Cyprus

Fig. 14.1: Thalassemia control: Effect

the school. It was recommended that screening thalassemia among school children may be successful if it is accompanied by continuous awareness, education and reminders to those who are thalassemia carriers.

Next group could be college students who are likely to get married over the next few years. These students will remember their thalassemia status provided they are given adequate information and are counseled and motivated for control of thalassemia. The major drawback of screening at this stage is that:

a. Many children do not enter the colleges for their higher studies in India.
b. Indian system of arranged marriages in which children often do not have their say especially in rural areas.

c. The possibility that they may forget their thalassemia status at the time of need cannot be excluded.

Screening of high-risk communities and relatives of affected children[8] (Family approach) is likely to yield good results. However, it may become discrimination against certain communities and relatives of thalassemic children. Though many thalassemic societies have conducted free thalassemia screening program but only few of their relatives have come forward for blood testing. It is from the index case that one proceeds backwards and follows up other family members to identify other carriers. Siblings have 1 in 2 risk of being carrier. Uncles and aunts have 1 in 4 while cousins have 1 in 8 risk of being carrier. However, under this program the first thalassemia baby in the family cannot be prevented.

Thalassemia screening during pregnancy seems to be most effective method as all pregnant ladies are most receptive to the obstetrician advice. Even if lady seeks medical attention during second trimester, it may not be possible to prevent thalassemia during that pregnancy but it will have an impact during their subsequent pregnancies. The major drawback of this screening method is that birth of thalassemic children will continue to be taking place as majority of women in India take medical advice during late second trimester and majority of deliveries are conducted in rural India at home. However, if screening during pregnancy is implemented strictly it is an effective method which will have immediate results.

Population screening: Other method is mass screening at schools, colleges, before marriage and during pregnancy. The target should be that everybody who is likely to reproduce, should know his or her thalassemic status. This is called prospective screening. It is easier to offer screening to a person when he or she comes in contact with a medical system for any problem. The screening program becomes integral part of medical infrastructure. Knowledge of blood group and thalassemia screening may be made mandatory like voter card. One needs to identify the existing system and incorporate the thalassemia screening data for thalassemia control. It requires an education program for the pediatricians, physicians, obstetrician, nurses, midwives, auxiliary nurses and health workers. All these groups need to be sensitized to the needs of thalassemia screening and control program. All schools, colleges and health centers need to be integral part of the program. If women attend the antenatal clinic early it will be easy to attend the couples at risk and to offer them prenatal diagnosis in time. This group will serve as the most efficient method for controlling thalassemia. It is unfortunate that only nearly 15% of population attended antenatal clinics during the first trimester while 47% and 38% attended in second and third trimester respectively, even in urban areas. This method appears to be the most effective method for screening and control program.

General population screening strategies: In India health is a state subject. Therefore, it is essential that central and state health departments need to work together for the success of the program. It will be desirable that also if all medical colleges are involved with the control program. The staff of these medical colleges will assist for the following besides providing the leadership role for conducting the program. They will be required to take the following responsibilities:

a. Education, training of all staff for the control program.
b. For external quality control program in their region.
c. For all confirmatory tests and counseling of families.
d. Centers for antenatal diagnosis which need very precise molecular diagnosis.
e. Abortion of the affected fetus.
f. Counseling and other facilities.

Two possible programs are being suggested. In the first program the state health program involving primary health centers, community health centers, district hospital, etc. is being used. The medical colleges are being kept above the district hospitals (Fig. 14.2). The advantages and disadvantages of central and state program are being given in Table 14.4. The staff of health program is well aware of local conditions, issues, areas, etc. Cooperation of the entire staff of the state health program is essential. Their commitment, dedication towards the program will be the keys for the success of the program. However, the present health staff, under primary health centers, is overburdened and is responsible for multiple government health programs.

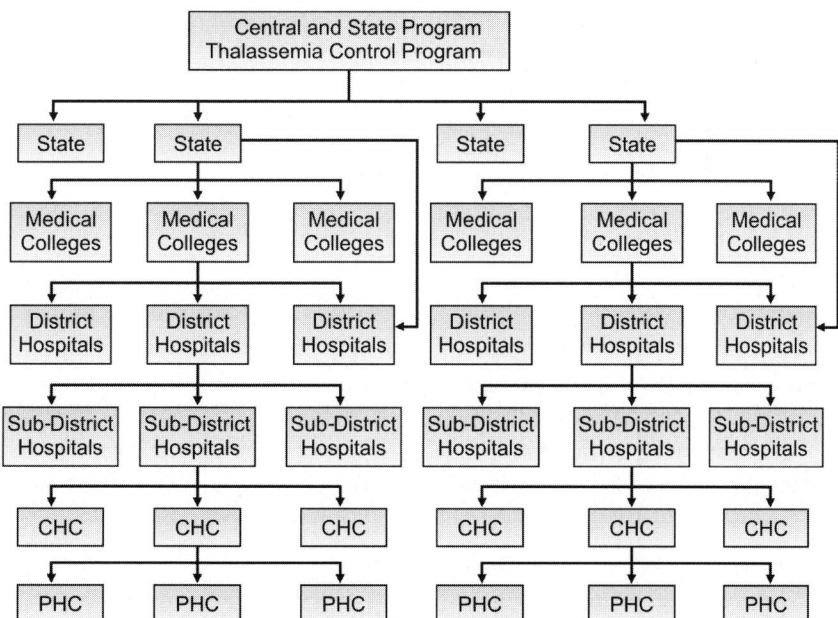

Fig. 14.2: Central government program

Table 14.4: Central and state screening program

Advantages:
1. Decreased central funds but states input essential
2. Use of existing health system
3. Decreased staff requirement
4. Staff—aware of local issues

Disadvantages:
1. Multiple administration
2. Decreased cooperation among agencies
3. Decreased accountability
4. Present staff—overburdened
5. Upgradation of district hospitals

The second possible way is that thalassemia screening and control program is made a national program like any other central program. A cell under Ministry of Biotechnology/ICMR/Ministry of Health is made the controlling body. Country may be divided in five regions ie east, west, north, south and central India. All medical colleges and district hospitals of state will be part of the program. However, under the districts, tehsils and the villages of tehsils form one unit (Fig. 14.3). The pros and cons of this approach are given in Table 14.5. This pattern is likely to be successful as the grass root staff will be responsible only for this program. Since this program will be under central government funds, though high, may not be a problem. Under the program the accountability need to be stressed at every level. The nonperforming staff needs to be changed. The entire staff

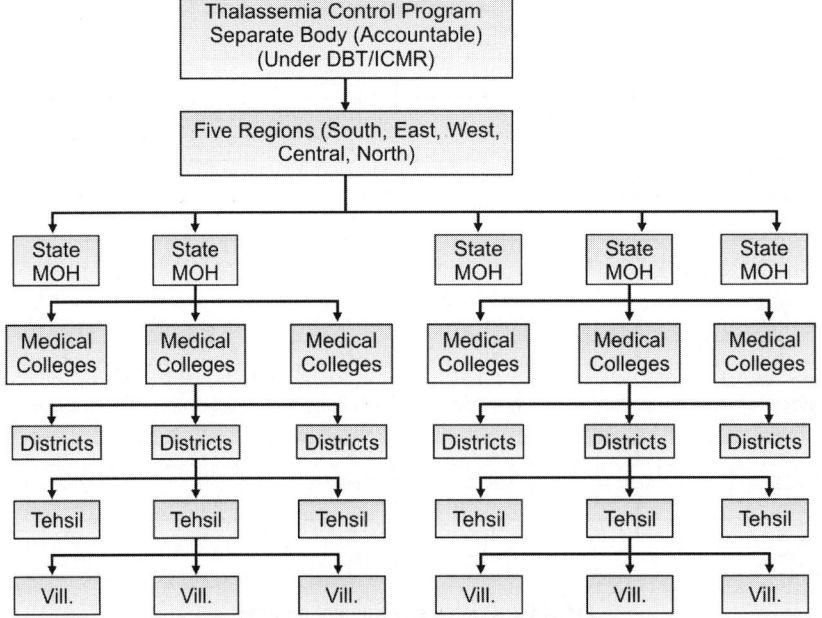

Fig. 14.3: Central Government Program (MOH)

Table 14.5: Thalassemia control program central government

Advantages:
1. Funds from central government
2. Control under central government
3. Better accountability
4. Higher success

Disadvantages:
1. Poor knowledge of local issues
2. Poor cooperation of state government
3. Separate staff at grass root
4. Higher financial input

will be newly appointed. The willing workers need to be appointed. The staff will need appropriate training and supportive material. Motivation of the staff needs to be maintained with accountability. Appropriate counseling will be given to the people in their native language by local health workers so that they understand the need for thalassemia control. All the states are likely to cooperate as their health burden will be reduced significantly with control of thalassemia. Secondly the entire funds for the program will come from central government. Program is likely to become successful as every person will be accountable for his job under one body.

Screening Tests (Table 14.6)

Hematologic Parameters

1. NESTROFT (Naked Eye Single Test Tube Red Cell Osmotic Fragility Test) (Table 14.7): This test has a very high specificity and sensitivity and being easy to perform, now increasingly being used in screening purposes. A positive test has to be followed by confirmatory test.[9,10]
2. Discrimination indices (Table 14.7): These are various formulas devised to differentiate between the iron deficiency anemia and beta thalassemia as both typically have microcytic hypochromic picture. But with the advent of modern cell counters they are now rarely used. Various discrimination factors which have been used are given in Table 14.6. MCV < 78 fl and MCH < 27 pg in presence of normal or high red cell count are suggestive of thalassemia trait. However, low MCV and MCH, in presence of low red cell count, is suggestive of iron

Table 14.6: Hemoglobinopathy screening tests

1. Population screening
   - Target population
   - NESTROFT
   - RBC indices
   - Hb electrophoresis/HPLC
2. Thalassemia control
   - Mutation studies
   - Genetic counseling
   - Antenatal diagnosis

Table 14.7: Discriminant factors

1. Mentzer: MCV/RBC
    If < 13   Thal minor
    If > 13   Iron deficiency
2. Shine-Lal: $(MCV)^2 \times MCH$
    If <1530   Thal minor
    If >1530   Iron deficiency
3. England-Fraser: MCV-(Hbx5)-RBC-3.4
    If negative Thal minor
    If positive Iron deficiency
    The England-Fraser formula is the most common one used.

Table 14.8: Comparative evaluation of NESTROFT and RBC indices

Test	No. of cases	BTT	Sensit (%)	Specific (%)	+ve predict value %	–ve predict value %
NESTROFT	177	133	98.5	78.8	75.1	98.7
MCV < 80 fl	217	131	97.03	63.47	62.98	97.05
MCH < 27 pg	224	134	99.2	56.73	54.8	99.1
Total RBC > 5 m	168	128	94.8	80.97	76.19	96.0

deficiency anemia which is widely prevalent in our country. Tests for screening include NESTROFT, MCV, MCH, red cell count. The specificity and sensitivity of these tests are given in Table 14.8. MCH and MCV along with red cell count can provide very high specificity and sensitivity.

3. Red cell distribution width: This is a measure of heterogeneity in the red cells. The value of RDW-CV > 17.1 indicates iron deficiency anemia. The problem with this value is that many coexistent conditions can alter the value making it less reliable. Since iron deficiency anemia is prevalent in India it may mask the underlying thalassemia trait as the RDW (red cell distribution width) will be higher in these cases.
4. Hemoglobin electrophoresis: Increase in Hb A2 fraction of more than 3.5% with a normal Hb pattern is diagnostic of thalassemic carriers.[11,12] It is considered as a gold standard in evaluation of thalassemia trait. An Hb A2 value of < 2% is normal and a value of > 3.5 indicates a carrier state.
5. Globin chain ratio: Beta/alpha chain ratio can be calculated by using radiolabelled amino acids. Usually it is 1.0 and any variation of this ratio indicates thalassemia state.

Biochemical Parameters[13-17]

DNA mutation studies: Worldwide over 200 mutations have been identified of which 6 common and 44 rare mutations have been identified in Indian population. These can be detected by DNA studies by various methods. Rapid tests have been developed which can be done at all medical colleges. However, in families where the definitive molecular diagnosis cannot be made, samples of the family could be analyzed for various mutations by using other molecular techniques such as Reverse Dot Blot Hybridization, ARMS, DGGE analysis, DNA sequencing, etc. at regional centers depending upon the available facilities.

Antenatal Screening

Preconceptional: Both partners should be tested for thalassemia trait. If both or either of them is normal, there is no need for further testing. But if both partners are thalassemia carriers, it is essential for the lady to undergo tests for determination of thalassemia status of fetus, preferably during first trimester. Family needs to be counseled regarding the possibility of thalassemic baby, carrier and normal along with the risk and benefit of the antenatal diagnosis. Couple needs to be counseled for termination of pregnancy if fetus is thalassemic.

The methods available for antenatal screening are: The first method here needs to be chorion villus sampling as this is the only technique applicable to first trimester testing.

1. Chorionic Villous Sampling (CVS): This is the standard and preferred method, as it is done at 10-12 weeks of pregnancy so that, if needed, pregnancy can be terminated safely.

    In this method, under ultrasonic guidance, a needle is inserted and a sample of chorionic villi is taken out. These cells can be analyzed further for the presence of thalassemia mutations. Couples with the affected mutations need to be counseled and prompt facilities need to be provided for safe and effective abortion at all centers even at village level for the success of the program.

2. Amniocentesis: In this method amniotic fluid is collected under ultrasonic guidance during second trimester and the shedded epithelial cells of fetus are analyzed for the presence of thalassemia mutations. It is applicable especially to patients who did not attend the antenatal clinic in their first trimester.

3. Cordocentesis: In this method under ultrasound guidance, a fine needle is inserted in fetal umbilical cord and 2-3 ml of fetal blood is obtained and run on a HPLC machine to know the variant Hb present in the fetal blood. It is now done only in selected cases usually in those in which CVS is not conclusive. This can also be undertaken in women who appear late for antenatal check-up, at 18-20 weeks of gestation. Adult hemoglobin levels are checked in cord blood and a level of less than 0.8% are suggestive of thalassemia major. This test can be done over one hour and the termination of pregnancy can be undertaken. However, this test cannot differentiate between thalassemia carrier and normal state. Also one has to be cautious for maternal blood contamination while interpreting the results. Hb A levels > 8.0% and the presence of any amount of HBA2 indicate maternal contamination and in these cases the procedure will need to be repeated.

Success of the program: Thalassemia screening and control program is the only acceptable method for controlling the birth of thalassemic children. It is well established that screening and control program is very much cost effective and countries like Cyprus,[18] Greece have completely controlled thalassemia in their country. Many other countries have adopted national program for the control.

It requires national program with involvement of people, their education, active participation of NGOs, religious bodies, medical staff at all levels from villages to metros. Most important is the willpower of politicians and availability of funds. Accountability of all, who are involved, coupled with time frame program are key to the success.

TAKE HOME MESSAGE

Comprehensive management of thalassemia is expensive and most children in India develop the complications of iron overload or its therapy. With the present technology the birth of thalassemia can be prevented. All hematologists, pediatricians, obstetricians and laboratory persons need to spread the massage and work together for control of thalassemia. The thalssemia control program is cost effective and can be easily implemented if there is political will.

REFERENCES

1. Weatherall DJ, Clegg JB. The thalassemia syndromes. 4th edn. Blackwell science, UK;2001.
2. Katewa S, Choudhry VP. Historical perspective and Introduciton to thalassemia in hemoglobinopathies. Sachdeva A, Lokeshwar MR, Shah N, Agarwal BR, Khanna VK, Yadav SP, Jain V (Eds) in Hemoglobinopathies. Jaypee Brothers Medical Publishers, New Delhi 2006: 3-7.
3. Thalassemia. Care and Control in the New Millennium. VP Choudhry and JS Arora (Eds) Novortes publications 2000.
4. Sood SK, Madan N, Colah R, Sharma S, Apte SV. Collaborative study on thalassemia. An ICMR Task Force Study, New Delhi. Indian Council of Medical Research, New Delhi 1993.
5. Verma IC, Choudhry VP, Jain PK. Prevention of Thalassemia: A necessity in India. Ind J Pediatr 1992;59:649-54.
6. Choudhry VP, Kotwal J, Saxena R. Thalassemia Screening and control program. Pediatr Today 1998;1:283-89.
7. Cao A, Rosatelli MC, Monni G, Galanello R. Screening of thalassemia: A model of success. Obstet Gynaecol clin north Am 2002;29:305-28.
8. Saxena A, Phadke SR. Feasibility of thalassemia control by extended family screening in India context. J Health Popul Nutr 2002;20:31.
9. Kotwal J, Saxena R, Choudhry VP and Bhargava M. Comparative evaluation of efficacy of NESTROF and red cell indices in screening for beta thalassemia trait. J Int Med Sci Acad 2001;14:92-94.

10. Sen AK, Kaur M. A Comparison of screening tests for beta thalassemia trait NESTROFT v/s MOFTI and confirmation of results by ion-exchange open colum chromatography. Indian Journal of Hematology and Blood Transfusion 1998 Mar; 16(1): 31-33.
11. Saraya AK, Kumar R, Choudhry VP, Tyagi RS and Sehgal AK. Diagnostic efficacy of haemoglobin A-2 in heterozygous beta thalassemia. Ind J Med Res 1984;80: 203-08.
12. Colah RB, Surve R, Sawant P, et al. HPLC Studies in hemoglobinopathies. Indian J Pediatr 2007;74(7);652-62.
13. Colah RB, Mohanti D. Beta thalassemia: Expression, molecular mechanism and mutations in Indians. Indian J Pediatr 1998;65:815-23.
14. Maheshwari M. Carrier screening and prenatal diagnosis of beta thalassemia. Indian Pediatrics 1999;36:1119-25.
15. Handoo A, Sood SK. Laboratory diagnosis of hemoglobinopathies and thalassemia syndromes. Sachdeva A, Lokeshwar MR, Shah N, Agarwal BR, Khanna VK, Yadav SP, Jain V (Eds) in Hemoglobinopathies. Jaypee Brothers Medical Publishers, New Delhi 2006:110-13.
16. Gupta N, Kabra M. Genetic counselling for thalassemia. Hemoglobinopathies. Sachdeva A, Lokeshwar MR, Shah N, Agarwal BR, Khanna VK, Yadav SP, Jain V (Eds) in Hemoglobinopathies. Jaypee Brothers Medical Publishers, New Delhi 2006:105-09.
17. Verma IC, Saxena R. Penatal diagnosis of beta thalassemia and related disorders. Hemoglobinopathies. Sachdeva A, Lokeshwar MR, Shah N, Agarwal BR, Khanna VK, Yadav SP, Jain V (Eds) in Hemoglobinopathies. Jaypee Brothers Medical Publishers, New Delhi 2006:85-93.
18. Angastiniotis MA. Cyprus Thalassemia program. Lancet 1990;336:1119-20.

SUGGESTED READING

1. Angastiniotis MA. Cyprus Thalassemia program. Lancet 1990;336:1119-20.
2. Choudhry VP. Thalassemia in Obstetrics and Gynaecology practice. Obs and Gynae Today 1997;2:27-29.
3. Gehlbach DL, Morgesten LL. Antenatal screening for thalassemia minor. Obstet Gynecol 1988 ;71:801-03.
4. Jain V, Lokeshwer MR, Sachdeva A. Prevention of thalassemia.Hemoglobinopathies. Jaypee Brothers Medical Publishers, New Delhi 2006.
5. Kashyap R, Choudhry VP. Management of Hemophilia in developing countries in Advances in Pediatrics-1. Editor Choudhry VP and Arya LS (Eds) 105-15.
6. Katewa S, Choudhry VP. Historical perspective and Introduciton to thalassemia in hemoglobinopathies. Sachdeva A, Lokeshwar MR, Shah N, Agarwal BR, Khanna VK, Yadav SP, Jain V (Eds) in Hemoglobinopathies. Jaypee Brothers Medical Publishers, New Delhi 2006.
7. Maheshwari M. Carrier screening and prenatal diagnosis of beta thalassemia. Indian Pediatrics 1999;36:1119-25.

Chapter 15

Pathophysiology of Bleeding in Dengue Virus Infection: A Holistic View

Kanjaksha Ghosh

INTRODUCTION

Approximately 50-100 million people are affected by dengue virus infection across the globe, living in tropical and subtropical countries.[1] The clinical manifestations in dengue virus infection can vary between asymptomatic viral infection to life threatening thrombocytopenia with hemorrhage and shock due to extensive capillary leakage, a phenomenon called dengue hemorrhagic fever/dengue shock syndrome (DHF/DSS).[2] Other clinical symptoms include severe backache, headache, skin rash, retro-orbital pain, hepatosplenomegaly, conjunctival infection and hepatitis in varying combinations along with mild to high grade fever. DHF and DSS are not synonymous. All DHF patients may not develop DSS and *vice versa*. Moreover even some dengue fever patients can have both, i.e. certain criteria of DSS fulfilled along with life threatening hemorrhage. Hence, World Health Organization (WHO) criteria of classifying four categories of DHF/DSS patients have been widely discussed and criticized.[3-7] It has also been found that ultrasonography (USG) evidence of thickened gallbladder wall could be a useful criteria for increased vascular permeability in children and it could be precursor to DHF/DSS.[8]

There are four serotypes of dengue virus (DEN 1-4), which probably evolved from a common ancestor in subhuman primate population around 500 years ago; all viruses probably have emerged separately and entered into human transmission cycle.[9] The reason for reiterating that there are four strains of dengue virus and they circulate in different time and space in different populations is linked to the peculiar property of dengue infection, i.e. secondary dengue infection causing more severe disease (ie more tendency to DHF/DSS) than the primary dengue infection.

Various studies conducted since 1960's have shown that dengue virus affects liver, vascular endothelial cells and platelets and in severe infection, the picture is typically of disseminated intravascular coagulation (DIC) in a small subset of patients.[10-12] Thus hemorrhage in dengue virus infection is a result of interaction of viral characteristics, humoral and cellular immune response of the host leading to cytokine storm, along with direct effect of the virus on bone marrow, platelets and vascular endothelial cells. Additional effects of the virus on the liver, T lymphocyte response to infected liver cells and cytokine storm—all cause liver dysfunction and abnormal coagulation. A holistic view of pathogenesis of thrombocytopenia and bleeding in dengue infection must take into account all these features, integrate this information into a testable hypothesis and generate some data to finally translate it to the treatment protocols so as to reduce the mortality from this common and cycling infection.

BLEEDING IN DENGUE FEVER AND DENGUE HEMORRHAGIC FEVER

Bleeding from various sites has been recorded in both dengue fever (DF) and dengue hemorrhagic fever (DHF). Bleeding occurs in the form of petechiae, purpura, epistaxis along with other extensive mucocutaneous bleeding like hematemesis and malena, depending on the severity of the disease. Abnormalities in platelet function, thrombocytopenia, hyperfibrinolysis, reduced synthesis of coagulation factors as a result of associated hepatitis, and DIC are the major causes of bleeding in dengue virus infection.[13-16] In case of DHF, substantial number of patients present with very low fibrinogen and reduced factor VIIIc levels (20-30%), which is reflected by prolongation of activated partial thromboplastin time (APTT) and prothrombin time (PT). Degree of prolongation of APTT or PT also correspond to the levels of serum transaminases. Severe gastrointestinal bleeding is generally attributed to concomitant hepatitis which is seen very often in these patients.

The major question is whether the abnormal coagulation, i.e thrombocytopenia, platelet dysfunction, reduced level of coagulation factors, increased fibrinolysis, capillary fragility due to endothelial damage is directly caused by some component of the virus or the level of viremia or whether some of these complications are related to immune disturbances or associated cytokine storm caused by the viral infection.

Thrombocytopenia and Platelet Dysfunction

Thrombocytopenia and platelet dysfunction have been shown to be common in dengue infection. Only the extent of this thrombocytopenia is much deeper in DHF cases. In general, there are two basic mechanisms of thrombocytopenia (i) reduced production of platelets, (ii) increased peripheral destruction of released platelets. The increased peripheral destruction could be due to (a) immunological destruction or (b) non-immunological destruction.

In vitro experiments conducted at National Institute of Immunohematology (NIIH) and National Institute of Virology (NIV) clearly showed that various strains of dengue virus, particularly DEN 2 strain, grown in C6/36 cell line (obtained from National Institute of Virology, Pune) when made to infect CFU-Mk colonies at various doses, i.e. multiplicity of Infection (MOI) of 0.1-10 led to a dose dependent inhibition of megakaryocytic progenitor cells leaving the other components of CFU-GEMM colonies intact. The CFU Meg assay showed that infection with dengue virus directly wiped away the megakaryocytic precursors from day 5 to day 12 of culture. Viruses could be demonstrated in the progenitor cells by immunofluorescent studies and using anti-caspase 3 and anti-annexin antibodies, and these megakaryocytic precursors also showed apoptosis.[17] These observations also confirm earlier reports from Thailand on bone marrow morphology, wherein degenerating or dying megakaryocytes were observed in patients with DHF.[18] Thus there is a direct *in vitro* proof that dengue viruses have the propensity to kill both CFU-Meg and mature megakaryocytes (Fig. 15.1). Several other studies have also shown that dengue virus can inhibit hemopoietic stem cells and they can be propagated in hemopoietic stem lines.[19,20]

Peripheral Activation of Platelets

Studies have shown that dengue virus can bind to human platelets and this can be enhanced by pre-existing antidengue antibodies.[21] Studies were conducted at NIIH, to see whether platelets obtained from individuals negative for antidengue antibodies can show some *in vitro* changes on addition of dengue virus at concentrations detected in the blood during the height of dengue viremia. Another similar flavivirus, i.e. Japanese encephalitis was used as the control virus as they are not known to cause any platelet dysfunction or bleeding manifestations. The study showed that dengue viruses can:

i. Directly activate platelets as shown by platelet aggregometry, CD-62P (P-Selectin) expression by flow cytometry and by striking morphological changes on scanning and transmission electron microscopy.[22]

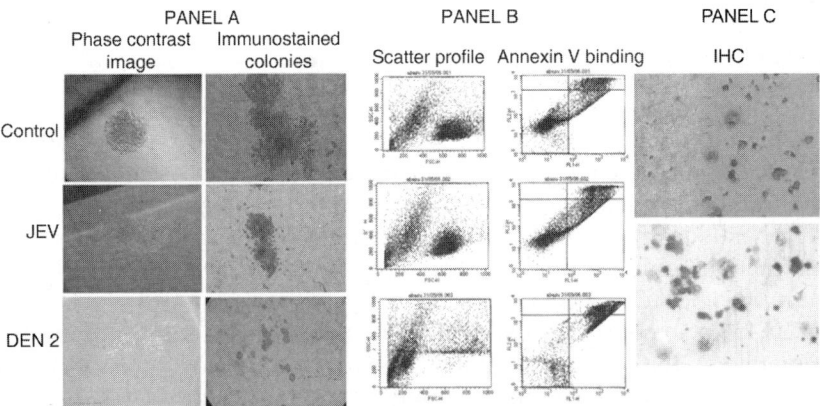

Fig. 15.1: Panel A: Total suppression of CFU-Meg by dengue virus infection *in vitro*. Panel B showing increased apoptosis and increased annexin binding in megakaryocyte precursors in culture on exposure to DEN-2 virus. Panel C showing immunohistochemistry of dengue virus positive Meg precursors. Upper figure is without infection *(For color version, see Plate 1)*

ii. These activated platelets subsequently were capable of further activation by other agonists like ADP and ristocetin.
iii. Japanese encephalitis virus had no action on platelets. These findings showed that at the height of viremia, the dengue virus itself can activate and remove platelets by activating them. Pre-existing dengue antibodies augment the binding of the virus to the platelets and destroy the platelets by activating complement on their surface.[23-24] Platelets have also been shown to have increased adhesiveness to dengue 2 virus infected human endothelial cells and these platelets have activated phenotype[25] and are likely to be destroyed.

Thus activation of platelets and its adherence to infected and damaged endothelium provides an important mechanism of removal of platelets from circulation without necessarily activating coagulation cascade. This part of pathophysiology is similar to falciparum malaria associated thrombocytopenia.

Immune Destruction of Platelets

In addition to complement activation on the surface of the platelets, immune complex formation with dengue viral antigen and their fixation on platelet surface leads to an innocent bystander kind of immune destruction.[23,24] Several reports of the presence of antiplatelet antibodies (APA) in dengue infected patients are available.[26,27] In our study of 35 patients with dengue hemorrhagic fever for APA, very high levels of antibodies to platelets ($4 \times 10^4 - 2 \times 10^6$ antibodies/platelet) were detected. It was also shown that nonstructural protein (NS1) from dengue virus can produce antibodies which can cross react with various integrin and adhesion molecules[28] common to human coagulation factors and platelets. The western blot analysis using mouse platelet lysate showed that dengue infected sera reacted strongly with a 29 kd protein from mouse platelet. This is likely to be one of the integrins from mouse platelet showing that autoimmune antiplatelet autoantibody generation is also an important component of dengue infection.

Thus a combination of suppression of production, immune and non-immune peripheral destruction contributes to thrombocytopenia in dengue virus infection. Another mechanism of nonimmune thrombocytopenia becomes important when in severe DHF, DIC ensues as a part of activation of blood coagulation and cytokine storm.

ACTIVATION OF ENDOTHELIAL CELLS

Several studies[29-31] including ours (unpublished) have shown that human endothelial cells or cell lines can be regularly infected with dengue virus. This infection leads to activation of endothelial cells leading to expression of tissue factor and up-regulation of certain coagulant, anticoagulant, fibrinolytic proteins and their inhibitors. Activated endothelial cells support platelet adhesion and ultra high molecular weight von Willebrand

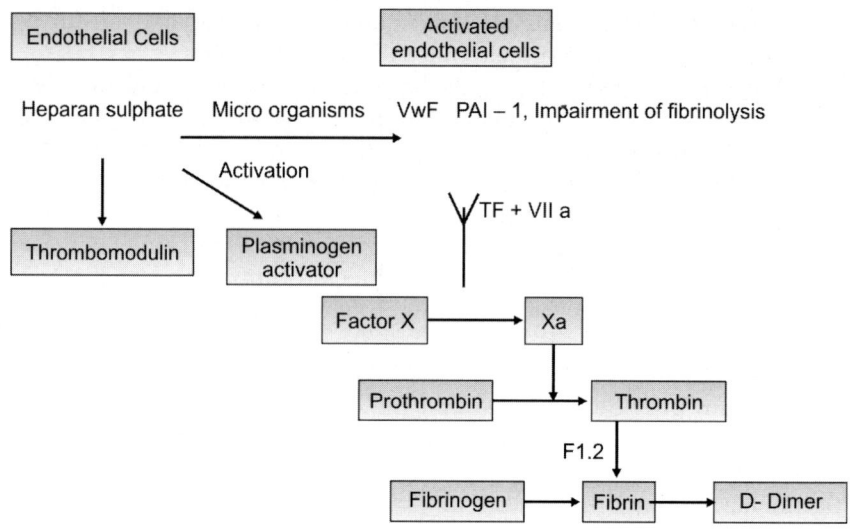

TF: Tissue factor, VwF: von Willebrand factor, F1.2: Fragment of prothrombin, PAI: Plasminogen activator inhibitor 1.
VIIa: Activated factor VII, Xa: Activated factor X, D-Dimer: Dimer of fragment D of fibrin.

Fig. 15.2: Endothelial cell activation in dengue virus infection

factor (VWF) supports spontaneous platelet aggregation. In addition, endothelial cells are the substrates where protease activated receptor –1 (PAR –1) is activated by tissue factor induced serine proteases and PAR-1 subsequently activates ERK 1/2/P, P38/MAPK-2 pathways leading to increased phosphorylation of NFKB and increased synthesis of various proteins augmenting pro-inflammatory cytokines and coagulant proteins.[32] Endothelial cell activation by dengue virus thus acts as a link between coagulation and inflammatory pathways. Infection and involvement of endothelial cells would drive the coagulation process (Fig. 15.2).[33]

Thus activation of coagulation on endothelial cells when excessive can lead to classical DIC with D-Dimer positivity. Liver involvement in dengue virus infection have been shown to specifically reduce factor VIII and factor XI levels[34] and may be a cause of prolonged APTT. Coagulation system and endothelial cell activation are further aggravated by a cytokine storm in dengue infection which mainly arises from monocytes, T lymphocytes, liver cells and endothelial cells while the monocytes bear the brunt of dengue virus infection.

CYTOKINE STORM IN DENGUE FEVER

A series of pro-inflammatory cytokines rise and fall at different stages of dengue fever with its complications.[1,13,35-37] Interferon γ, TNFα, IL 2, IL 4, IL 6, IL 8, IL 10, IL 1b are elevated at different stages of the disease and some, i.e. IL 8 is correlated strongly with capillary leak[38] leading to DSS

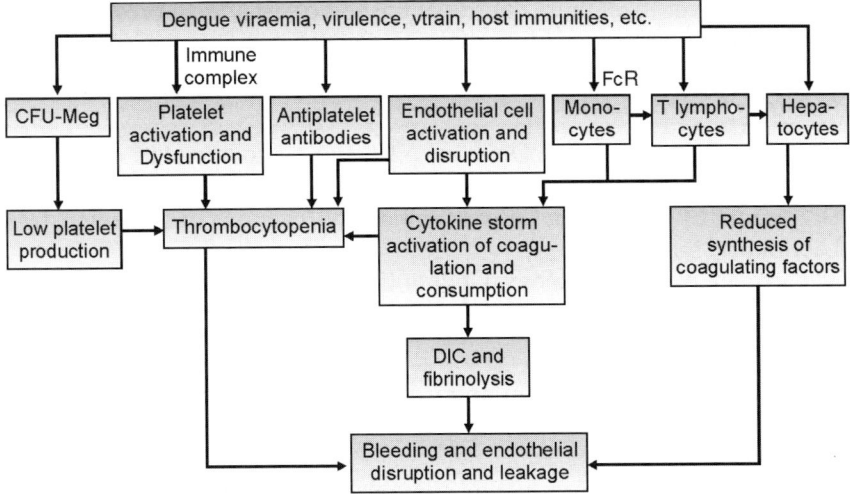

Fig. 15.3: Holistic view of development of coagulation abnormalities in dengue virus infections

so also CCL2 chemokine, i.e. chemokine C-C motif ligand 2 (Synonyms: GDCF-2, HC11, HSMCR30, MCAF, MCP-1, MCP1, MGC9434, SCYA2, SMC-CF).[39] IL 6 and IL 1 receptor alpha has been correlated with marker of coagulation, i.e. F1.2 (Prothrombin fragment 1.2) or thrombin-antithrombin complex (TATc), yet other like TNFα has been correlated with markers of fibrinolysis like D-Dimer.[40] Higher cytokine storm during secondary infection with different strains of dengue virus is explained by higher load of viral infection in monocytes and macrophages related to higher level of viruses in the cell due to antibody dependent enhancement.[1] Finally a holistic view of development of coagulation abnormality is presented in Figure 15.3.

CONCLUSION

Though pathogenesis of abnormal coagulation in DF and DHF is broadly understood as multifactorial, yet several questions still remain unanswered, i.e. (i) Why only certain viruses show antibody dependent enhancement phenomenon but others do not and if this is true for dengue virus then vaccine development will have its own limitations? (ii) Why only few patients in a community develop clinical dengue fever and few of them develop DHF/DSS and others do not? (iii) Whether antibody dependent enhancement affects megakaryocytes too? (iv) Would it be possible to prevent DHF if we can prevent activation of endothelial cells and platelets? As capillary leak syndrome is short lasting, will it be possible to block the capillary leak by blocking specific cytokines without interfering with immunity to this infection?

Future research work on this common and occasionally devastating infection may try to answer some of these questions and we may have a definite answer to all these queries at the end of decade, to prevent DHF/DSS at least in a large majority of the patients!

ACKNOWLEDGMENTS

Dr Atanu Basu, Assistant Director, NIV, Pune and the staff of electron Microscopy Department of NIV.
Dr Shrimati Shetty, Senior Research officer, NIIH and Staff of Haemostasis Laboratory, NIIH.
Department of Biotechnology, Govt of India for funding this study.

TAKE HOME MESSAGE

Dengue virus related coagulation abnormality are multifactorial and includes:
Direct effect of the virus as:
  i. Virulence of the virus – DEN 2 is considered to be most hemorrhagic though American strain of DEN 2 is relatively nonhemorrhagic.
  ii. Activation of platelet and removal of activated platelets.
  iii. Endothelial cell activation triggering platelet consumption and coagulation.
  iv. Directly infecting and causing apoptosis of megakaryocytic precursors leading to reduced production of platelets.
  v. Infecting liver and reducing synthesis of coagulation proteins.

Indirect effect on coagulation by:
  i. Antibody dependent – enhancement of infection.
  ii. Immune complex and complement activation leading to thrombocytopenia.
  iii. T lymphocyte dependent liver cell injury.
  iv. Cytokine storm generated at liver, monocytes, T cells, liver and endothelial cells.
  v. Disseminated intravascular coagulation.

REFERENCES

1. Halstead SB. Pathogenesis of dengue: Challenges to molecular biology 1988; 239:476-81.
2. Halstead SB. Dengue Lancet 2007;370:1644-52.
3. Deen JL, Harris E, Wills B, et al. The WHO dengue classification and case definitions: Time for a reassessment. Lancet 2006;368:170-73.
4. Rigau-Perez JG. Severe dengue: The need for new case definitions. Lancet infect. Dis 2006;6:297-302.
5. Balasubramanian S, Janakiraman L, Kumar SS, Murlinath S, Shivbalan S. A reappraisal of the criteria to diagnose plasma leakage in dengue haemorrhagic fever. Indian Pediatr 2006;43:334-39.
6. Balmaseda A, Hammond SN, Perez MA, et al. Short report: Assessment of world health organization scheme for classification of dengue severity in Nicaragua. Am J Trop Med Hyg 2005;73:1059-62.
7. Bandyopadhyay S, Lum LCS, Kroeger A. Classifying dengue! A review of the difficulties in using WHO case classification for dengue haemorrhagic fever. Trop Med Int Health 2006;11:1238-55.

8. Colbert JA, Gordon A, Roxelin R, et al. Ultrasound measurement of gallbladder wall thickening as a diagnostic test and prognostic indicator for severe dengue in pediatric patients. Pediatr Infect Dis J 2007;26:850-52.
9. Wang E, Ni H; XuR, et al. Evolutionary relationships of epidemic/endemic and Sylvatic dengue viruses. J Virol 2000;74:3227-34.
10. Nimmannitya S, Halshead SB, Cohen SN, Margotta MR. Dengue and Chikunguniya virus infection in Thailand 1962-64. Observations in hospitalized patients with haemorrhagic fever. Am J Trop Med Hyg 1969;18:954-57.
11. Pongphanich B, Kumponopant S. Studies on dengue haemorrhagic fever. Hemodynamic studies of clinical shock associated with dengue haemorrhagic fever. J Pediatr 1973;83:1073-77.
12. Bhamaraparavati N, Tuchinda P; Boonyaapaknavik V. Pathology of Thailand Haemorrhagic fever: A study of 100 autopsy cases. Ann Trop Med Parasitol 1967;61:500-10.
13. Lei H-Y, Yeh T-M; Liu H-S; Lin Y-S, et al. Immunopathogenesis of dengue virus infection. J Biomed Sc 2001;8:377-88.
14. Willis BA, Oragui EE, Stephen AC, et al. Coagulation abnormalities in dengue haemorrhagic fever: Serial in investigations in 167 Vietnamese children in the dengue shock syndrome. Clin Infec Dis 2002;35:277-85.
15. Sri Chaikul T, Nimmannitya S. Hematology in dengue and dengue haemorrhagic fever Bailleres Best Practice and Research in clinical hematology 2000;13(2): 261-76.
16. Carlos C, Oishi K, Cinco MTDD, et al. Comparison of clinical features and hematologic abnormalities between Dengue fever and Dengue haemorrhagic fever among children in Philippines. Am J Trop Med Hyg 2005;73:435-40.
17. Basu A, Jain P, Gangodkar SV, Shetty S, Ghosh K. Dengue 2 virus inhibits *in vitro* megakaryocyte colony formation and induces apoptosis in thrombopoietin – inducible megakaryocytic differentiation from Cord blood CD 34 + Cells. FEMS Immunol Med Microbiol 2008;53:46-51.
18. Na-Nakorn S, Suindumrong A, Pootrakul S, Bhamarapravati N. Bone marrow studies in Thai haemorrhagic fever. Bull WHO 1966;35:54-60.
19. Murgue B, Cassar O, Guigon M, Chungue E. Dengue virus inhibits human hematopoietic progenitor growth *in vitro*. J infect Dist 1997;175:1497-1501.
20. Nakao S, Lai CJ, Young NS. Dengue virus, a flavivirus propagates in human bone marrow progenitors and hematopoietic cell lives. Blood 1989;74:1235-40.
21. Wang S, HeR, Patarapotikul J, Innis BL, Anderson R. Antibody enhanced binding of dengue – 2 virus to human platelets. Virology 1995;213:254-57.
22. Ghosh K, Gangodkar S, Jain P, Shetty S, Ramjee S, Poddar P, Basu A. Imaging the interaction between dengue 2 virus and human blood platelets using atomic force and electron microscopy. J Electron Micros 2008;57:113-18.
23. Malasit P. Complement and dengue haemorrhagic fever/shock syndrome. SE Asian J Trop Med Pub Health 1987;18:316-20.
24. Malasit P, Mongkolsapaya J, Kalayanarooj S, Nimmannitya S. Surface associated complement fragments (C3a) on platelets from patients with dengue infection. SE Asian J Trop Med Pub Health 1990;21:705.
25. Krishnamurti C, Peat RA, Cuting MA, Rothwell SW. Platelet adhesion to Dengue – 2 virus infected endothelial cells. Am J Trop Hyg 2002;66:435-41.
26. Huang KJ, Li SYJ, Chen SC, et al. Manifestation of thrombocytopenia in dengue 2 virus infected mice. J Gen Vriol 2000;81:2177-82.
27. Lin CF, Lei HY, Liu CC, et al. Generation of IgM antiplatelet autoantibody in dengue patients. J Med Virol 2001;63:143-49.

28. Falconar AKI. The dengue virus nonstructural 1 protein (NS1) generates antibodies to common epitopes on human blood clotting, integrin/adhesive proteins and binds to human endothelial cell: Potential implications in haemorrhagic fever pathogenesis. Arch Virol 1997;142:897-916.
29. Avirutnan P, Malasit P, Seliger B, Bhakdi S, Husmann M. Dengue virus infection of human endothelial cells leads to chemokine production, complement activation, and apoptosis. J Immunol 1998;161:6338-46.
30. Andrews BS, Theofilopoulos AN, Peters CJ, et al. Replication of dengue and Junin viruses in cultured rabbit and human endothelial cells. Infect Immun 1978; 20:776-81.
31. Jiang Z, Tang X, Xiao R, Jiang L, Chen X. Dengue virus regulates the expression of hemostasis – related molecules in human vein endothelial cells. J Infec 2007; 55:e23-e28.
32. Huerta - Zepada A, Carbello-Gutierrez C, Cime-Cartillo J, et al. Crosstalk between coagulation and inflammation during dengue virus infection Thromb Haemost 2008:99:936-43.
33. Mairuhu ATA, Mac Gillavry MR, Setiati TE, et al. Is clinical outcome of dengue virus infections influenced by coagulation and fibrinolysis? A critical review of the evidence. The lancet infect. Dis 2003;3:33-41.
34. Van Gorp ECM, Minnema Moniqne C, Sharti C, et al. Activation of coagulation factor XI without detectable contact activation in dengue haemmrohgic fever. Br J Haemat 2001;113:94-99.
35. Chakravarti A, Kumar R. Circulating levels of tumor necrosis factor alpha and inter feron – gamma in patients with dengue and dengue haemerrhagic fever during an outbreak. Ind J Med Res 2006; 123:25-30.
36. Hung TN, Lei HY, Lan NT, et al. Dengue hemorrhagic fever in infants: A study of clinical and cytokine profiles. J Infect Dis 2004; 189:221-32.
37. Sosothikul D, Seksarn P, Pongsewalak S, et al. Activation of endothelial cells, coagulation and fibrinolysis in children with Dengue Virus infection. Thromb Haemost 2007; 97:627-34.
38. Raghupathy R, Chaturvedi UC, Al-Sayer H, et al. Elevated levels of IL8 in dengue haemorrhagic fever. J Med Virol 1998; 56:280-85.
39. Lee YR, Liu MT, Lei HY, et al. MCP – 1 a highly expressed chemokine in dengue haemorrhagic fever/dengue/shock syndrome patients, may cause permeability change, possibly through reduced tight Junctions of vascular endothelial cells. J Gen Virol 2006; 87:3623-30.
40. Suharti C, Vangorp ECM, Setiatti TE, et al. The role of cytokine in activation of coagulation and fibrinolysis in dengue shock syndrome. Thromb Haemost 2002; 87:42-46.

Chapter 16

Approach to Polycythemia

Manoranjan Mahapatra, Shyam Rathi

SUMMARY

Patients with high hemoglobin need investigations to differentiate true from apparent erythrocytosis. Those with true erythrocytosis, deserve further work-up to differentiate polycythemia vera from secondary erythrocytosis. The diagnostic criteria for polycythemia vera are complex. Recently an activating point mutation in the JAK2 gene (JAK2-V617F) has been detected in majority of PV patients, but is not specific, and needs more evaluation. Patients may present with plethora, thrombosis in arterial or venous circulations, erythromelalgia, pruritus, hemorrhage, splenomegaly, gout, leukocytosis or thrombocytosis. Patients with polycythemia vera have significant morbidity and mortality due to thrombosis and hemorrhage. All patients deserve cytoreduction to hematocrit of 0.45 or less, preferably by venesection. Low dose aspirin (75 mg/day) is a universal recommendation, unless contraindicated. Those with high-risk disease or a progressive disease deserve cytoreduction using hydroxyurea or interferon alpha. Anagrelide may be used for thrombocytosis. With appropriate therapy, survival has improved from an average of 2 years to more than 10 years.

KEYWORDS
Polycythemia vera, JAK2, Thrombosis, Hydroxyurea, Venesection.

INTRODUCTION

Patients with raised hematocrit need evaluation for presence of polycythemia. The term polycythemia has been used in relation to a group of disorders with an increase in circulating red cells. It is recommended that the term erythrocytosis be used where only the red cells are involved, while polycythemia is preferred for the clonal disorder involving three cell lineages, polycythemia vera (PV). Secondary erythrocytosis is far more common and is usually consequent to increased erythropoietin production. It is important to diagnose PV, as it has a high morbidity and mortality.

Evaluation of Erythrocytosis

Hematocrit values more than 0.51 in males and 0.48 in females are considered elevated and require further evaluation.[1] Erythrocytosis may

Table 16.1: Classification of erythrocytosis

1. Apparent erythrocytosis (normal red cell mass)
   (a) Relative erythrocytosis: Decreased plasma volume (dehydration, stress erythrocytosis or Gaisbock's syndrome)
   (b) Extreme "high normal" values
2. True erythrocytosis (increased red cell mass)
   (a) Primary: Polycythemia vera
   (b) Secondary erythrocytosis
   - Congenital: High O_2 affinity hemoglobin, von Hippel Lindau (VHL) gene mutation, activating mutation of erythropoietin (EPO) receptor
   - Increased EPO related to central or peripheral hypoxia: High altitude, chronic lung disease, right to left cardiac shunts, sleep apnea syndrome, renal artery stenosis (local hypoxia)
   - Increased EPO production by malignant or benign conditions: Hepatocellular carcinoma, renal cell carcinoma, cerebellar hemangioblastoma, uterine leiomyoma, phaeochromocytoma, renal cysts
   - Drug associated: Exogenous EPO, androgens
   (c) Unknown mechanism: Postrenal transplant erythrocytosis

be seen in a number of conditions (Table 16.1). Once true erythrocytosis is confirmed, tests should be carried out to differentiate between the more common secondary erythrocytosis, from primary polycythemia or PV. It is then necessary to establish the etiology. It can be either due to congenital and acquired causes.

Congenital Erythrocytosis (Flow Chart 16.1)

These cases usually present at young age. They may have family history of erythrocytosis. The defect can be either in erythropoietin (EPO) signaling pathway or high oxygen affinity hemoglobin.[2] EPO levels are below normal in erythropoietin receptor defect and elevated or normal with Chuvash polycythemia and high oxygen affinity hemoglobin.

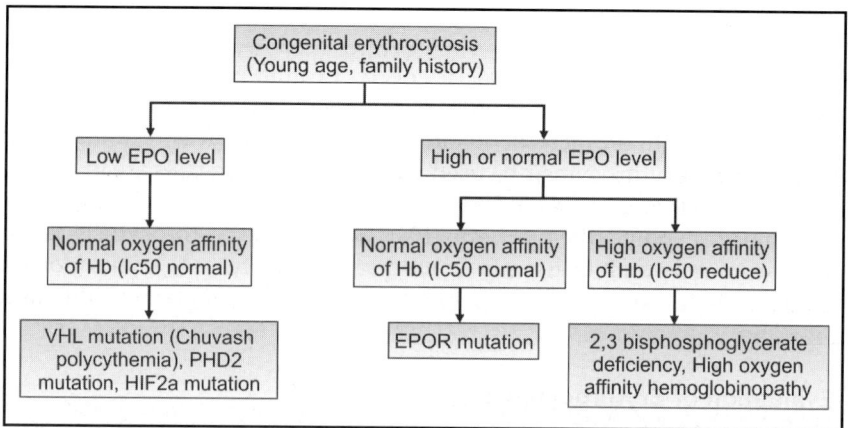

Flow chart 16.1: Approach to patients with congenital erythrocytosis

EPO Signaling Pathway Defect

Chuvash polycythemia (VHL mutation):[3] First described in Chuvash region in Russia. Inheritance is autosomal recessive. VHL gene has an important role in hypoxia sensing where cells sense a decrease in oxygen and allow organism to adopt. Mutation in VHL gene leads to abnormal VHL protein that no longer combines with HIF-proteins, thus impairing proteasomal degradation. This ultimately results in increased erythrocytosis. HIF2a, PHD2 and EPO receptor are other rare mutations associated with congenital polycythemia.[4]

High Oxygen Affinity Hemoglobin[5]

The capacity of hemoglobin to deliver oxygen to the tissues is expressed by the shape of the hemoglobin-oxygen dissociation curve and shift of the curve to the left indicates abnormal hemoglobin which has increased affinity for oxygen (High oxygen affinity hemoglobin). As they do not release oxygen to the tissues the resulting hypoxia drives EPO production and thus erythrocytosis. There are two conditions:
- High oxygen affinity hemoglobinopathy
- Bisphosphoglycerate mutase deficiency

The 2,3-Bisphosphoglycerate (BPG) binds the hemoblobin tetramer and converts the hemoglobin molecule to a low oxygen affinity state. Deficiency of 2,3 BPG would shift the curve to left and increase the oxygen affinity of hemoglobin.

Polycythemia Vera

Polycythemia vera (PV) is a clonal disorder of unknown etiology involving a multipotent hematopoietic progenitor cell giving rise to increase in erythrocytes, granulocytes and platelets. The World Health Organization groups PV under the title chronic myeloproliferative neoplasm. PV is most common of these MPNs and only one with absolute erythrocytosis. Classically two phases of PV can be recognized: (a) an initial proliferative polycythemic phase and (b) a spent or post-polycythemic phase, in which cytopenias are associated with ineffective hematopoeisis, bone marrow fibrosis, extramedullary hematopoesis and hypersplenism. The WHO criteria[6] are given in Table 16.2. The discovery of JAK2 mutation is major achievement in last three decades in diagnosis of myeloproliferative neoplasm (MPN). Presence of JAK2 mutation indicates the clonal erythrocytosis and helps to differentiate from nonclonal causes of erythrocytosis. More than 95% of polycythemia vera patients are JAK2 V617F positive. Small percentage of patients who are JAK2 V617F negative polycythemia vera demonstrated to have JAK2 exon 12 mutation.[7] So a JAK2 negative PV is very unlikely.

Table 16.2: WHO criteria (2009) for polycythemia vera[6]

Major Criteria
1. Hb > 18.5 g/100 ml in men or 16.5 g/100 ml in women or Hb > 17 g/100 ml in men or 15 g/100 ml in women if associated with 2 g/100 ml increase from baseline that is not attributed to correction of iron deficiency anemia. Hb or Hct > 99 percentile of reference range for age/sex/altitude or red cell mass > 25% above mean normal predicted value.
2. Presence of JAK2 V617F or JAK2 exon 12 mutation.

Minor Criteria
1. BM biopsy hypercellular for age with panmyelosis with prominent erythroid, granulocytic and megakaryocytic proliferation.
2. Serum EPO level below the reference range for normal.
3. Endogenous erythroid colony formation *in vitro*.

For diagnosis of polycythemia vera requires the presence of both major criteria and one minor criteria or the presence of first major criteria and two minor criteria.

Lab Evaluation of Patients with Erythrocytosis or Suspected PV

The aim of evaluating a patient with erythrocytosis is to identify true erythrocytosis and then decide if it is secondary, or primary (PV). Confirmation of erythrocytosis is mandatory to diagnose PV.

Primary Investigations (to be done in all patients)

a. *Complete blood count/film:* For other features of PV. Thrombocytosis occurs in about 50% and neutrophilia, often with mild basophilia, occurs in approximately 60% of PV.
b. *Arterial oxygen saturation (SaO_2):* A pulse oximeter can be used. If ≤ 92%, erythrocytosis secondary to hypoxia is likely.
c. *Serum erythropoeitin level:* A low erythropoeitin level is a minor criterion for PV. An elevated level excludes PV but a normal level excludes neither PV nor hypoxia.
d. *Serum ferritin:* Low ferritin levels are more often seen in PV than in secondary erythrocytosis.
e. *Renal and liver function tests:* Secondary erythrocytosis may be associated with renal and liver disease.
f. *Abdominal ultrasound:* To exclude secondary causes in the liver, kidneys and uterus. A nonpalpable splenomegaly on ultrasound (in absence of liver disease) is a minor criteria for PV.
g. *Chest X-ray:* To exclude lung pathology, which may suggest secondary erythrocytosis.

Secondary Investigations are Selectively Indicated, after Primary Work-up and Clinical Evaluation

a. *Bone marrow studies:* Bone marrow aspirate and biopsy studies are not essential to diagnose PV. Bone marrow may be sent for cytogenetic studies to establish clonality. Characteristically, the marrow is hypercellular with trilineage involvement and the iron stores are absent. The investigation is also useful as a baseline for future studies for evolution into myelofibrosis.

b. *Cytogenetics:* Cytogenetic abnormalities are detected in about 10-20% of cases of PV at diagnosis, limiting its diagnostic utility. The common abnormalities are trisomy of chromosome 8 and 9, del (20q), del (13q) and del (1p).
c. *Culture studies for BFU-E:* For normal *in vitro* culture of erythroid progenitors, addition of erythropoietin is needed for growth of erythroid burst-forming units (BFU-E). In PV, endogenous growth occurs in absence of erythropoietin.
d. *JAK2 mutation:* Till recently, there was no biological marker for polycythemia vera. A number of studies in the year 2005 have shown that a single somatic activating point mutation in the Janus kinase 2 (JAK2) gene is found in the great majority of patients with PV (65-97%). The mutation (V617F) may also be present in 23 to 57% with essential thrombocytosis or primary myelofibrosis and rarely in other myeloproliferative disorder. Thus presence of the JAK2 mutation can distinguish PV from secondary erythrocytosis but not from related myeloproliferative disorders. Further work is in progress for possible development of molecular targeted therapy.
e. *Other selected tests:* Oxygen dissociation curve (p50) studies may be done to exclude high affinity hemoglobins in unexplained erythrocytosis; Sleep studies are indicated in suspected sleep apnea; Lung function tests are required for pulmonary disease; Erythropoeitin receptor gene analysis may be done to exclude a rare erythropoietin receptor mutation.

Clinical Features of Polycythemia Vera

The peak age of onset is between 50 to 60 years. The clinical features are given in Table 16.3.

Management

The aim of therapy is to decrease the risk of thrombosis and hemorrhage and manage complications. In summary, all patients should undergo

Table 16.3: Clinical features and complications of polycythemia vera

Feature	Characteristic
Thrombosis (15-60%)	Arterial (coronary, cerebral) or venous (hepatic, portal venous)
Hemorrhage	Mucosal, gastrointestinal
Pruritis (20-25%)	Characteristically aquagenic
Erythromelalgia	Red burning toes, feet, fingers
Splenomegaly	In 50-75%
Hepatomegaly	In 30%
Peptic ulcer	3 to 5 times more common than general population
Hyperuricemia (40%), gout	About 5% with hyperuricemia develop gout
Myeloid metaplasia	Increasing heptosplenomegaly, leucocytosis, anemia
Acute leukemia	Mainly non-lymphoblastic
Facial plethora, headache, vertigo, tinnitus, visual disturbances	May not be present in early cases

venesection to achieve a target hematocrit of less than 0.45 and take low dose aspirin (unless contraindicated). In selected cases cytoreductive therapy may be added.

The choice of cytoreductive therapy is age related:
a. < 40 years: First line interferon alpha (IFN); second line hydroxyurea or anagrelide.
b. 40-75 years: First line hydroxyurea; second line IFN or anagrelide.
c. > 75 years: First line hydroxyurea; second line ^{32}P or intermittent low dose busulphan.

Conventional risk factors for atherosclerosis such as hypertension, diabetes, and hyperlipidemia should be corrected and smoking discouraged.

Prognosis

Survival of untreated patients historically has been poor with a 2 years survival of less than 50%. Adequately treated PV now have a life expectancy of more than 10 years from diagnosis. Causes of death are thrombotic events, transformation to acute leukemia, myelofibrosis, myelodysplasia or hemorrhage.

General Approach for a Patient with Acquired Erythrocytosis (Flow chart 16.2)

Most important is to establish whether erythrocytosis is clonal (primary) or secondary. A raised hemoglobin or hematocrit is the first criterion for diagnosis of erythrocytosis. The measurement of red cell mass is not required in those who have a raised Hct/Hb and JAK2 mutation. Red cell mass measurement is more useful in JAK2 negative patients to differentiate absolute from apparent erythrocytosis.

JAK2 mutation should be evaluated in all patients with erythrocytosis. It is a relatively simple test and easily available. JAK2 negative patients should be evaluated for JAK2 exon 12 mutations. Serum EPO level is raised in hypoxic conditions and certain EPO producing tumor, while in PV usually EPO level is low. In PV bone marrow biopsy is hypercellular

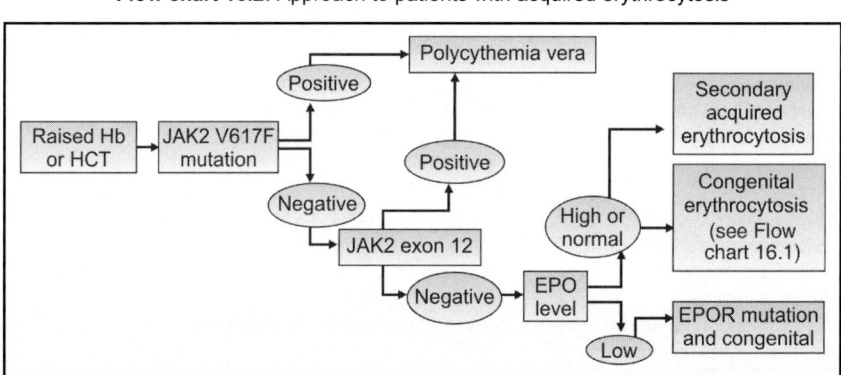

Flow chart 16.2: Approach to patients with acquired erythrocytosis

with erythroid, megakaryocytic and granulocytic proliferation. In WHO classification bone marrow examination is included as minor criteria. In a patient with raised Hb, JAK2 positive and low EPO level one can skip bone marrow examination (As per criteria for diagnosis). Bone marrow examination is more useful in JAK2 negative patient to distinguish from secondary and reactive causes.

TAKE HOME MESSAGES

1. Patients with raised hemoglobin merit detailed evaluation to determine presence of true or apparent erythrocytosis.
2. Polycythemia vera has a high morbidity and mortality due to thrombosis and hemorrhage.
3. All patients should undergo reduction of hematocrit to less than 0.45, preferably by venesection. Aspirin in low doses (75 mg/day) is recommended in all, unless contraindicated.
4. Cytoreductive therapy is indicated in high-risk or progressive disease with hydroxyurea or interferon alpha, while in elderly patients busulphan or radioactive phosphorus have a role. Anagrelide may be used for thrombocytosis.
5. Discovery of the JAK2 mutation is promising as a new diagnostic modality.

REFERENCES

1. McMullin MF, Bareford D, Campbell P, et al. Guidelines for the diagnosis, investigation and management of polycythaemia/erythrocytosis. Br J Haematol 2005;130(2):174-95.
2. Gordeuk V R, et al. Congenital polycythemia. Haematologica 2005;90:109-16.
3. Ang SO et al. Endemic Polycythaemia in Russia: Mutation in VHL gene. Bld cells molec dis 2002;28:57-62.
4. Percy MJ. Genetically heterogeneous origins of idiopathic erythrocytosis. Haematology 2007;12:131-39.
5. Charache S, et al. Polycythemia associated with a hemoglobinopathy. J of clin Inves 1996;45:813-22.
6. World Health Organization. Pathology and genetics of tumors of Haematopoietic and lymphoid Tissues. Lyon, France : IARC press 2009.
7. Cazzola M. Somatic mutations of JAK2 exon 12 as a molecular basis of erythrocytosis. Haematologica 2007;92:1585-89.

Chapter 17

Aplastic Anemia: Issues in Management

Manoranjan Mahapatra, Tuphan Kanti Dolai, Niranjan Rathod

SUMMARY

Aplastic anemia is an uncommon but potentially serious hematological disorder. It is characterized by pancytopenia secondary to a hypocellular bone marrow. Its exact incidence in India is not known, but it is more commonly seen in Asia than west. Investigations should include a bone marrow aspirate and biopsy. In children and young adults, Fanconi's anemia should be excluded by chromosomal breakage studies. In most cases no cause can be found. Supportive therapy is needed in most patients to correct anemia, prevent bleeding and treat any infections. Due to prolonged neutropenia, these patients are prone for fungal infections.

The specific therapy varies with the age of the patient and availability of an HLA identical sibling. Allogeneic hematopoietic stem cell transplantation is curative in majority of young patients, if an HLA identical related donor is available. In those without a donor, or the elderly, the best treatment is with immunosuppressive therapy. A combination of anti-thymocyte globulin (ATG) and cyclosporine offers the best results with about 60-65% response. Unfortunately, the response is often incomplete, relapses are common and evolution into clonal disorders like PNH, myelodysplastic syndrome and leukemias can occur over period of time. Androgens are much less effective, but are often the only form of therapy offered to patients due to cost constraints. There is no primary role of corticosteroids or hematopoietic growth factors, except as adjunctive therapy in special circumstances. New immunosuppressive therapies are being evaluated for refractory patients.

KEYWORDS

Bone marrow failure, ATG, Bone marrow transplant, Immunosuppression.

INTRODUCTION

Aplastic anemia (AA) is a life-threatening bone marrow failure disorder, if untreated, is associated with very high mortality. The incidence of AA is 2 to 3-fold more common in Asia than in Europe.[1] Aplastic anemia is defined as pancytopenia with a hypocellular bone marrow (BM) without infiltration or fibrosis. To diagnose AA at least two of the following must be present: (i) hemoglobin < 10 g/dl, (ii) platelet count < 50,000/μl, (iii) neutrophil count <1,500/μl (International Agranulocytosis and Aplastic Anemia Study Group, 1987).

The assessment of disease severity is important in treatment decisions and has prognostic significance. The severity of the disease is graded according to the blood count parameters and bone marrow findings as summarized in Table 17.1.

Table 17.1: Criteria for severity of aplastic anemia

Severe AA (Camitta et al, 1976) [SAA]
- Bone marrow cellularity < 25%, or 25-50% with < 30% residual hemopoietic cells.
- Two out of three of the following:
    - Neutrophils < 500/µl,
    - Platelets < 20,000/µl,
    - Reticulocytes < 20,000/µl,

Very severe AA (Bacigalupo et al, 1988) [VSAA]
As for severe AA but neutrophils < 200/µl,

Nonsevere AA [NSAA]
Patients not fulfilling the criteria for severe or very severe aplastic anemia.

Natural History of Aplastic Anemia

The natural history of AA is heterogeneous with a more benign outcome in nonsevere AA patients and fatal outcome in other group of patients like severe and very severe AA. The one-year mortality for patients with SAA treated with transfusion only was > 80% in an older, retrospective series.[3] Early spontaneous remissions of SAA in childhood are reported but rare, often associated with the identification and treatment of infection such as Hepatitis A. In a large cohort of (mostly) SAA patients diagnosed in the 1980s and treated only with androgens, mortality was 58% at 2 years, 60% at 5 years and 65% at 12 years.[4] The actuarial risk of death related to AA in those that survived to 5 years was 14% at 15 years after diagnosis; some had late spontaneous recovery of cytopenias: Most reported good quality of life.[5] AA may relapse or occur *de novo* during pregnancy, and may improve spontaneously after delivery or termination.

Supportive Care

The benefits of definitive therapies will be unrealized if the patient succumbs to early clinical complications. A haphazard and inadequate transfusion policy can jeopardize the patient's life and increase morbidity. The ultimate possibility of cure depends on better supportive care.

Transfusional Support

Support with red cell and platelet transfusions is essential for patients with AA to maintain a safe blood count. Blood products from close relatives such as a sibling or a parent (who share histocompatibility antigens) should be avoided. In presence of bleeding manifestations, platelets should be transfused irrespective of platelet count. It is recommended to give prophylactic platelet transfusions when the platelet count is < 10,000/µl (or < 20,000/µl in the presence of fever). Irradiated blood products should be used routinely in all patients with AA who are transplant candidates and also the routine leukocyte depletion of all blood and platelet transfusions may be at least as important in reducing the risk of allo-immunization.

Hemopoietic Growth Factors

There are currently no effective and safe hemopoietic growth factors to support red cells and platelets in patients with AA. The serum erythropoietin level is elevated in the majority of patients with AA, so erythropoietin (rHuEpo) is ineffective. Interleukin-6 (IL-6) and stem cell factor were shown to stimulate hemopoiesis in some patients with AA, but subsequent results are conflicting. There have been no clinical studies of recombinant human thrombopoietin (rHu-TPO) in AA and in other studies the development of anti-TPO antibodies resulted in prolonged thrombocytopenia and discontinuation of its use in clinical trials. Newer second generation thrombopoietin analogues are promising, but not yet tried in AA. There are no roles of GCSF and granulocyte macrophage-colony stimulating factor (GM-CSF) in AA as a routine treatment. A short course of subcutaneous G-CSF at a dose of 5 µg/kg/d may be considered for severe systemic infections that are not responding to intravenous antibiotics and antifungal treatment.[2]

Prevention of Infection

Patients with AA are at risk of bacterial and fungal infections. Aspergillus infections have a very high mortality in patients with SAA because of prolonged neutropenia (and monocytopenia). Dental hygiene is important, and sources of infection should be removed under antibiotic and platelet coverage. Early attention to the signs of infection can avert many of the complications of initially minor infectious episodes. Prophylactic antibiotics and antifungals can be used to prevent severe infections. There is no indication for routine prophylactic measures against *Pneumocystis carinii* pneumonia (PCP) or antiviral prophylaxis in untreated patients with AA.

Treatment of Infection

As for all neutropenic patients, fever may require immediate hospitalization and treatment before the results of bacterial investigations are available. A combination of antibiotics such as aminoglycoside and β-lactam penicillin is commonly used. The duration of neutropenia, the patient's infection history and recent antibiotics, will also influence the antibiotic choice, including the early introduction of amphotericin. Once a patient with AA is colonized with aspergillus, it is usually difficult to treat successfully as the neutrophil count may not recover for a long period of time. A short course of subcutaneous G-CSF at a dose of 5 µg/kg/d may be considered for severe systemic infections that are not responding to intravenous antibiotics and antifungals. It may produce a temporary neutrophil response but usually only in those patients with residual marrow granulocytic activity (that is, those with nonsevere disease). G-CSF should be stopped if there is no response by 1 week.

Immunosuppressive Therapy (IST)

Antithymocyte Globulin (ATG) and Ciclosporin (CSA)

IST is indicated in (1) patients with non-SAA who are dependent on red cell and/or platelet transfusions, (2) patients with SAA or very SAA who are > 40 years of age, (3) patients with severe or very severe disease who lack an HLA-compatible sibling donor. Children with non-SAA with an HLA-identical sibling donor and who are transfusion dependent, particularly if the blood count is falling, may be considered for BMT. For those patients with non-SAA who are not dependent on either red cell or platelet transfusions, and maintain safe blood counts, it is reasonable to observe the blood count and monitor the patient regularly without initially instigating immunosuppressive therapy.[2]

The ATG is a pan-antilymphocyte immunoglobulin composed of purified animal polyclonal antibodies directed against human lymphocytes. In India, the standard preparation of ATG is horse ATG [ATG-Thymogam (Bharat serum, India) and ATG-ATGAM (Pharmacia-Upjohn, Kalamazoo, Michigan, USA)]. The rabbit preparation (Thymoglobuline, Genzyme, Cambridge, MA, USA) is usually reserved for second or subsequent courses. ATG is given as a daily intravenous infusion over 6-8 hours. The dose is 40 mg/kg/body weight × 4 days for horse ATG (one vial of horse ATG, Lymphoglobuline, contains 250 mg protein). The dose is 3.75 mg/kg body weight × 5 days for rabbit ATG (one vial of rabbit ATG, Lymphoglobuline, contains 25 mg protein). A test dose (1 mg in 100 ml N saline as an intravenous infusion over 1 hour) must be given beforehand and, if a severe systemic reaction or anaphylaxis occurs, further doses of that preparation of ATG must not be given. Platelet transfusions should be given to maintain a safe platelet count (ideally > 30,000/µl), but should not be given concurrently with ATG administration because of the anti-platelet activity of ATG.[2] On the fifth day of ATG, prednisolone at 1 mg/kg/d is commenced to prevent serum sickness and continued for 2 weeks. Oral CSA should be commenced after 2 weeks at 5 mg/kg/d, aiming to keep the trough CSA blood level between 150 and 250 mg/L for adults and between 100 and 150 mg/L for children. Because response to ATG is delayed until 3 months, patients will need to continue with regular blood product support during this time. A second course of ATG is recommended if there is no response or relapse after the first course. This should not be given earlier than 3 months after the first course because it usually takes around 3 months before a response occurs.[2] One can either use rabbit ATG or horse ATG again, although there is a higher incidence of allergic reactions and earlier serum sickness if the same preparation is used again. It is possible to consider giving a third course of ATG if there has been no response to two courses and BMT is not an option.

The combination of ATG and CSA remains the currently recommended immunosuppressive regimen for both severe AA and transfusion-dependent non-severe AA. IST using the combination of ATG and CSA is associated with response rates of between 60 and 80% with current 5-year survival rates of around 75%.[11,12] For SAA and even non-SAA, the response rate to ATG alone is significantly less than with the combination of ATG and CSA.[7,8,13] Relapse may occur after IST. This was previously reported to be around 30%[14] but with longer use and slower tailing of CSA the rate is closer to 10%.[8] For the one-third of patients who are refractory to h-ATG/CsA, repeated courses of immunosuppression have yielded response rates varying from 30-70%.[16-18] Re-treatment with ATG/CsA in relapsed AA has resulted in response rates of 50-60%.[10,16,18] A third course of ATG – containing IST is a reasonable option in previous responders but those are refractory to first two courses of ATG have a much lower response rate and may be suitable for noval therapeutic options.[19] In a recent Japanese prospective study, the risk of relapse was significantly higher in patients receiving ATG plus CSA (42%) compared with that of patients receiving ATG plus CSA with the addition of granulocyte colony-stimulating factor (G-CSF; 15%) (P =.01),[28] although 4-year survival was not significantly different (88% vs 94%).[19] A large multicenter randomized European trial is under way that compares ATG and CSA with or without G-CSF, which will more definitively address the benefits and possible pitfalls of cytokine addition in SAA.

Horse vs Rabbit ATG

The standard first-line IST is currently horse ATG plus CSA and second-line treatment is r-ATG plus CSA, although the latter has been successfully used also as first-line therapy. Rabbit-ATG is similar to h-ATG except that gamma immunoglobulin is obtained by immunization of rabbits with human thymocytes. Clinically, r-ATG appears to be more immunosuppressive as a more prolonged lymphopenia is observed with this agent compared to h-ATG.[20] This enhanced lymphocytotoxicity of r-ATG may be explained by higher affinity IgG subtype to human lymphocytes, less batch-to-batch variability, longer half life, and more efficient lymphocyte depletion.[21] The response rates of re treatment with r-ATG (3.5 mg/kg/d for five consecutive days) in refractory patients or relapsed patients have varied significantly, from 30 to 77%.[22,17]

Ciclosporin Dependence and Relapse

CSA dependency is observed in 26-62% of patients, necessitating long-term maintenance of the drug. Current IST regimens including CSA call for a full CSA dose (5 mg/kg orally per day) for 6 months; after this time point, CSA is tapered, and it is unclear exactly when and how fast this should be done.[10] A recent, as-yet-unpublished study of the Italian pediatric group has addressed these two questions.[23] In this study, 42 children were divided into three groups: Very slow tapering (< 0.3 mg/kg/month), slow CSA tapering (0.4-0.7 mg/kg/month) and rapid tapering (≥ 0.8 mg/kg/month). The cumulative incidence of relapse was 8% in the slow/very slow taper group and 60% in the rapid taper group. Among patients who eventually discontinued CSA, the median duration of CSA treatment at full therapeutic dose (4-6 mg/kg) was 12 months (range 3-45 months), and tapering was completed in a median of 19 months (range: 4-64 months). In that study, the actuarial probability of discontinuing CSA was 21% at 5 years, 38% at 7 years, and 60% at 10 years, respectively.[23] This study suggests that (1) it is safe to start taper CSA at 12 months of treatment (rather than 6 months) and (2) that taper should be very slow (less than 10% of the dose/month) for at least 1 year, to minimize the risk of relapse.

Clonal Evolution and Second Malignancies

After long-term follow-up some patients with AA may proceed to frank PNH, acute leukemia and MDS. Patients are at risk of later clonal disease, between 5-10% for MDS/AML and 10-15% for hemolytic PNH.[15] The overall risk of developing a clonal cytogenetic abnormality/MDS at 10 years is set between 5% and 20% and may depend on the degree of response to IST.[12] The risk of MDS/acute myeloid leukemia (AML) was significantly higher for patients who underwent IST as compared with those who underwent BMT, suggesting that MDS/AML follows IST rather than being present at diagnosis, because 200 mg/kg cyclophosphamide (CY) used in transplantation, would be unlikely to eradicate a neoplastic clone.[24] Second tumors were frequent in patients receiving radiation before BMT, and radiation is currently not recommended in HLA-identical sibling transplantations. Very low dose (2 Gy) total body irradiation (TBI) is being explored in patients undergoing an alternative donor transplantation.[25]

Factors Predicting Survival After IST

Despite better understanding of the pathogenesis of SAA, methods to predict response to IST are lacking. In a recent study on almost 1000 patients treated in Europe between 1991 and 2002, the strongest negative predictor was age (older than 16 years) [relative risk (RR), 1.76; P =.0009], followed by an IST protocol other than ATG plus CSA (RR, 1.29; P =.02) and interval between diagnosis and treatment over 23 days (RR, 1.32; P =.04).[26] Of interest is the fact that severity of the disease, as identified by PMN counts (< 0.2, 02-0.5, and > 0.5 × 10^9/L), had no impact on survival, in contrast to results from the original analysis of the EBMT showing that PMN count was the strongest predictor of survival.[27]

A recently completed retrospective analysis of over 300 patients treated with h-ATG/CsA (Scheinberg P at el ASH Annual Meeting

Abstracts 2007; 110:504a) showed that baseline absolute reticulocyte count (ARC) and absolute lymphocyte count (ALC) combined served as a good predictor of response to IST: Patients with an ARC of at least 25000/mL and ALC of at least 1000/ml at baseline had an 80 percent response rate compared with 40 percent with those with an ARC less than 25000/mL and ALC less than 1000/ml. An age less than 18 years also correlated to improved response (about 75%).

Other Immunosuppressive Drugs

High Dose Cyclophosphamide without Stem Cell Support

High-dose cyclophosphamide has been used as a form of immunosuppression. The use of high dose cyclophosphamide (45 mg/kg/day for 4 days) without stem cell support has been proposed by one center as treatment for patients with newly diagnosed aplastic anemia.[29] However, a prospective randomized study comparing its use in combination with CSA against the gold standard of ATG and CSA was terminated prematurely because of an excess of early deaths and systemic fungal infections in the cyclophosphamide arm. The use of cyclophosphamide was associated with profound and very prolonged pancytopenia resulting in a significant increase in use of blood and platelet transfusions, days of intravenous antibiotics and amphotericin and in-patient days in hospital.[30] The use of high dose cyclophosphamide without stem cell support cannot be recommended in either newly diagnosed patients or patients who have failed ATG and ciclosporin in view of its serious toxicity and high mortality.[2]

Corticosteroids

Marrow recovery can occur after very high doses of glucocorticoids. Methylprednisolone in modest doses (1 mg/kg/day) is usually administered during ATG and ALG therapy to ameliorate the symptoms of serum sickness. Methylprednisolone in the range from 500 to 1000 mg daily for 3 to 14 days has been successful in some trials but the side effects can be severe and life-threatening.

Androgens

Androgens no longer have a primary role in the management of AA and are generally reserved for patients who have failed immunosuppressive therapy. In the past, early reports of responses to androgens were not supported by subsequent studies that found low rates of remission and no improvement in survival.

Useful androgens include nandrolone decanoate, oxymetholone, danazol and stanazolol. Nandrolone decanoate administered at 400 mg intramuscularly per week is one approach.

Oxymetholone (2 mg/kg/day) has been used extensively in the treatment of AA for many decades before the availability of ATG and

CSA. In combination with ATG, it increases the response compared with ATG alone.[31]

Danazol, a type of synthetic anabolic steroid, has unique properties similar to those of corticosteroids, such as inhibition of both interleukin-1 and TNF-α production. Several case reports have documented the efficacy of danazol in the treatment of AA refractory to IST. A recently prospective clinical trial of over 16 patients AA refractory to IST and those who relapsed after IST treated with danazol, at 300 mg/day for 12 weeks showed that the rate of response between males and females are 17% and 75% respectively.[32] Marwaha et al from PGIMER Chandigarh reported that Stanazolol (1 mg/kg/day) is ineffective for severe and very severe AA in children and it induced remission in 38% of nonsevere AA patients. So, it can be tried in this group if other methods of treatment are unaffordable or have failed.[33]

The mechanism of action by which male hormones improve hematopoietic failure states remains unclear. The hemoglobin response frequently is more impressive than improvements in granulocyte or platelet levels. Androgens, if used, should be continued for at least 3 to 6 months because responses may require prolonged treatment.

When the effects of androgens are compared in patients with severe and moderate AA, the response rate (8% vs 56%)[34] and subsequent survival (20% vs 58%)[35] have generally been lower in those patients with severe diseas. Complications occur infrequently, although some are serious and may limit effective therapy, especially in the elderly. Virilization, hirsutism and acne, fluid retention, and psychological alterations are seen. The associated liver cholestasis is usually reversible. Hepatotoxicity (e.g. bile duct proliferation, peliosis, atypical hepatocyte hyperplasia, tumors) can occur but is less common with parenteral formulations. Children appear to tolerate high doses of androgens without lasting effects on growth or maturation. It must, therefore, be used with caution, with regular monitoring of liver function tests and liver ultrasound. Because the drug causes virilization, it is often unacceptable to women. Long-term survivors after androgen therapy have essentially the same progression to clonal hematologic disorders as patients treated with immunosuppressive agents.

Other Immunosuppressive Agents

Other immunosuppressive agents currently under investigation include an anti–IL-2 receptor monoclonal antibody (Daclizumab), mycophenolate mofetil (MMF; Cell-Cept), FK506 and rapamycin, etc.

Bone Marrow Transplantation (BMT)

HLA-identical Sibling Donor Transplantation

Indications: Patients with severe AA, if they are < 40 years old and have an HLA compatible sibling, should be transplanted up front, and should not receive prior immunosuppressive therapy.[2] Delay in transplantation also increases the risk of life-threatening infections.

Conditioning and GVHD prophylaxis regimen: GVHD prophylaxis should be the combination of CSA and methotrexate (MTX), since this has been shown to be superior to CSA alone. Therefore, standard cyclophopshamide 50 mg/kg/day for 4 days, with 3 days of ATG, followed by unmanipulated marrow and CSA plus MTX is still standard of care for patients with aquired AA undergoing an HLA-identical sibling transplantation.[2] The conditioning regimen used for patients aged < 30 years is a nonmyeloablative, highly immunosuppressive regimen which includes fludarabine to help prevent graft rejection and GVHD.

Results: Transplantation for SAA from an HLA-identical sibling donor is now very successful with a 75-90% chance of long-term cure.[11] The incidence of graft rejection has fallen from > 30% before 1980 to around 5-10%. Graft-versus-host disease (GVHD) remains a problem: The probability of acute GVHD grade II–IV is 18 ± 3% and chronic GVHD of any grade is 26 ± 5%, for patients transplanted after 1990, as reported to the International Bone Marrow Transplant Registry (IBMTR).[36]

EBMT recently (2007) analyzed 1567 patients allografted in the period 1991 through 2002. Favorable predictors of survival were year of transplantation after 1997, matched sibling donor (MSD), age younger than 16 years, an interval between diagnosis and transplantation of less than 83 days, and a conditioning regimen without radiation.[26]

The current survival for patients with AA younger than 16 years who have received a BMT from an HLA-identical sibling after conditioning with 200 mg/kg CY is 91%[26] and it does not cause infertility or second tumors. For older patients, results are less encouraging, and peripheral blood (PB) transplantations have been introduced with the aim of reducing rejection and infections. A recent EBMT/IBMTR study suggests that PB transplantations actually reduce survival compared with marrow transplantations, in patients with AA younger than 20 years, from 85 to 73%, and in patients older than 20 years, from 64 to 52%:[37] The major cause of excess mortality in the PB arm is chronic graft-versus-host disease (GVHD). This study suggests that PB transplantations are not recommended in patients with acquired AA, possibly because increased chronic GVHD is not beneficial, as may be the case in leukemia. CY alone remains the best conditioning regimen for young patients, and ATG would seem to reduce the risk of graft failure:[38] A recent randomized trial has shown a nonsignificant survival advantage for patients receiving ATG.[39]

Source and dose of stem cells: It is recommended that bone marrow stem cells, and not G-CSF-mobilized peripheral blood stem cells (PBSC), should be used. Earlier engraftment occurs with PBSC but there is serious concern about more chronic GVHD and worse outcome after PBSC transplantation for SAA. In a recent combined retrospective International Bone Marrow Transplant Registry (IBMTR)/EBMT study there was no difference in graft failure rates amongst AA patients receiving MSD BM or PBSC. However, BM recipients had significantly less chronic GvHD and better overall survival.[14] It is important to give at least 3×10^8 nucleated marrow cells/kg because at lower doses the risk of graft rejection increases significantly.[40]

Post-transplant management: There is a significant risk of late graft failure in AA following allogeneic BMT, which is most commonly associated with discontinuing CSA too early or low CSA blood levels. Therapeutic CAS should be continued for at least 9 months before gradually reducing the dose to zero over the following 3 months. For adults, CSA trough blood levels should be maintained between 250 and 350 g/l. For children, lower CSA levels are often used (150-200 lg/l), to avoid toxicity.

Chimaerism should be monitored particularly closely during the time of CSA withdrawal. If there is evidence of significant mixed chimaerism (> 20% recipient cells) or a rising proportion of recipient cells, as assessed with sensitive techniques such as polymerase chain reaction of short tandem repeats, there is a high-risk of late rejection, and CSA should not be reduced or withdrawn at that time.

Unlike intensive AHSCT regimens that frequently perturb growth and development, non-TBI containing regimens for AA often result in normal growth, attainment of predicted adult heights and well-preserved fertility.[41] Nonetheless, routine assessments of growth and development, dermatological status, endocrine and pulmonary function and bone mineral density should be made and appropriate counseling, including that related to fertility, should be provided to patients and families. Attention to immunization status is important. Delayed infectious complications, dermatological issues (including scleroderma), cataracts, pulmonary insufficiency and bone and joint problems may present after MSD AHSCT for AA.[42] The development of secondary malignancies is another concern after AHSCT for AA.

Matched Unrelated Donor Bone Marrow Transplantation

Results: The role of matched unrelated donor (MUD) BMT in the treatment of SAA remains controversial due to the continued high morbidity and mortality from this procedure. A large number of patients analyzed retrospectively from combined sources (IBMTR, EBMTR, Seattle and a large UK study) show long-term survival of around 30% with a high incidence of graft rejection, GVHD and severe infections. A matched sibling donor is available in only 20-30% of cases. Data from large retrospective studies suggest that the outcome for an unrelated donor HSCT remains less favorable compared with a matched-related transplant, due to more GVHD, a mortality rate that is about twice that observed in matched sibling transplants, and long-term survival of about 50%.[43,44] In many cases a myeloablative regimen incorporating, most frequently, irradiation has been employed. More recent data from relatively small numbers of patients show reduced transplant related mortality when (i) only fully matched donors or donors matched for HLA-DRB1 are used and (ii) non-myeloablative and therefore, less toxic conditioning is employed, such as low dose total body irradiation (Deeg et al, 1999, 2001; Vassiliou et al, 2001; Elebute et al, 2002) or more immunosuppressive regimens incorporating fludarabine (Bacigalupo et al, 2002).

A multicenter prospective study compared the outcomes of a second course of IST to a MUD HSCT in children who failed initial course of IST: Among the 60 initial ATG failures, 21 underwent a MUD HSCT and 31 received a second course of IST. Those who underwent a MUD HSCT had a higher failure free survival (defined as survival with response) compared with those who underwent a second course of IST, although no difference in overall survival was observed between the two groups.[45] There have been no prospective randomized studies of MUD BMT in AA due to the rarity of the disease, but the EBMT SAA Working Party has recently proposed a standard conditioning protocol of fludarabine, low dose cyclophosphamide and ATG, with short course of both CSA and methotrexate as GVHD prophylaxis, based on the pilot study of Bacigalupo et al (2002). A similar protocol has been recommended by the BSBMT, the only difference being the option to use Campath-1H instead of ATG.

Indications: MUD BMT may be considered when patients fulfill all the following criteria.[2] They should:
1. Have a fully matched (at DNA level for both class I and II antigens) donor,
2. Be < 40 years old,
3. For adults, have failed at least two courses of ATG and ciclosporin and for children, at least one course,
4. Have SAA, and
5. Have no evidence of active infection and or acute bleeding at time of BMT.

MUD versus mismatched donor transplantation: Alternate donors include MUDs, mismatched (MM) UDs and mismatched related donors (MMRDs). While a retrospective analysis of 318 AA patients receiving low resolution HLA typed alternate donor transplants demonstrated no significant differences in multivariate analysis in rates of graft failure, GvHD or overall survival according to donor type (MUD, MMUD or MMRD;[43] superior survival of AA patients with use of fully matched UDs (by high resolution HLA typing) rather than HLA class I MMUDs has been reported. Thus, the prognostic importance of single-antigen donor mismatches may therefore vary according to the HLA typing technology used as well as the locus of individual HLA antigen mismatch. It seems prudent to select a fully matched UD; however, mismatched donors should be considered if a MUD is unavailable.

Umbilical Cord Blood Transplantation from Matched Sibling Donors

Umbilical cord blood as an alternative source of stem cells for transplantation has been used in a small number of patients with aplastic anemia. Its use, however, is limited to small recipients because of the low number of hemopoietic cells that can be obtained from a donation, despite their higher proliferative potential compared with bone marrow cells. Compared with bone marrow transplants, umbilical cord blood transplants are associated with a lower risk of acute and chronic GVHD. Umbilical cord blood transplantation may also be considered in children who lack an HLA-identical sibling donor or a fully matched unrelated adult donor. The first reported use of UCB was from a sibling donor to transplant a patient with FA (Gluckman et al, 1989). Although, most subsequent reported experience is with unrelated donors, there is limited experience with MSD UCB transplants in children with both malignant and nonmalignant disorders (Wagner et al, 1995). Better rates of engraftment (> 80%) have been achieved with higher doses of nucleated cells (Locatelli et al, 1999). Unfortunately there is no potential for additional cells doses to be obtained if graft failure occurs. A joint study by Eurocord and the IBMTR compared the outcome of 113 children who received UCB transplants from MSDs to children receiving MSD BM transplants. In this study (which contained eight children with idiopathic AA who received UCB transplants) MSD UCB transplantation was associated with slower neutrophil engraftment but less acute and chronic GvHD, although overall survival was the same in both groups (Rocha et al, 2000). Arrangements should be made to store UCB from siblings of children with severe AA wherever possible for potential future use, particularly in those who lack existing MSDs and/or matched unrelated donors (MUDs). Antenatal HLA typing can be performed but this strategy is most commonly employed in families of children with inherited bone marrow failure syndromes.

Unrelated Donor Umbilical Cord Blood Transplantation

Unrelated donor UCB transplantation has been used extensively in children with both malignant and nonmalignant conditions (Rubinstein et al, 1998). In a matched pair analysis combining children with hematological malignancies and AA, the use of MUD UCB was associated with a similar outcome to MUD marrow, suggesting that unrelated UCB should be considered as a possible alternative to unrelated marrow.[46]

Management of Aplastic Anemia in Pregnancy

Aplastic anemia can present in pregnancy although this may be due to chance and other possible causes should always be sought. The disease may remit spontaneously after termination, whether spontaneous or therapeutic, and after delivery, but not in all cases and much support may be needed. The disease often progresses during pregnancy and there is a significant risk of relapse in pregnancy in patients who have previously responded to immunosuppressive therapy.[2] So, if a young woman is in complete remission, off therapy, and aware of the risk of relapse of the disease, a pregnancy is a possibility.[10]

Supportive care is the mainstay of treatment of AA in pregnancy and the platelet count should, if possible, be maintained above 20,000/μl with platelet transfusions. There is an increased risk of alloimmunization to red cell and platelet transfusions during normal pregnancy and this risk is increased further in AA. ATG is too hazardous to give during pregnancy, although there is one reported case of its use in late pregnancy in a patient with very SAA who delivered a normal healthy baby (Aitchison et al, 1989). One can consider the use of CSA

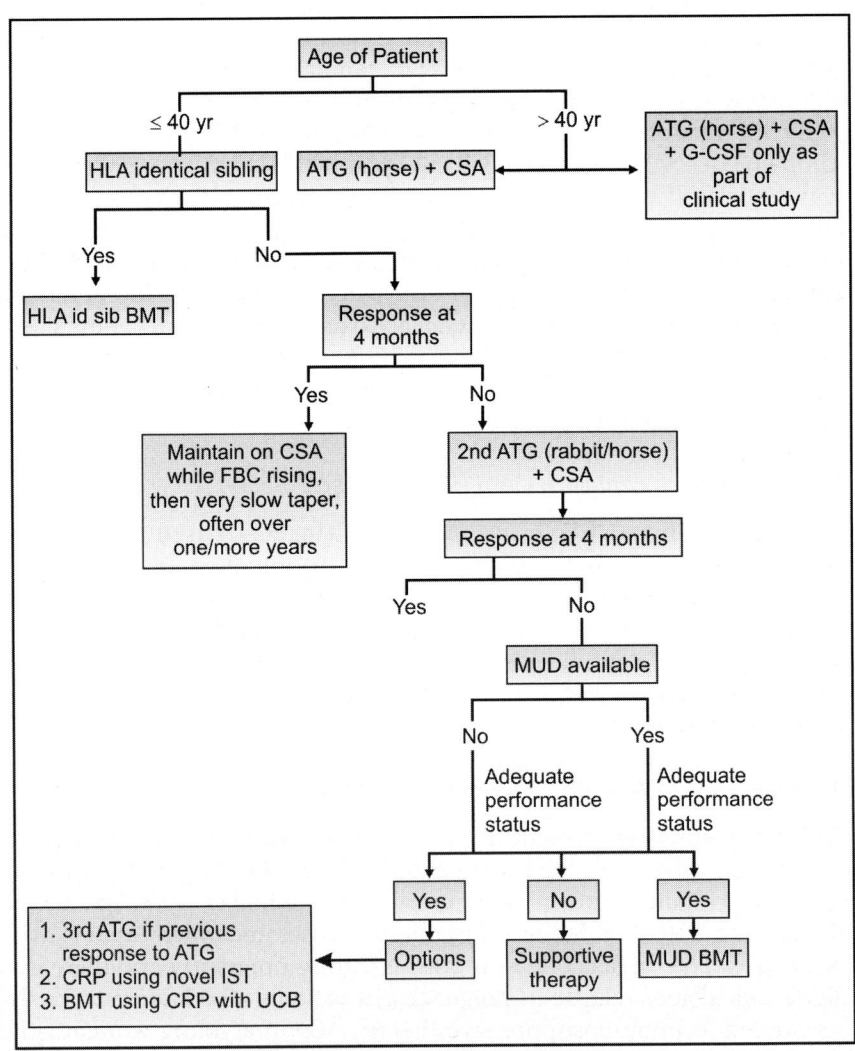

Flow chart 17.1: Algorithms for treatment of acquired aplastic anemia (adult SSA)[48]

Flow chart 17.2: Algorithms for treatment of acquired aplastic anemia (Adult NSAA)[48]

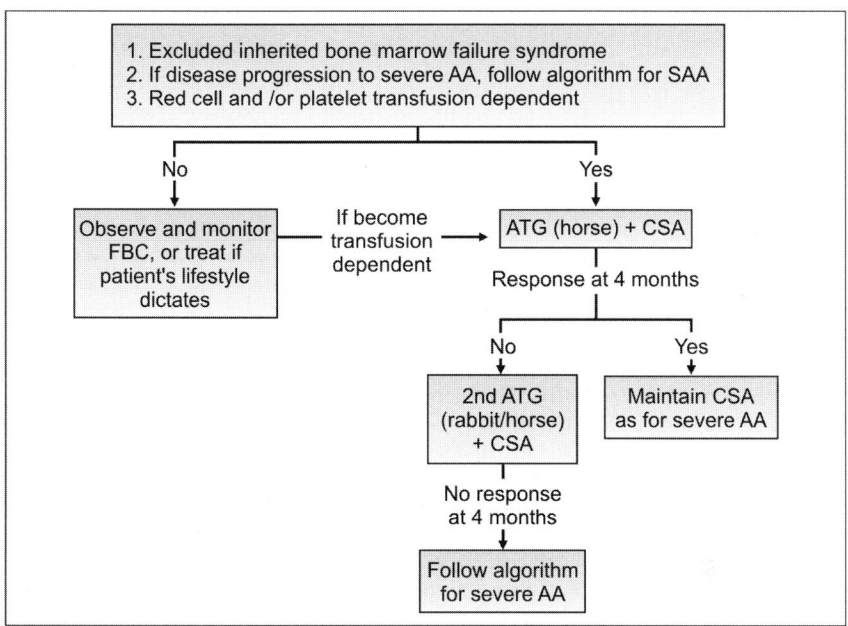

in pregnancy. If a patient needs transfusions or if the blood counts are falling towards levels that will soon require transfusional support, it is recommended to start oral CSA 5 mg/kg/d to maintain levels between 150 and 250 ng/l.[2] Response to CSA is delayed and may take between 6 and 12 weeks. Finally, it is essential that the patient and her blood counts are monitored frequently throughout pregnancy and very close liaison with the obstetric team and general practitioner is essential.

Management of Aplastic Anemia in Older Patients

The patients with AA over the age of 70 years can be treated with ATG and CsA, although response rates and survival are lower compared with young patients:[47] the actuarial 10-year survival is 45% for patients aged 51 to 70 years and 25% for patients over the age of 70 years.[47] Nevertheless, the standardized mortality ratio (SMR), indicating the ratio between mortality of patients and of an age matched population, is 33, 14, and 9, respectively, for the age groups younger than 50, 50-70, and older than 70 years.[47] These data suggest that the corrected risk of death in AA is highest in young patients and becomes progressively lower with increasing age (Flow charts 17.1 and 17.2).

CONCLUSION

Early intervention is associated with a significantly better outcome and is strongly recommended, whatever the first line therapy. Acquired SAA can be treated successfully with either IST or BMT. IST can be readily administered to all patients but is not curative. BMT produces rapid and long-lasting hematologic recovery without the long-term risk of MDS, but requires a suitable donor and appropriate financial resources, and may cause long-lasting chronic GVHD. Age remains a major predictor and requires careful consideration when deciding the treatment strategy. Due to financial constraint most of the patients in the developing countries do not receive definite form of therapy.

REFERENCES

1. Young NS, Kaufman DW. The epidemiology of acquired aplastic anemia. Haematologica 2008;93(4):489-92.
2. Marsh JC, Ball SE, Darbyshire P, et al. Guidelines for the diagnosis and management of acquired aplastic anaemia. Br J Haematol 2003;123(5):782-801.
3. Williams DM, Lynch RE, Cartwright GE. Prognostic factors in aplastic anaemia. Clin Haematol 1978;7(3):467-74.
4. Davies JK, Guinan EC. An update on the management of severe idiopathic aplastic anaemia in children. Br J Haematol 2007;136(4):549-64.
5. Najean Y, Haguenauer O. Long-term (5 to 20 years) Evolution of nongrafted aplastic anemias. The Cooperative Group for the Study of Aplastic and Refractory Anemias. Blood 1990;76(11):2222-28.
6. Keidan AJ, Tsatalas C, Cohen J, Cousins S, Gordon-Smith EC. Infective complications of aplastic anaemia. Br J Haematol 1986;63(3):503-08.
7. Camitta BM. What is the definition of cure for aplastic anemia? Acta Haematol 2000;103(1):16-18.
8. Fuhrer M, Burdach S, Ebell W, et al. Relapse and clonal disease in children with aplastic anemia (AA) after immunosuppressive therapy (IST): The SAA 94 experience. German/Austrian Pediatric Aplastic Anemia Working Group. Klin Padiatr 1998;210(4):173-79.
9. Matloub YH, Smith C, Bostrom B, et al. One course versus two courses of antithymocyte globulin for the treatment of severe aplastic anemia in children. J Pediatr Hematol Oncol 1997;19(2):110-14.
10. Bacigalupo A. Aplastic anemia: pathogenesis and treatment. Hematology Am Soc Hematol Educ Program 2007;23-28.
11. Bacigalupo A, Brand R, Oneto R, et al. Treatment of acquired severe aplastic anemia: Bone marrow transplantation compared with immunosuppressive therapy—The European Group for Blood and Marrow Transplantation experience. Semin Hematol 2000;37(1):69-80.
12. Bacigalupo A, Bruno B, Saracco P, et al. Antilymphocyte globulin, cyclosporin, prednisolone, and granulocyte colony-stimulating factor for severe aplastic anemia: An update of the GITMO/EBMT study on 100 patients. European Group for Blood and Marrow Transplantation (EBMT) Working Party on Severe Aplastic Anemia and the Gruppo Italiano Trapianti di Midolio Osseo (GITMO). Blood 2000;95(6):1931-34.
13. Marsh J, Schrezenmeier H, Marin P, et al. Prospective randomized multicenter study comparing cyclosporin alone versus the combination of antithymocyte globulin and cyclosporin for treatment of patients with nonsevere aplastic anemia: A report from the European Blood and Marrow Transplant (EBMT) Severe Aplastic Anaemia Working Party. Blood 1999;93(7):2191-95.
14. Schrezenmeier H, Marin P, Raghavachar A, et al. Relapse of aplastic anaemia after immunosuppressive treatment: A report from the European Bone Marrow Transplantation Group SAA Working Party. Br J Haematol 1993;85(2):371-77.

15. Socie G, Rosenfeld S, Frickhofen N, Gluckman E, Tichelli A. Late clonal diseases of treated aplastic anemia. Semin Hematol 2000;37(1):91-101.
16. Scheinberg P, Nunez O, Wu C, Young NS. Treatment of severe aplastic anaemia with combined immunosuppression: Anti-thymocyte globulin, ciclosporin and mycophenolate mofetil. Br J Haematol 2006;133(6):606-11.
17. Di Bona E, Rodeghiero F, Bruno B, et al. Rabbit antithymocyte globulin (r-ATG) plus cyclosporin and granulocyte colony stimulating factor is an effective treatment for aplastic anaemia patients unresponsive to a first course of intensive immunosuppressive therapy. Gruppo Italiano Trapianto di Midollo Osseo (GITMO). Br J Haematol 1999;107(2):330-34.
18. Tichelli A, Passweg J, Nissen C, et al. Repeated treatment with horse antilymphocyte globulin for severe aplastic anaemia. Br J Haematol 1998;100(2):393-400.
19. Gupta V, Gordon-Smith EC, Cook G, et al. A third course of anti-thymocyte globulin in aplastic anaemia is only beneficial in previous responders. Br J Haematol 2005;129(1):110-17.
20. Scheinberg P, Fischer SH, Li L, et al. Distinct EBV and CMV reactivation patterns following antibody-based immunosuppressive regimens in patients with severe aplastic anemia. Blood 2007;109(8):3219-24.
21. Young NS, Scheinberg P, Calado RT. Aplastic anemia. Curr Opin Hematol 2008;15(3):162-68.
22. Scheinberg P, Nunez O, Young NS. Retreatment with rabbit anti-thymocyte globulin and ciclosporin for patients with relapsed or refractory severe aplastic anaemia. Br J Haematol 2006;133(6):622-27.
23. Saracco P, Quarello P, Iori AP, et al. Cyclosporin A response and dependence in children with acquired aplastic anaemia: A multicentre retrospective study with long-term observation follow-up. Br J Haematol 2008;140(2):197-205.
24. Socie G, Henry-Amar M, Bacigalupo A, et al. Malignant tumors occurring after treatment of aplastic anemia. European Bone Marrow Transplantation-Severe Aplastic Anaemia Working Party. N Engl J Med 1993;329(16):1152-57.
25. Kojima S, Matsuyama T, Kato S, et al. Outcome of 154 patients with severe aplastic anemia who received transplants from unrelated donors: The Japan Marrow Donor Program. Blood 2002;100(3):799-803.
26. Locasciulli A, Oneto R, Bacigalupo A, et al. Outcome of patients with acquired aplastic anemia given first line bone marrow transplantation or immuno-suppressive treatment in the last decade: A report from the European Group for Blood and Marrow Transplantation (EBMT). Haematologica 2007;92(1):11-18.
27. Bacigalupo A, Hows J, Gluckman E, et al. Bone marrow transplantation (BMT) versus immunosuppression for the treatment of severe aplastic anaemia (SAA): A report of the EBMT SAA working party. Br J Haematol 1988;70(2):177-82.
28. Teramura M, Kimura A, Iwase S, et al. Treatment of severe aplastic anemia with antithymocyte globulin and cyclosporin A with or without G-CSF in adults: A multicenter randomized study in Japan. Blood 2007;110(6):1756-61.
29. Brodsky RA, Sensenbrenner LL, Smith BD, et al. Durable treatment-free remission after high-dose cyclophosphamide therapy for previously untreated severe aplastic anemia. Ann Intern Med 2001;135(7):477-83.
30. Tisdale JF, Dunn DE, Geller N, et al. High-dose cyclophosphamide in severe aplastic anaemia: A randomised trial. Lancet 2000;356(9241):1554-59.
31. Bacigalupo A, Chaple M, Hows J, et al. Treatment of aplastic anaemia (AA) with antilymphocyte globulin (ALG) and methylprednisolone (MPred) with or without androgens: A randomized trial from the EBMT SAA working party. Br J Haematol 1993;83(1):145-51.

32. Chuhjo T, Yamazaki H, Omine M, Nakao S. Danazol therapy for aplastic anemia refractory to immunosuppressive therapy. Am J Hematol 2008;83(5):387-89.
33. Marwaha RK, Bansal D, Trehan A, Varma N. Androgens in childhood acquired aplastic anaemia in Chandigarh, India. Trop Doct 2004;34(3):149-52.
34. Pizzuto J, Conte G, Sinco A, et al. Use of androgens in acquired aplastic anaemia. Relation of response to aetiology and severity. Acta Haematol 1980;64(1):18-24.
35. Najean Y. Long-term follow-up in patients with aplastic anemia. A study of 137 androgen-treated patients surviving more than two years. Joint Group for the Study of Aplastic and Refractory Anemias. Am J Med 1981;71(4):543-51.
36. Passweg JR, Socie G, Hinterberger W, et al. Bone marrow transplantation for severe aplastic anemia: Has outcome improved? Blood 1997;90(2):858-64.
37. Schrezenmeier H, Passweg JR, Marsh JC, et al. Worse outcome and more chronic GVHD with peripheral blood progenitor cells than bone marrow in HLA-matched sibling donor transplants for young patients with severe acquired aplastic anemia. Blood 2007;110(4):1397-400.
38. Storb R, Leisenring W, Anasetti C, et al. Long-term follow-up of allogeneic marrow transplants in patients with aplastic anemia conditioned by cyclophosphamide combined with antithymocyte globulin. Blood 1997;89(10):3890-91.
39. Champlin RE, Perez WS, Passweg JR, et al. Bone marrow transplantation for severe aplastic anemia: A randomized controlled study of conditioning regimens. Blood 2007;109(10):4582-85.
40. Niederwieser D, Pepe M, Storb R, Loughran TP, Jr, Longton G. Improvement in rejection, engraftment rate and survival without increase in graft-versus-host disease by high marrow cell dose in patients transplanted for aplastic anaemia. Br J Haematol 1988;69(1):23-28.
41. Eapen M, Ramsay NK, Mertens AC, Robison LL, DeFor T, Davies SM. Late outcomes after bone marrow transplant for aplastic anaemia. Br J Haematol 2000;111(3):754-60.
42. Deeg HJ, Leisenring W, Storb R, et al. Long-term outcome after marrow transplantation for severe aplastic anemia. Blood 1998;91(10):3637-45.
43. Passweg JR, Perez WS, Eapen M, et al. Bone marrow transplants from mismatched related and unrelated donors for severe aplastic anemia. Bone Marrow Transplant 2006;37(7):641-49.
44. Horowitz MM. Current status of allogeneic bone marrow transplantation in acquired aplastic anemia. Semin Hematol 2000;37(1):30-42.
45. Kosaka Y, Yagasaki H, Sano K, et al. Prospective multicenter trial comparing repeated immunosuppressive therapy with stem-cell transplantation from an alternative donor as second-line treatment for children with severe and very severe aplastic anemia. Blood 2008;111(3):1054-59.
46. Barker JN, Davies SM, DeFor T, Ramsay NK, Weisdorf DJ, Wagner JE. Survival after transplantation of unrelated donor umbilical cord blood is comparable to that of human leukocyte antigen-matched unrelated donor bone marrow: Results of a matched-pair analysis. Blood 2001;97(10):2957-61.
47. Tichelli A, Socie G, Henry-Amar M, et al. Effectiveness of immunosuppressive therapy in older patients with aplastic anemia. European Group for Blood and Marrow Transplantation Severe Aplastic Anaemia Working Party. Ann Intern Med 1999;130(3):193-201.
48. Marsh J. Making therapeutic decisions in adults with aplastic anemia. Hematology Am Soc Hematol Educ Program 2006:78-85.

Chapter 18

Secondary Leukemia

Seema Tyagi, Prashant Sharma

DEFINITION

The term secondary leukemia refers to malignant hematopoietic neoplasms of the blood and bone marrow arising in patients who have received chemotherapy, radiotherapy or other treatments for any indication. The indication for the primary therapy may have been a hematopoietic neoplasm or a solid malignancy. A smaller number of patients have suffered from initial nonmalignant disorders, usually diseases treated with cytotoxic or immunosuppressive therapy like autoimmune disorders. Another significant group is patients who have undergone hematopoietic stem cell transplantation following marrow ablation by high-dose chemoradiotherapy who subsequently develop another distinct leukemia.[1-3] Table 18.1 lists some common associations.

The underlying presumption in this definition is that the secondary leukemia is a direct consequence of the iatrogenic intervention. However, this may be difficult to prove in each individual case. Additionally, host factors may influence susceptibility to the development of these sequelae of therapy.

Adopting this definition of secondary leukemia, we restrict discussion in this chapter to essentially therapy-related neoplasms. Not included in this discussion are the accelerated and blast phases of chronic myeloproliferative neoplasms, leukemias in persons with inherited bone marrow failure syndromes or PNH, leukemias-lymphomas associated with infectious agents like Epstein-Barr virus and HIV and leukemias arising following environmental toxin and radiation exposures.

Table 18.1: Underlying primary disorders treated with drugs associated with risk of development of secondary leukemia

Hematologic neoplasms: Hodgkin lymphoma, non-Hodgkin lymphoma, multiple myeloma, acute lymphoblastic leukemia, acute myeloid leukemia, chronic myeloproliferative neoplasms
Solid tumors: Carcinomas of breast, ovary, prostate, lung, cervix, testicular tumors, Ewing sarcoma, primitive neuroectodermal tumor, neuroblastoma, osteosarcoma, Wilms tumor, rhabdomyosarcoma
Nonmalignant disorders: Rheumatoid arthritis, Wegener granulomatosis, seizure disorders, psoriasis, multiple sclerosis, severe congenital neutropenia

Relevance of secondary leukemia: The development of a secondary neoplasm is one of the most devastating sequelae of cancer. Secondary tumors may be of any histologic subtype, ranging from benign and low-grade tumors to high-grade malignant ones. Acute leukemias are the commonest secondary neoplasms, and include acute myeloid leukemia (AML)/myelodysplastic syndrome (MDS) and acute lymphoblastic leukemia (ALL). Rarer are therapy related chronic myeloid leukemia and other leukemias. These sequelae of treatment assume increasing importance as current therapeutic regimens increase the life spans and quality of life of patients with malignant disorders.[1-3]

Therapy-related MDS and t-AML are in particular important to study for several reasons:
1. They represent the most serious long-term complications to current cancer chemoradiotherapy and are, in most cases, uniformly fatal.
2. They are directly induced by well-characterized chemical agents or irradiation with well-known cellular and genomic effects.
3. They possess similar chromosomal aberrations and genetic mutations as *de novo* MDS and AML, allowing better insights into both types of disease.
4. An early stage of MDS with refractory cytopenia is often diagnosed in therapy-related disease, because most patients are followed thoroughly after intensive chemotherapy or irradiation. In *de novo* AML, such information is often lacking.[4,5]

These disorders are therefore dealt with first.

Therapy-related Myeloid Neoplasms

Therapy-related myeloid neoplasms (t-MDS/t-AML) are the better characterized of all the therapy-related acute leukemias. They represent 10 to 20% of all acute leukemias, MDS, and myelodysplastic/myeloproliferative neoplasms. They were first reported in the 1970s following combination chemotherapy and radiotherapy for lymphoma and myeloma. During the early 1970s, several groups reported an excess risk of s-AML in adults and children with Hodgkin lymphoma who received combined mechlorethamine, vincristine, procarbazine, and prednisone (MOPP) chemotherapy or similar alkylating agent regimens. The Late Effects Study Group observed that survivors of Hodgkin lymphoma who had been treated with alkylating agents at age 16 years had a relative risk of leukemia that was nearly 80 times that of population controls.

Knowledge in this field has expanded over the years with insight into the diverse genetic pathways leading to their development. Cases arise roughly equally after treatment of hematologic and nonhematologic malignancies. Latency periods and clinical manifestations vary depending on the cytotoxic drug, cumulative dose, and dose intensity.[2,4-8]

Etiology and clinical characteristics of t-AML/t-MDS: A variety of cytotoxic agents have been implicated in the development of t-MDS/t-AML

(Table 18.2). The classical examples are alkylating agents (e.g. busulfan, cyclophosphamide, chlorambucil) and topoisomerase II inhibitors (e.g. etoposide, daunorubicin, mitoxantrone) responsible for 2 distinct clinical syndromes. Additionally, antimetabolites (e.g. methotrexate, 6-mercaptopurine, fludarabine) have been linked to the genesis of t-MDS/ t-AML. Alkylating agents are often combined with other drugs or with radiotherapy and are also used as myeloablative therapy, thereby resulting in additive effects.[5-7] The pathogenesis and clinical characteristics of the two major groups, i.e. alkylating agent versus topoisomerase II inhibitor associated acute leukemia are described in Table 18.3. Their pathological features are discussed later.

Other drugs implicated in the development of t-MDS/t-AML include platinum-based agents and histone deacetylase inhibitors like valproic acid, hydroxyurea (Table 18.2) and miscellaneous drugs frequently used to treat hematopoietic and solid tumors. G-CSF in patients treated with chemotherapy or in patients with severe congenital neutropenia also increases risk of therapy-related leukemia.[1-7]

Table 18.2: Cytotoxic and other chemotherapeutic and supportive agents implicated in the development of t-MDS/t-AML

Alkylating agents: Busulfan, Carboplatin, Carmustine, Chlorambucil, Cisplatin, Cyclophosphamide, Dacarbazine, Dihydroxybusulfan, Lomustine, Mechlorethamine, Melphalan, Mitomycin C, Nitrogen mustard, Procarbazine, Semustine, Thiotepa

Topoisomerase II inhibitors: Amsacrine, Bimolane, Dactinomycin, Daunorubicin, Doxorubicin, 4-Epi-doxorubicin, Etoposide, Mitoxantrone, Razoxane, Teniposide

Antimetabolites: Fludarabine, 6-Mercaptopurine, Methotrexate

Antimicrotubule agents: Docetaxel, Paclitaxel, Vinblastine, Vincristine, Vindesine

Radiotherapy: Usually large fields involving active bone marrow, e.g. conditioning before HSCT, large-field therapeutic irradiation

Growth factors: G-CSF and GM-CSF in context of radiochemotherapy

Immunomodulator: Azathioprine

Pathogenesis of t-AML/MDS

In *de novo* AMLs, two types of genetic lesions cooperate in leukemogenesis. Activating *class I mutations* lead to constitutive activation of receptor tyrosine kinases or the downstream RAS-BRAF-MEK-ERK signal transduction pathway with resultant increase in cell proliferation and survival. These are accompanied by inactivating *class II mutations* involving genes encoding for hematopoietic transcription factors that disturb cellular differentiation. Inactivating mutations of the p53 tumor suppressor gene may represent a third class of mutations.[7,9]

Similar pathways have been mapped in t-MDS/t-AMLs. Leukemias following *alkylating agents* which induce centromeric chromosome breakage are characterized by complex karyotypes (Table 18.3). There is loss of either entire chromosomes 5 and 7 or the loss of their long arms. The primary mechanism of action is induction of double-stranded DNA

Table 18.3: Alkylating agent versus epipodophyllotoxin-associated t-AML

	Alkylating agent associated t-AML	Topoisomerase II inhibitors (mainly epipodophyllotoxins) associated t-AML
Relative frequency	~50% of t-AML/t-MDS	~30% of t-AML/t-MDS
Commonly associated drugs	Busulfan, Chlorambucil, Cisplatin, Mitomycin C, Cyclophosphamide, Dacarbazine, Melphalan	Etoposide, Tenoposide, Mitoxantrone, Actinomycin D, Daunorubicin, Doxorubicin
Latency	Average 5-10 years (range 1-20 years)	Median 2-3 years (range 1-10 years)
Relation to increasing age	Incidence increases with increasing age	Mostly age independent incidence
Nature of relation with drug	Cumulative dose determines evolution period	Administration schedule (frequent, intermittent dosing) likely to influence risk. Less clear relationship with total dose.
Synergism with concurrent L-asparaginase or G-CSF	Not established	Yes
Synergism with ionizing radiation	Established relationship	Less well established
Preceeding myelodysplastic phase	Frequent, bone marrow failure is usual presentation, leading to frank dysplasia with < 5% blasts.	Usually not seen, especially with prior G-CSF therapy also.
Morphological correlations	Panmyelosis, multilineage dysplasia, blasts often < 5% in initial phases, ring sideroblasts in up to 60% cases, fibrosis in 15%.	Blasts often ≥ 20% at first suspicion of secondary leukemia. Significant monocytic component is characteristic. Most cases are FAB AML-M4/M5. M2, M3, MDS and M7 are seen but uncommon. ALL with t(4;11) also reported.
Immunophenotypic correlations	No clear pattern. Multiple subtle or marked abnormalities of maturation are common even in cases with < 20% blasts. Increased expression of MDR-1 glycoprotein on blasts.	Usually corresponds to the subtype of AML recapitulated. Aberrant expressions are common.
Common genetic abnormalities	High incidence of clonal cytogenetic abnormalities, primarily monosomy or unbalanced translocations or deletions of chromosomes 5 and 7, nonrandom involvement of chromosomes 1, 4, 12, 14 and 18 with complex cytogenetics being very common.	Predominantly balanced translocations involving 11q23 (*MLL* gene), often t(9;11) and t(6;11). Others include t(8;21), t(15;17), t(3;21), inv(16), t(8;16)(p11;p13) and t(6;9). Rarer recurrent genetic abnormalities include 3q21q26, 11p15, t(9;22) (q34;q11)
Prognosis	Usually treatment refractory, associated with short survival.	Most cases respond to chemotherapy similar to *de novo* AML with similar risk profile. Long-term outcome poor.

breaks with a propensity to the centromeric and pericentromeric regions of chromosomes 1, 5, 7, 13, 17, 21, and 22. Two genetic pathways have been defined for this group of diseases. One group with deletion of long arm of chromosome 7 or monosomy 7 is often accompanied by AML1 mutations and abnormalities of RAS or p53. Another group is characterized by loss of chromosome 5 (monosomy 5 or 5q–) and, in a proportion of cases, is accompanied by –7/7q–. The majority of these leukemias show mutations of the p53 tumor suppressor gene or abnormalities of chromosome 17 that affect p53 function.[5-7,9]

In contrast, cases arising in the context of *topoisomerase II inhibitors* show predominantly balanced translocations (Table 18.3). Topoisomerase II inhibitors prevent the re-ligation of DNA and stabilize the topoisomerase-DNA complex, facilitating crossover recombination of nonhomologous DNA strands. The topoisomerase II cleavage sites include MLL/11q23, AML1, ETO, core-binding factor (CBF) β and NUP98. RAS or BRAF mutations frequently accompany MLL/11q23 translocations. Therapy-related leukemias with involvement of CBF-β, especially those with AML1 involvement are also associated with defects of chromosome 7. A group of therapy-related leukemias with a PML-RARa translocation show relatively high frequency of FLT3 mutations.[7,9]

Approximately 20% of patients with t-MDS/t-AMLs possess a normal karyotype by conventional cytogenetics. Similar to *de novo* normal cytogenetics AML, this group frequently has mutations of the FLT3, RAS, and AML1 genes. There is no clear cut association with a specific therapy. These may represent truly sporadic cases with only coincidental exposure to cytotoxic therapies.[10]

Impact of concomitantly administered chemotherapeutic agents: L-asparaginase administration possibly enhances the risk of epipodophyllotoxin induced t-AML. The precise mechanism is unknown, but it is speculated that the asparaginase enzyme downregulates the synthesis of specific proteins that protect from etoposide-induced recombinogenesis. This was used to explain the high incidence of t-AML in clinical studies with chronic exposure to high-dose asparaginase (25,000 IU/m^2) weekly for up to 20 weeks. Some of these investigators subsequently postulated that asparaginase exposure immediately before epipodophyllotoxin administration accounted for the increased incidence of t-AML. The combination of epipodophyllotoxins and alkylating agents (e.g. cisplatin) or antimetabolites (e.g. mercaptopurine or methotrexate) also has been associated with an increased incidence of t-AML.[11,12]

Hematopoietic stem cell transplantation: Various second malignancies including leukemias have been reported in hematopoietic stem cell transplant recipients. Estimated incidence of t-AML/t-MDS among non-Hodgkin and Hodgkin lymphoma patients undergoing autologous transplants ranges between 1 to 14% at 3-15 years. Patients undergoing autologous hematopoietic cell transplants for breast cancer, germ cell tumors or myeloma appear to be at lower risk.[13,14]

Recognized risk factors for a second malignancy include age, extent of prior therapy and exposure to certain agents before and during the transplantation procedure. Genotoxic damage and stresses imposed on hematopoietic stem cells during the priming or mobilizing chemotherapy and engraftment also play a role. Pre-transplantation preparative conditioning chemotherapy and total body myeloablative irradiation for autologous transplantation are likely potent contributors along with DNA repair during the extensive cellular proliferation associated with engraftment. Clonal hematopoiesis has been identified in some patients prior to development of overt secondary disease. The inherited polymorphisms in genes governing drug metabolism and DNA repair likely contribute to leukemogenesis and are discussed later.[12,14,15]

Studies of the latency periods between first cytotoxic exposure, the autologous HSCT itself, and the emergence of therapy-related leukemia suggest that the initial malignant event occurs prior to HSCT in most patients. However, the cytotoxic therapy delivered during the HSCT is likely additive to previous genomic damage and contributes to the etiology by cooperating mutations. Post-transplant t-AML/t-MDS often shows features of alkylating agent-associated disease, although it is unclear whether these alkylating agents or other factors play an exclusively causative role.[12-15]

Therapy-related leukemia after breast cancer therapy and an adjunctive role for G-CSF: These are dealt with separately as several large studies have examined the risks for women receiving adjuvant chemoradiotherapy for breast cancer. In six trials by the National Surgical Adjuvant Breast and Bowel Project, the relative risk of therapy-related leukemia was 6.7 times higher among patients receiving intensified doses of daunomycin and cyclophosphamide who required G-CSF support. Breast radiotherapy further increased the risk 2.38 times. In another study, 1.8% of the women who received chemotherapy for breast cancer who also received G-CSF or GM CSF developed therapy-related leukemia as compared to 1.0% of those who did not receive growth factors. A case-control study matched 182 patients who developed therapy-related leukemia after breast cancer treatment with 534 controls. The risk of leukemia was markedly increased after topoisomerase-II inhibitors and was higher after mitoxantrone than after conventional anthracyclines. The risk was increased 3.9-fold after breast radiotherapy. The risk was increased still further among those who received G-CSF even after controlling for chemotherapy doses.[16-18]

Genetic Susceptibility to t-MDS/AMLs

t-MDS/t-AMLs develop in only a small proportion of patients exposed to cytotoxic agents. This suggests there may be host's predispositions to leukemogenic potentials of chemotherapy and radiotherapy. Detoxification and DNA repair protect organisms against harmful environmental influences, including endogenous and exogenous oxidants, drugs and other xenobiotic chemicals. Polymorphisms in detoxification and DNA repair enzymes have been correlated with an increased risk of therapy-related neoplasms. These gene polymorphisms are responsible for individual differences in susceptibility to DNA damage and ability to repair potentially carcinogenic genetic aberrations including those caused by chemotherapy.[7,10,15]

Two major enzyme systems are involved in detoxification: The cytochrome P450 family (phase 1) and the metabolizing/conjugating enzymes involved in phase 2 metabolism. Several polymorphisms of the cytochrome P450 enzyme system have been implicated in metabolizing cytotoxic drugs and environmental pollutants. CYP11 has a role in bioactivation of polycyclic aromatic hydrocarbons and its CYP1A1*2A polymorphism is associated with increased enzyme expression. Even though the individual contribution of this polymorphism to the development of t-MDS/t-AMLs is yet to be established, this variant, in combination with other enzyme polymorphisms is associated with an increased risk of t-MDS/t-AML.[10,19,20]

CYP3A4 is another cytochrome P450 system enzyme involved in the metabolism of epipodophyllotoxins, cyclophosphamide and vinblastine. A CYP3A4-V polymorphism results in decreased production and lower levels of the toxic metabolites of these drugs. Studies have shown a significant difference in the frequency of this polymorphism between therapy-related versus *de novo* pediatric AML. However, the significance of this association has been questioned by other reports.[10,20-22]

Phase II drug-detoxifying enzymes include sulfonyl transferase, glucuronosyl transferase, NADPH:quinone oxidoreductase NQO1, eposide hydrolase, glutathione S-transferase (GST) and N-acetyl transferases. These are responsible for conjugation and enhanced secretion of xenobiotics and toxic metabolites into bile and urine. Polymorphisms of these enzymes are reportedly associated with both *de novo* and t-MDS/t-AMLs. For instance, a higher degree of homozygous and heterozygous NQO1*2 polymorphisms are seen in patients with t-MDS/t-AML that are associated with abnormalities of chromosomes 5 and 7. Similarly, GSTs metabolize many cytotoxic drugs including alkylators and topoisomerase II inhibitors through conjugation to reduced glutathione. Their main function is to prevent DNA damage following cytotoxic therapy. There is a significant variation in the GSTs across populations. Various *GST polymorphisms* (e.g. GSTM1, GSTT1 and GSTP1) either solely or in association with other metabolic pathway polymorphisms are over-represented in people with t-MDS/t-AMLs.[10,20]

DNA repair safeguards the integrity of the genome by preventing persistence of potentially carcinogenic mutations and gene rearrangements. Double stranded DNA breaks that arise following chemotherapy or exposure to radiation result in cell death or in gene rearrangements contributing to leukemogenesis. Individual capacities to repair damaged DNA vary widely. RAD51 is a central gene involved in the repair of double-stranded DNA breaks that is essential for maintenance of genomic stability. Polymorphisms in RAD51 (and its paralog gene XRCC3) are linked to susceptibility to breast and bladder cancers as well as t-MDS/t-AML.[7,10,20]

Nucleotide excision repair is another pathway with a role in DNA repair after environmental or iatrogenic genotoxin exposure. Polymorphisms in one component of the nucleotide excision repair pathway, the xeroderma pigmentosum complementation group D (XPD) gene has been reported to be associated with high-risk cytogenetic changes involving chromosomes 5 and 7 in t-AML. Defects in the *DNA mismatch repair genes* detected by microsatellite instability are described in t-MDS/t-AMLs arising in patients with prior malignancy and in organ-transplant recipients treated with azathioprine.[23,24]

Current understanding of gene polymorphisms and other potential factors predisposing to therapy-related myeloid neoplasms is rapidly expanding. Even though select pathways are implicated, identification of individuals with a propensity to develop therapy-related leukemia is not yet feasible. High throughput gene array techniques may help identify susceptible phenotypes in the future. Prototype models of such genome-wide approaches have identified novel pathways and novel candidate genes in patients at high-risk for t-MDS/t-AML.[25]

Pathological Features of t-AML/t-MDS

Pathological Definition

The 2008 WHO classification groups t-AML, t-MDS and t-MDS/MPN in a single unique clinical syndrome of "therapy related myeloid neoplasms, ICD-O code 9920/3" described as late complications of cytotoxic chemotherapy and/or radiotherapy administered for a prior neoplastic or non-neoplastic disorder. Nearly equal numbers of patients have a past history of treatment for hematological and for nonhematological disorders. Between 5-20% patients have a past history of non-neoplastic diseases and HSCT each.[26]

Morphology of Therapy Related Myeloid Neoplasms

The peripheral blood shows cytopenias. Anemia is almost always present and the RBCs show macrocytosis, poikilocytosis and cytoplasmic basophilia. Dysplastic changes in the neutrophils include abnormal nuclear lobation, especially hypolobation, and cytoplasmic hypogranularity.

The bone marrow in the majority of patients present with t-AML/t-MDS shows multilineage dysplasia. It may be hypo-, normo- or hypercellular, and shows mild to marked fibrosis in about 15% cases. Dysgranulopoiesis and dyserythropoiesis are seen in most patients, and ring sideroblasts are present in up to 60% cases. Megakaryocytes are often reduced but show dyspoietic features including widely separated nuclei, small hypolobate forms and micromegakaryocytes.

The blast percentage varies and differentiation between t-AML (blasts more than or equal to 20%) and t-MDS (blasts <20%) may not always be useful. t-AML following epipodophyllotoxins frequently lacks a preceeding myelodysplastic phase.

Immunophenotype

There is no distinctive immunophenotypic abnormality that distinguishes *de novo* from t-MDS/t-AML. Immunophenotypic studies reflect the underlying disease heterogeneity and are often similar to their *de novo* counterparts. Blasts are CD34 positive, and show pan-myeloid antigens like CD13 and CD33. Aberrant expression of CD7 and CD56 is common. Maturing non-blast cells may show light scatter and signal intensity different from their normal counterparts.

Genetic Pathways

Over 90% of t-MDS and t-AML show abnormal karyotypes. And about 70% have unbalanced chromosomal translocations, mainly involving chromosomes 5 or 7. The remainder 20-30% have balanced translocations, often involving 11q23 and other common recurring abnormalities.

In an attempt at classification of therapy-related myelodysplasia (t-MDS) and acute myeloid leukemia (t-AML), at least eight alternative genetic pathways have been defined based on characteristic recurrent chromosome abnormalities. Patients presenting as t-MDS and patients presenting as overt t-AML cluster differently in these pathways. The cytogenetic pattern depends on the type of leukemogenic therapy received: Alkylating agents, topoisomerase II inhibitors, or radiotherapy. These eight alternative genetic pathways in t-MDS and t-AML are outlined in Table 18.4.[8,27]

Factors Influencing Outcome in t-MDS/t-AML

Therapy-related leukemia is unfortunately mostly a terminal disease. Its life-threatening nature is the result of persistent and profound multilineage cytopenias due to the failure of normal hematopoiesis. Supportive care is still considered by most centers as standard management. A number of factors may explain the poor outcome of patients with therapy-related leukemia. The persistence of the primary malignant disease, particularly metastatic cancer or lymphoma, causes morbidity and mortality independent of the bone marrow failure caused by leukemia.

Injury to organs and their vascular supply from prior treatment compromises the ability of these patients to tolerate intensive chemotherapy or stem cell transplantation. Normal hematopoietic stem cells are depleted from previous therapy, hence these patients suffer prolonged cytopenias after induction chemotherapy. The marrow stroma is damaged especially by therapeutic radiation to fields that include the pelvis or lumbosacral spine. Regeneration of normal hematopoiesis is therefore defective. Patients with t-AML are often also chronically immunosuppressed from prior disease or ongoing therapy and have defective phagocyte function. They are thus often hosts to pathogenic antibiotic-resistant bacteria and fungi.

Table 18.4: Alternative genetic pathways in t-MDS and t-AML

Pathway I. Patients with 7q–/–7 but normal chromosomes 5 and without balanced aberrations. Characteristically present as t-MDS. Occur following therapy with alkylating agents. Point mutations of AML1 are frequent. Significantly associated with subsequent progression to overt t-AML.

Pathway II. Patients with 5q–/–5, but without balanced aberrations. Present as t-MDS or t-AML. Most cases show p53 mutations and complex chromosome rearrangements. Primarily observed after alkylating agents. Occasionally, also have 7q–/–7.

Pathway III. Patients with overt t-AML and balanced translocations involving 11q23, resulting in chimeric rearrangements between the MLL gene and one of its numerous alternative partner genes. Overt leukemias, often of FAB subtypes M4 or M5. Significantly associated with previous therapy with topoisomerase II inhibitors, primarily epipodophyllotoxins. NRAS, KRAS or BRAF mutations are common.

Pathway IV. Patients with balanced translocations to chromosome band 21q22 or inv(16). Lead to chimeric rearrangement between the core binding factor genes AML1 or CBFB. Except for cases with the t(3;21), such patients characteristically present as overt t-AML. Frequently follow therapy with anthracyclines. Patients of this type with de novo AML show point mutation of the receptor tyrosine kinase cKIT as the most common additional mutation.

Pathway V. Patients with acute promyelocytic leukemia and chimeric rearrangement of the RARa gene at 17q21. Responsive to retinoic acid with favorable prognosis, they are grouped separately. In t-AML, often relate to previous therapy with mitoxantrone for breast cancer. Like patients with *de novo* acute promyelocytic leukemia, they often present with FLT3-ITD duplications.

Pathway VI. Patients with t-MDS or t-AML and chimeric rearrangement of the NUP98 gene on 11p15. Most are related to therapy with topoisomerase II inhibitors. So far, no other specific mutations have been observed to cluster in patients belonging to this pathway.

Pathway VII. Patients with a normal karyotype. Point mutations of NPM1 gene, CEBPA and FLT3-ITD have been observed: contribute differently to the prognosis of the disease. Also, point mutations of RAS and internal tandem duplications of MLL are occasionally observed in t-AML with a normal karyotype. In t-MDS and t-AML, a normal karyotype is often observed in clinically atypical cases without association to any specific type of previous therapy.

Pathway VIII in t-MDS and t-AML. Comprises other, often unique chromosome aberrations. Trisomy 8 may belong to this pathway or represent a separate entity. Patients in pathway VIII with "other aberrations" are not associated with any specific type of previous therapy. Only rarely show mutations of RAS-BRAF signal transduction pathway or of transcription factors.

Following prior supportive care, patients may be refractory to additional transfusion support. These are particularly suboptimal candidates for intensive myelosuppressive chemotherapy. The high frequency of unfavorable cytogenetic aberrations arising during or after chemoradiotherapy appears to result in the rapid emergence of chemotherapy resistance in t-AML stem cells.[1,3,6,15]

Treatment and Outcome of Secondary AML

The poorer prognosis of t-AML than that of *de novo* AML, the disease refractoriness to chemotherapy and low tolerance of these patients to treatment because of prior therapies limit the use of curative (i.e. highly intensive) therapies. Survival rates of patients with t-AML are difficult to predict and are often affected by recurrence of the primary cancer. In one study treated patients with t-AML had lower rates of remission induction, survival and event-free survival than patients with *de novo* AML. Outcomes were better among patients (including patients with t-AML) assigned randomly to receive intensively timed induction therapy than among those receiving standard-timed induction.[1,3,6,15,28,29]

Other investigators have speculated that the comparatively low survival rate of t-AML patients results from the predominance of t-AML with unfavorable karyotypes. Poor survival also correlates with advanced age, lower performance status and the presence of comorbidities with t-AML in adults. After adjustment for risk factors, the outcomes of pediatric and adult patients with t-AML are comparable to outcomes in *de novo* AML after hematopoietic stem cell transplantation.[1,3,6,15,28,29]

A management algorithm for adult t-AML using performance status, age, comorbidities, primary disease status, complications of primary therapy and karyotype has been proposed (Fig. 18.1). According to this algorithm, patients with t-AML who have a good performance status should be treated in a manner similar to the treatment for patients with *de novo* AML with the same cytogenetic abnormalities, i.e. chemotherapy alone for favorable genetic features such as t(15;17), inv(16), and t(8;21); intensive chemotherapy and hematopoietic stem cell transplantation for other karyotypes; and investigational therapy in clinical trials for unfavorable karyotypes. Supportive care alone may be warranted for those with very poor performance status. The applicability of this approach to pediatric patients is not known.[30]

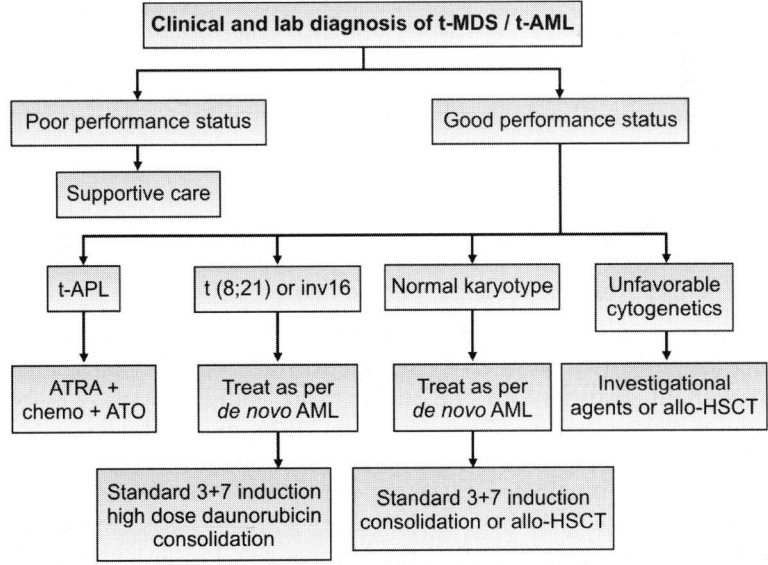

Fig. 18.1: Proposed treatment algorithm for t-MDS/t-AML (Larson, 2007)

ALL as a Secondary Malignancy

Although t-MDS/t-AML are well described, ALL after primary cancer is very rare. It is often unclear whether cases are secondary to the primary cancer or represent a second primary cancer. Herein, cases of ALL after cancer are termed 'secondary ALL' (s-ALL). These comprise 5 to 10% of all secondary acute leukemias. S-ALL has been reported after primary ALL, as well as after various other malignancies. The apparent rarity of s-ALL after primary ALL may also be due to the majority of cases being misdiagnosed as recurrence of the primary ALL. Epipodophyllotoxins can be associated with therapy-related ALL as well. These frequently show a t(4;11)q21;q23) abnormality.[31-34]

Molecular level studies of immunoglobulin and T-cell receptor gene rearrangements facilitate identification of s-ALL. Using these methods, Zuna et al estimated that between 0.5 to 1.5% of their 366 cases of 'recurrent' ALL were actually s-ALL. The malignant clones in all s-ALL cases differed from those at the time of diagnosis. The duration of first complete remission ranged from 1.7 years to 6.5 years. The authors proposed diagnostic criteria for s-ALL, but acknowledge obstacles to definitive diagnosis (Table 18.5). Another study identified different T-cell receptor gene rearrangement at diagnosis and late 'recurrence' of T-ALL in 5 of 16 patients, suggesting the diagnosis of secondary T-cell ALL rather than relapse. However, all their patients remained in complete remission after retrieval therapy, which is an unexpectedly good outcome for patients with recurrent T-ALL. Knowledge is likely to increase as more cases of s-ALL are identified using modern technologies.[31-34]

Table 18.5: Proposed diagnostic criteria for secondary ALL (Zuna et al, 2007)

A. **Essential factor:** No relation between ALL clones at diagnosis and at disease recurrence (immunoglobulin/T-cell receptor gene arrangements, fusion genes at DNA level, cytogenetic markers)

B. **Additional factors:**
   1. Significant immunophenotypic shift
   2. Significant cytogenetic shift
   3. Gain or loss of a fusion gene

For secondary ALL: A plus at least 1 B criterion should be fulfilled.

Other Therapy Related Secondary Leukemias

An increased incidence of chronic leukemia has also been observed among the patients who received therapeutic radiation for malignant and nonmalignant disorders. In one study 15,000 patients with ankylosing spondylitis treated with radiation between 1935 and 1954 were followed for almost 50 years. The updated results published in 1994 revealed seven patients with CML and seven with CLL. Another international case-controlled study of over 30,000 women treated with radiation for carcinoma cervix found that that the relative risk for all leukemias rose twofold, and the relative risk for CML was 4.2.[35,36] The risk is believed to be negligibly low with modern involved field radiotherapy.

CONCLUSION

Numerous studies confirm that treatment with the topoisomerase II inhibitors (epipodophyllotoxins and anthracyclines) and alkylating agents increases the probability of t-AML. The risk of t-AML is influenced by treatment factors, including the schedule of administration and concomitant medications. The role of host factors such as polymorphisms of detoxification enzymes and primary tumors should also be considered. The risks and benefits of using epipodophyllotoxins in frontline pediatric cancer treatment regimens are often unclear. The benefit of epipodophyllotoxins may outweigh the risk of s-AML in some cases of high-risk childhood ALL, although more studies are needed to confirm this possibility. In addition, the probability of t-AML may be reduced by controlling or considering other risk factors, such as concomitantly administered drugs, administration schedule, and host characteristics. Recent studies have demonstrated that the outcome of adults with t-AML does not differ from that of those with *de novo* AML when data are adjusted for unfavorable cytogenetic findings. More studies are needed to determine whether the same approach can be applied to pediatric patients. S-ALL has been reported very rarely, but more cases may be identified as modern technologies emerge.

REFERENCES

1. Dann EJ, Rowe JM. Best Pract Res Clin Haematol. Biology and therapy of secondary leukaemias 2001;14:119-37.
2. Leone G, Mele L, Pulsoni A, Equitani F, Pagano L. The incidence of secondary leukemias. Haematologica 1999;84:937-45.
3. Rowe JM. Therapy of secondary leukemia. Leukemia 2002;16:748-50.
4. Larson RA, Le Beau MM. Therapy-related myeloid leukaemia: A model for leukemogenesis in humans. Chem Biol Interact 2005;153-154:187-95.
5. Felix CA. Secondary leukemias induced by topoisomerase targeted drugs. Biochem Biophys Acta 1998;1400:233-55.
6. Smith MA, McCaffrey RP, Karp JE. The secondary leukemias: Challenges and research directions. J Natl Cancer Inst 1996;88:407-18.
7. Pedersen-Bjergaard J, Andersen MK, Andersen MT, et al. Genetics of therapy-related myelodysplasia and acute myeloid leukemia. Leukemia 2008;22:240-48.
8. Scholl C, Gilliland DG, Frohling S. Deregulation of signalling pathways in acute myeloid leukemia. Semin Oncol 2008;35:336-45.
9. Bhatia S, Robison LL, Oberlin O, et al. Breast cancer and other second neoplasms after childhood Hodgkin's disease. N Engl J Med 1996;334:745-51.
10. Czader M, Orazi A. Therapy-Related Myeloid Neoplasms. Am J Clin Pathol 2009;132:410-25.
11. Pui CH, Relling MV, Behm FG, et al. L-asparaginase may potentiate the leukemogenic effect of the epipodophyllotoxins. Leukemia 1995;9:1680-84.
12. Amylon MD, Shuster J, Pullen J, et al. Intensive high-dose asparaginase consolidation improves survival for pediatric patients with T cell acute lymphoblastic leukemia and advanced stage lymphoblastic lymphoma: A Pediatric Oncology Group study. Leukemia 1999;13:335-42.
13. Friedman DL, Leisenring W, Schwartz JL, Deeg HJ. Second malignant neoplasms following hematopoietic stem cell transplantation. Int J Hematol 2004;79:229-34.

14. Hake CR, Graubert TA, Fenske TS. Does autologous transplantation directly increase the risk of secondary leukemia in lymphoma patients? Bone Marrow Transplant 2007;39:59-70.
15. Hijiya N, Ness KK, Ribeiro RC, Hudson MM. Acute leukemia as a secondary malignancy in children and adolescents: Current findings and issues. Cancer 2009;115:23-35.
16. Le Deley MC, Suzan F, Cutuli B, et al. Anthracyclines, mitoxantrone, radiotherapy, and granulocyte colony-stimulating factor: Risk factors for leukemia and myelodysplastic syndrome after breast cancer. J Clin Oncol 2007;25:292-300.
17. Hershman D, Neugut AI, Jacobson JS, et al. Acute myeloid leukemia or myelodysplastic syndrome following use of granulocyte colony-stimulating factors during breast cancer adjuvant chemotherapy. J Natl Cancer Inst 2007;99:196-205.
18. Patt DA, Duan Z, Fang S, Hortobagyi GN, Giordano SH. Acute myeloid leukemia after adjuvant breast cancer therapy in older women: Understanding risk. J Clin Oncol 2007;25:3871-76.
19. D'Alo F, Voso MT, Guidi F, et al. Polymorphisms of CYP1A1 and glutathione S-transferase and susceptibility to adult acute myeloid leukemia. Haematologica 2004;89:664-70.
20. Bolufer P, Collado M, Barragan E, et al. Profile of polymorphisms of drug-metabolising enzymes and the risk of therapy-related leukaemia. Br J Haematol 2007;136:590-96.
21. Rund D, Krichevsky S, Bar-Cohen S, et al. Therapy related leukemia: Clinical characteristics and analysis of new molecular risk factors in 96 adult patients. Leukemia 2005;19:1919-28.
22. Collado M, Barragan E, Bolufer P, et al. Lack of association of CYP3A4-V polymorphism with the risk of treatment-related leukemia. Leuk Res 2005;29:595-97.
23. Seedhouse C, Foulkner R, Ashraf N, et al. Polymorphisms in genes involved in homologous recombination repair interact to increase the risk of developing acute myeloid leukemia. Clin Cancer Res 2004;10:2675-80.
24. Smith AG, Worrillow LJ, Allan JM. A common genetic variant in XPD associates with risk of 5q- and 7q-deleted acute myeloid leukemia. Blood 2007;109:1233-36.
25. Hartford C, Yang W, Cheng C, et al. Genome scan implicates adhesion biological pathways in secondary leukemia. Leukemia 2007;21:2128-36.
26. WHO Classification of tumours of Haematopoietic and Lymphoid tissues, 4th edn. Swerdlow SH et al (Eds.). IARC press (Lyons) 2008.
27. Pedersen-Bjergaard J, Christiansen DH, Desta F, Andersen MK. Alternative genetic pathways and cooperating genetic abnormalities in the pathogenesis of therapy-related myelodysplasia and acute myeloid leukemia. Leukemia 2006;20:1943-49.
28. Kern W, Haferlach T, Schnittger S, Hiddemann W, Schoch C. Prognosis in therapy-related acute myeloid leukemia and impact of karyotype. J Clin Oncol 2004;22:2510-11.
29. Abdelhameed A, Pond GR, Mitsakakis N, et al. Outcome of Patients Who Develop Acute Leukemia or Myelodysplasia as a Second Malignancy After Solid Tumors Treated Surgically or With Strategies That Include Chemotherapy and/or Radiation. Cancer 2008;112:1513-21.
30. Larson RA. Etiology and Management of Therapy-Related Myeloid Leukemia. Hematology 2007:453-59.
31. Zuna J, Cave H, Eckert C, et al. Childhood secondary ALL after ALL treatment. Leukemia 2007;21:1431-35.

32. Geetha N, SreedeviAmma N, Kusumakumary P, Lali VS, Nair MK. Acute lymphoblastic leukemia occurring as a second malignancy: Report of a case and review of literature. Pediatr Hematol Oncol 1999;16:267-70.
33. Hunger SP, Sklar J, Link MP. Acute lymphoblastic leukemia occurring as a second malignant neoplasm in childhood: Report of 3 cases and review of the literature. J Clin Oncol 1992;10:156-63.
34. Szezepanski T, van der Velden VHJ, Van Vlierberghe PV, et al. Late relapses of childhood T-ALL are frequently second T-ALL [abstract]. Blood 2007;110:430a.
35. Weiss HA, Darby SC, Fearn T, Doll R. Leukemia mortality after X-ray treatment for ankloysing spondylitis. Radiat Res 1995;142:1-11.
36. Boice JD Jr, Blettner M, Kleinerman RA, Stovall M, Moloney WL, Engholm G, et al. Radiation dose and leukemia risk in patients treated for Cancer of the cervix. J Natl Cancer Inst 1987;79:1295-311.

Chapter 19

Current Pathogenesis and Therapy in Essential Thrombocythemia

VP Choudhry

SUMMARY

There are now clear evidences that essential thrombocytosis is a clonal disorder as shown by identification of JAK-II mutation in majority of patients. Currently its annual incidence has been estimated between 1 to 2.5 per 100,000 individuals. Arterial thrombosis is three times more common than venous thrombosis. Common sites for arterial thrombosis include CNS, cardic system. Hepatosplenomegaly is secondary to extramedullary hematopoiesis. It is paradoxical that patients have bleeding symptoms when platelet counts are above 1000-1500 × 10^9/L. It may also evolve into myelofibrosis. The etiopathogenesis of myelofibrosis could be secondary to busulfan/hydroxyurea therapy or as a result of the natural progression of the disease. Its current pathogenesis along with molecular studies have been reviewed. The treatment depends upon the risk stratification. Current modalities of treatment include hydroxyurea, anagrelide, interferon alpha along with futuristic therapies have been reviewed. Pregnancy associated with essential thrombocytosis is a special condition which has adverse effects on the mother and fetus. There is a need for collaborative studies to determine the safe and effective therapy of ET during pregnancy.

KEYWORDS

Essential thrombocythemia, Pathogenesis, Management.

Essential thrombocythemia (ET) is characterized by increase in peripheral platelet count and is associated with increase in megakaryocytes without erythrocytosis or leukoerythroblastosis. It had been recognized as one of the myeloproferative disorders (MPD). As per WHO a platelet count of 600 × 10^9/L along with megakaryocytic hyperplasia without clinical, pathological or molecular evidences of polycythemia vera (PV), primary myelofiberosis (PMF), chronic myeloid leukemia (CML), myelodysplastic syndrome (MDS) or reactive thrombocytosis was essential for diagnosis of ET (Table 19.1).[2] The identification of Janus Kinase 2 (JAK2) mutation (JAK2 V617F an exon 14 somatic 1849 G > T mutation) in PV in 95% of cases and 50% of cases with ET and PMF lead to the belief that these are clonal disorders.[3-7] More recently JAK2 (exon 12 mutations) and MPL W515L/K have been identified in individuals who were negative for JAK2. (exon14) mutation.[8,9]

Table 19.1: World Health Organization criteria for essential thrombocythemia, 2001

Positive criteria
1. Sustained platelet count > 600 × 10^9/L.
2. Bone marrow biopsy showing proliferation of megakaryocytic lineage with large number of mature megakaryocytes.

Exclusion criteria
1. No evidence of polycythemia vera
   a. Normal red cell mass or Hb. < 18.5 gm/dl in men, < 16.5 gm/dl in women.
   b. Normal MCV/ Serum ferritin or stainable iron in bone marrow.
2. No evidence of chronic myeloid leukemia, absence of philadelphia chromosome or BCR-ABL fusion gene.
3. No evidence of chronic idiopathic myelofibrosis
   a. Collagen fibrosis absent
   b. Minimal/absent reticulin fibrosis.
4. No evidence of myelodysplastic syndrome.
   a. No del (5q), + (3:3)(q21: q26), inv(3) (q21 : q26)
   b. No significant granulocytic displasia.
5. No evidence of reactive thrombocytosis
   a. Underlying inflammation/infection
   b. Prior splenectomy
   c. Presence of any neoplasm.

Table 19.2: Revised WHO criteria for essential thrombocythemia

1. Sustained platelet count > 450 × 10^9/L
2. Bone marrow biopsy showing proliferation of megakaryocytic lineage with increase in mature megakaryocytes. No significant increase or left shift of myelopoiesis or erythropoiesis.
3. Demonstration of JAK 2617 V > F or other clonal marker. In absence of clonal marker reactive thrombocytosis must be excluded.
4. Absence WHO Criteria for PV, PMF, MDS, or CML.

With these developments WHO has revised the diagnostic criteria's and now any patient with platelet count of more than 450 × 10^9/L can be classified as ET (Table 19.2).[1] In spite of detailed clinical, pathological and molecular investigations at times it is difficult to distinguish between ET and cellular phase of PMF.[11] In the present review the epidemiology and clinical features are being described briefly while the emphasis will be in the current pathogenesis and therapy.

EPIDEMIOLOGY

ET was earlier regarded as the least common among the various myeloproferative disorders. With frequent use of cell counters in all laboratories and current WHO criteria, ET is now more common than CML.[12] Annual incidence of ET is 1 to 2.5 per 100,000 individuals.[13] It is believed that annual incidence may be higher than estimated as most patients with ET generally are asymptomatic and thus are never diagnosed. Presently nearly 50% of patients with ET are symptomatic and are diagnosed as cases of ET. ET is a disease of elderly (over 50 years of age with equal incidence among men and women). However, there is second peak around 30 years which affects women more frequently.[13] The reasons why it is more common in women at younger age are not well understood.

Clinical Features

Predominant clinical features are secondary to thrombotic events in the microvessels/~ beds.[14,15] In the uncontrolled studies cumulative rates for thrombosis and bleeding range from 7 to 17% and 8 to 14% respectively.[16] In a control population study thrombotic episodes were seen in 6.6% per patient year in ET versus 1.2% of control subjects while hemorrhagic complications was observed in 0.33% per patient per year.[17] Arterial thrombosis is three times more common than venous which occur as deep venous thrombosis, portal and hepatic vein thrombosis. Common sites for arterial thrombosis include brain, heart and extremities.[14] Microvascular thrombi may result in headache, paresthesia, and digital ischemia. These microvascular phenomena may occur in ET even when platelet counts are as low as $400 \times 10^3/L$.

Extramedullary hematopoiesis may occur in liver or spleen. Splenomegaly is observed in 20-50% of cases while hepatomegaly may be seen in 15-20% of cases. When the platelet count is more than 1000-1500 $\times 10^9/L$ patients are at higher risk of bleeding.[18,19] Bleeding commonly occurs in the skin, mucous membrane and gastrointestinal tract. It has been observed that in some cases, ET may evolve into myelofibrosis or leukemia.[13] Most common type of leukemia to occur in association with ET is acute myeloid leukemia (M_4 or M_7).[20] It has been reported that hydroxyurea therapy may be responsible for development of acute leukemia. However, recent studies support the above hypothesis that busulfan, hydroxyurea either alone or in combination may have some leukemogenic effect.[21,22]

Reactive thrombocytosis, hereditary and neoplastic conditions need to be excluded before making a diagnosis of ET (Table 19.3 and Fig. 19.1). Reactive thrombocytosis commonly occurs in iron deficiency anemia, acute blood loss, hemolytic anemia, postsplenectomy, various inflammatory conditions (tuberculosis), drug reactions (vincristine, cytoklines, growth factors).[25] Thus it is essential to have detailed clinical history, hematological

Table 19.3: Difference between essential thrombocythemia and reactive thrombocytosis

Features	Essential thrombocythemia	Reactive thrombocytosis
Anemia	–	+
Thrombotic/hemorrhagic events	+	–
Splenomegaly	+	–
Iron deficiency	–	+
Clonal hematopoiesis	+	–
Increased megakaryocytes clustering/hyperlobulation	+	–
Abnormal cytogenetics	+	–
Abnormal platelet aggregation	+	–
Increased acute phase reactants	–	+

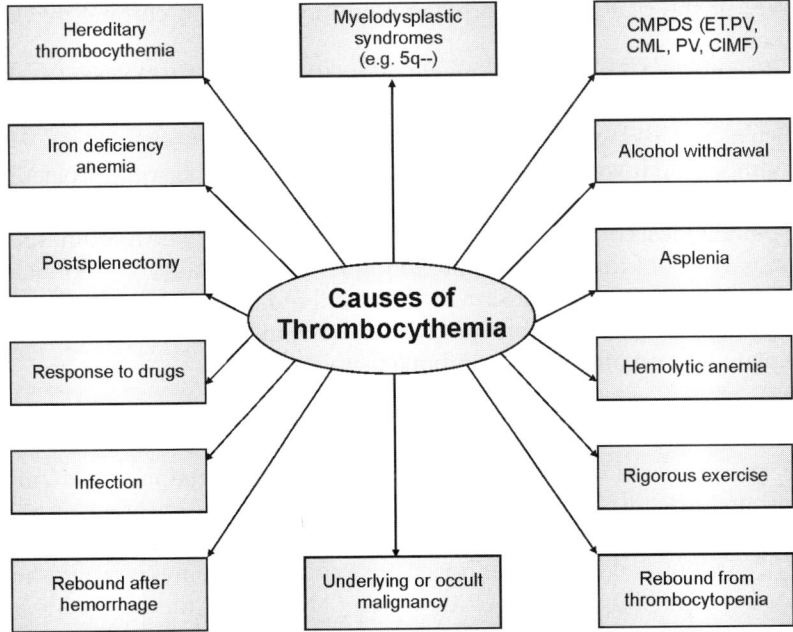

Fig. 19.1: Causes of thrombocythemia

tests, bone marrow, bone biopsy, molecular and other relevant tests for definitive diagnosis of ET.

PATHOGENESIS

Currently it is believed that ET is a clonal proliferation of stem cells with predominately megakaryocytic differentiation. DNA and RNA, X-chromosome inactivation studies have revealed that nearly half of cases have polyclonal hematopoiesis while the rest have monoclonal hematopoiesis.[14,23,24] Increased risk of thrombosis has been observed in patients with monoclonal group. While no significant differences were observed in platelet count, age at diagnosis or presence of splenomegaly when the data was compared between monoclonal vs polyclonal hematopoiesis in ET. Thrombopoietin (TPO) levels may be high or normal which is in contrast to erythropoietin level in PV. The elevated TPO level in ET may be secondary to abnormal TPO receptor (MPL). Normally TPO binds to MPL receptor in order to stimulate proliferation of megakaryocytes.[20] Increased MPL and mRNA expression has been observed in bone marrow cells.[26]

Defective platelet aggregations have been observed in over 70% of cases with ET. Abnormal response to epinephrine in 58%, collagen in 38% and adenosine diphosphate in 11% of cases. However, these abnormalities did not co-relate with bleeding time or bleeding episodes.[27] Alpha- granules are decreased in platelets which normally contain platelet factor IV, factor V and XIII and fibrinogen. In addition deficiency of von Willebrand factor

(VWF) in the platelets is more common in ET than in chronic myeloid leukemia.[28]

Patients of ET with very high platelets (1000-1500 × 10^9/L) are at higher risk of bleeding which is paradoxical[18,19] and it has been attributed to VWF deficiency or dysfunction of VWF termed as AvWS (loss of large VWF multimers).[14] However, the exact pathogenesis of higher risk of bleeding associated with very high platelet counts is not well understood. Similarly the pathogenesis of thrombosis in ET is ill-understood. The hypothesis for increased risk of thrombosis is based upon increased polymorphonuclear leukocytes (PMN) activation. PMN also bind with platelets through increased CDIIb expression on activated cell membrane which activate the platelets and other prothrombotic factors.[10,29,30]

MOLECULAR STUDIES

Several studies identified mutation in PV in which guanine to thymine transversion leading to valine to phenylalanine substitution at codon 617 is acquired as a somatic mutation (JAK2 V617F).[31,32] However, this allele has not been identified in the germline of any patients with myeloproliferative disorders. Two largest studies identified JAK2 V617F mutations in 53 to 55% of patients with ET.[33,34]

Subsequent studies revealed that JAK2 V617F mutant erythroid colonies are present in nearly all patients with polycythemia vera, but rarely in patients with ET.[35,36] These studies indicated that homozygosity is a common pathogenetic event in PV but not in ET. More studies are required to determine if cells with heterozygous and homozygous for JAK2 V617F have differential signaling characteristics. The possibility of additional mutations which play an important role in phenotype of JAK2 V617F positive hemopoietic progenitor cells, cannot be excluded.

Presuming that JAK2 has central role in cytokine receptor signaling, several investigators felt whether mutation in cytokine receptor can activate signaling in JAK2 V617F negative ET. Recently Beer and his colleagues identified somatic MPL mutation in ET.[37] Vannucchi and his colleagues screened 994 ET patients for MPL W515L/K mutation identified in 3% of all ET patients and in 5% of JAK2 V617F negative ET patients.[34] MPL W515 studies have shown that MPL W515L is a gain of function allele since expression of MPL W515L induces hematopoietic cells to cytokine- independent growth and activation of JAK2 along with other signaling pathways such as STAT3, STAT5, MAPK and P13K/AKT.[38] Further studies are essential to determine the clinical, molecular and therapeutic correlates. Presently there are evidences of increased risk of arterial thrombosis in patients with JAK2 V617F positive mutation when treated with anagrelide as compared with patients who were negative for this mutation.[33] Recent studies have indicated that hydroxyurea therapy was more effective in patients who were positive for JAK2 V617F mutation there by suggesting that these cells are more sensitive to hydroxyurea.[39]

Diagnosis

A platelet count of > 450 × 10^9/L is required as per WHO diagnostic criteria (on 2 occasions and 2 months apart) with exclusion of other causes of thrombocytosis. Platelets show anisocytosis, bizzare shapes and hypogranulation. White blood cells may be normal or mildly increased. Bone marrow biopsy is an important tool for diagnosis of ET. It may be normocellular to hypercellular. Presence of stainable iron and normal red cell mass is helpful in excluding iron deficiency anemia and PV. Megakaryocytes in ET are increased in number and size along with hyperlobated nuclei. The megakaryocytes are often in small clusters which are better appreciated on bone biopsy. Dysplastic and bizarre megakaryocytes are often seen in MDS and not in ET. Erythroid and myeloid series are normal. Reticulin fibrosis is minimal.

As stated earlier ET is a diagnosis of exclusion. Other causes of thrombocytosis need to be excluded (Table 19.3 and Fig. 19.1). Disorders such as myelodysplastic syndrome (MDS) particularly –5q syndrome, PV, iron deficiency anemia, hemolytic anemia, postsplenectomy, occult malignancy, acute or chronic infections need to be excluded.

MANAGEMENT

It is essential to evaluate the history of thrombotic or hemorrhagic events along with the presence of cardiovascular risk factors such as hypertension, smoking, diabetes and hypercholesterolemia as ET is disease of elderly people. ET has been classified into various risk categories based upon the risk of thrombosis and hemorrhages (Table 19.4).

Table 19.4: Risk categorization in essential thrombocytosis

Low-risk	Age < 60 years and
	No past history of thrombosis, absence of risk factors and
	Platelet count <1500 × 10^9/L.
Intermediate risk	Age 40-60 years and
	Presence of any cardic risk factors or
	Positive family history of thrombophilia and
	Platelet count < 1500 × 10^9/L.
High-risk	Age > 60 years or
	A previous history of thrombosis or major bleeding or
	Platelet count > 1500 × 10^9/L.

Low-risk

Cytoreduction therapy is an option in patients with low-risk group. In age and sex matched study with a median follow-up of 41 years the incidence of thrombosis was not significantly higher in controls (1.91% vs 1.5%).[40] Similarly there were no major bleeding episodes. Therefore, it is not essential to use cytoreduction therapy in ET in patients with low-risk.

Aspirin at different dose is able to control microvascular symptoms, transient neurologic and occular disturbance. Collaborative studies on low dose aspirin in PV(ECLAP study) clearly indicated that aspirin alone significantly lowered the cardiovascular deaths, nonfatal stroke and major venous thromboembolism.[41] Presently there are no control studies on use of aspirin in ET. If above evidences are considered then patients with low-risk can be easily managed with low dose aspirin alone.

Intermediate Risk

In a review Elliott and Tefferi concluded that in patients below 60 years with no previous history of thrombosis and platelet counts below 1500 × 10^9/L and absence of any cardic risk factors such as hypertension, diabetes, smoking, etc. should be treated with aspirin definitively, however, there was no consensus on cytoreduction therapy.[42] Patients with presence of any cardic risk factors or in presence of family history of thrombophilia need to be treated with cytoreduction therapy along with aspirin.

High-risk

There is consensus that all patients at high-risk of thrombosis (Table 19.3) need to be treated with cytoreduction along with low dose aspirin. Among the various drugs hydroxyurea and anagrelide have been evaluated in randomized clinical trials.

Hydroxyurea

It has emerged as the treatment of choice in high-risk patients with ET because of its efficacy and minimal toxicity. Its dose need to be adjusted to maintain platelet count around and 600 × 10^9/L. The main concern is its leukemogenic effect. In an analysis of 25 patients with ET who were younger than 50 years under went hydroxyura (HU) therapy, there was no leukemia or neoplastic transformation occurred after a median follow-up of 8 years (range 5-14 years).[43] In ECLAP prospective study on 1638 patients, hydroxyurea alone did not enhance the risk of leukemia.[44] However, it has been observed that the risk of acute leukemia transformation is higher in patients of ET who have cytogenetic abnormalities.[45] The 17 p deletion was observed in patients of ET who developed MDS or acute leukemia following HU treatment.[46] In a long-term study of 112 patients with ET none of 20 patients who never received any chemotherapy developed any malignancy as compared with 3 of 77 patients who received HU Therapy alone (3.9% p = not significant).[47] Guide Fianzzi and Clarie Harrison in their review concluded that HU remains the first drug of choice for patients of ET who require cytoreductive therapy.[48]

Anagrelide

It reduces platelet count but the exact mechanism of inducing thrombocytopenia is not well understood. In high doses, it inhibits the platelet aggregation by inhibition of phosphodiesterase III. The side effect of this drug includes palpitation, headache, and congestive cardic failure besides hyperacidity. In a large study over 7 years on 934 patients with ET, there was no evidence of increased risk for development of acute leukemia or myelofibrosis.[49] In another study of 35 young patients of ET who were treated with anagrelide for a median follow-up of 10.7 years, it was observed that 20% of patients had thrombotic complication. When the platelet counts were above $400 \times 10^9/L$.[50] It is good, effective and safe drug but it is essential that platelet count should be maintained below $400 \times 10^9/L$. Its dose should be so adjusted to maintain the platelet count at safe levels.

Interferon-alpha

It has been evaluated in several studies on patients with ET.[51] Platelet count could be reduced below $600 \times 10^9/L$ at least after 3 months of therapy with daily dose of 3MIU daily. Interferon-alpha is not known to cause any malignancy and does not cross the placenta. Therefore, it is very safe during pregnancy. The only draw back is its prohibitive cost and the side effects. The therapy was discontinued in 55% of cases because of its side effects. Therefore, it is not a drug of choice for treatment of ET. However, it is safe for patients with ET during pregnancy as compared with other agents.

Pregnancy and ET

ET is common in women during child bearing age. There are retrospective series of ET in which it has been reported that live birth rate varies between 50-57%, first trimester loss varied 26 to 36% and late pregnancy loss was observed between 5 to 9.6% of cases. In the same study the preterm delivery occurred between 5.6 to 8% of pregnant women and intrauterine growth retardation was observed between 4 to 5.1% of cases.[52,53] Thrombotic episodes involved sagittal sinus and deep vein thrombosis along with transient ischemic attacks. Most of these events were observed in postpartum period.[54] Thus there is a need of prophylaxis therapy during the postpartum period.

The management of ET during pregnancy is essential to decrease the morbidity, mortality and to improve the neonatal outcome. Patients with low-risk should be treated with aspirin and postpartum prophylaxis should be with low molecular weight heparin along with aspirin. Various options of treatment such as aspirin, low molecular heparin and alpha interferon need to be considered for patients with high-risk or disease related complications such as previous loss, severe intrauterine or thrombotic events. All these patients need to be monitored closely for any complications fatal and successful outcome. Presently there is no large study to form the basis of optimal treatment for pregnant women with ET. Therefore, there is a need for an international collaboration to define the best care during pregnancy and postpartum prophylaxis for these patients.

Future Therapies

Identification of somatic mutation which activates JAK2 signal transduction is the basis to develop novel therapies. Specific inhibitors of JAK2 will be safe and effective. Specific inhibitors of JAK2 kinase activity have been developed and have used for clinical phase I/II trrals.[55] Activation of multiple cellular processes is dependent upon JAK2 signaling system. Therefore, it is expected that there may be significant toxicities. Signal JAK2 specific inhibitor ICNB 018424 is orally bioavailable and inhibits JAK1 and JAK2 but not JAK3 or TYK2 signals. This agent has produced clinical improvement with modest reduction in JAK2 V617F allele burden. In higher doses it resulted in thrombocytopenia which reversed on withdrawal or reduction of therapy. Many question such as prevalence and severity of thrombocytopenia, modest reduction of JAK2 V617F allele burden, the optimal dose and duration of therapy, side effects of therapy, etc. need to be evaluated.

Studies are in progress towards development of other JAK2 inhibitors. However, other agents such as HDAC also selectively inhibitis JAK2 V617F positive cell growth.[56] Recently it has been observed that pegylated interferon alfa 2a resulted in complete hematological response and marked reduction in JAK2 V617F allele burden.[57] With all these development the newer therapies either singly or in combination will provide much better management strategies for patients with ET.

TAKE HOME MESSAGE

Essential thromocythemia is one of myeloproliferative disorder. It is being recognized more frequently because of wide use of cell counters. Its presentations are wide spread and are secondary to thrombotic events in the microvasculature. Its early recognition and appropriate management can prevent its complications and mortality. The treatment is life long and thus it is essential to monitor these patients regularly.

REFERENCES

1. Tefferi A, Thiele J, Orazi A, et al. Proposals and rationale for revision of the World Health Organization diagnostic criteria for polycthemia vera, essential thrombocythemia, and primary myelofibrosis: Recommendations from an ad hoc international expert panel. Blood 2007;110:1092-97.
2. Vardiman JW, Harris NL, Brunning RD. The World Health Organigation (WHO) classification of the myeloid neoplasms. Blood 2002;100:2292-2302.
3. Landolfi R, Cipriani MC, Novarese L. Thrombosis and bleeding in polycythaemia vera and essential thrombocythemia: Pathogenetic mechanisms and prevention. Best Pract Res Clin Haematol 2006;19:617-33.
4. Elliott MA, Tefferi A. Thrombosis and haemorrhage in polycythaemia vera and essential thrombocythemia. Br J Haematol 2005;128:275-90.
5. Carobbio A, Finazzi G, Guerini V, et al. Leukocytosis is a risk factor for thrombosis in essential thrombocythemia: Interaction with treatment, standard-risk factors, and Jak2 mutation status. Blood 2007;109:2310-13.

6. Landolfi R, Di Gennaro L, Barbui T, et al. Leukocytosis as a major thrombosis risk factors in patients with polycythaemia vera. Blood 2007;109:2446-52.
7. Carobbio A, Antonioli E, Guglielmelli P, et al. Leukocytosis and risk stratification assessment in essential thrombocythemia. J Clin Oncol 2008;26:2732-36.
8. Kralovics R, Passamonti F, Buser As, et al. A gain-of-function mutation of JAK2 in Myeloproliferative disorders. N Engl J Med 2005;352:1779-90.
9. Baxter EJ, Scott LM, Campbell PJ, et al. Acquired mutation of the tyrosine kinase JAK2 in human Myeloproliferative disorders. Lancet 2005;365:1054-61.
10. Marchetti M, Castolidi E, Spronk M.H, et al. Thrombin generation and activated protein C resistance in patients with essential thrombocythemia and polycythemia vera. Blood 2008;112:4061-68.
11. WilkinsBS, Erber WN, Bareford D, et al. Bone marrow pathology in essential thrombocythemia: Interobserver reliability and utility for identifying disease subtypes. Blood 2008;111:60-70.
12. Sanchez S, Ewton A, A review of diagnostic and pathologic features; Arch Pathol Lab Med 2006;130:1144-50.
13. Jaffe ES, Harris NL, Stein H, Vardiman JW. World Health Organization Classification of Tumours. Pathology and Genetics of Tumours of Haematopoietic and Lymphiod Tissues. IARC Press: Lyon 2001,39-42.
14. Elliot MA, Tefferi A. Thrombosis and haemorrhage in polycythaemia vera and essential thrombocythemia. Br J haematol 2005;128:275-90.
15. Cortelazzo S, Viero P, Finazzi G, D'Emilio A, RodeghieroF, Barbui T. Incedence and risk factors for thrombotic complications in historical cohort of 100 patients with essential thrombocythemia. J Clin Oncol 1990;8:556-62.
16. Barbui T, Barosi G, Grossi A, Guglitta L, Liberato LN, Marchetti M, et al. Evidence- and consensus-based practice guidelines for the therapy of essential thrombocythemia. A statement from the Italian Society of Hematology. Haematologica 2004;89:215-32.
17. Cortelazzo S, Viero P, Finazzi G, D'Emilio A, Rodeghiero F, Barbui T. Incidence and risk factors for thrombotic complication in a historical cohort of 100 patients with essential thrombocythemia. J Clin Onco 1990;l8:556-62.
18. Barbui T, Barosi G, Grossi A, et al. Practice guidelines for the theraphy of essential thrombocythemia: A statement from the Italian Society of hematology, the Italian Society of Haematologica 2004;89:215-32.
19. Michiels JJ, Berneman ZN, Schroyens W, Van Vliet HH. Pathophysiology and treatment of platelet-mediated microvascular disturbances, major thrombosis and bleeding complications in essential thrombocythemia and polycythaemia vera. Platelets 2004;15:67-84.
20. Shibata K, Shimamoto Y, Suga K, Sano M, MatsuzakiM, Yamagucjhi M. Essential thrombocythemia terminating in acute leukemia with minimal myeloid differentiation: A brief review of recent literature. Acta Haematol 1994;91:84-88.
21. Finazzi G, Barbui T. Treatmnet of essential thrombocythemia with special emphasis on leukemogenic risk. Ann Hematol 1999;78:389-92.
22. Mavrogianni D, Viniou N, MichaliE, et al. Leukogenic risk of hyroxyuera therapy as a single agent in polycythemia vera and essential thrombocythemia: N- and K-ras mutations and microsatellite instability in chromosomes 5 and 7 in 69 patients. Int J Hematol 2002;75:394-400.
23. Finazzi G, Harrison C. Essential thrombocythemia. Semin Hematol 2005;42:230-38.
24. Shih LY, Lin TL, Lai CL, et al. Predictive values of X-chromosome inactivation patterns and clinicohematologic parameters for vascular complications in female patients with essentail thrombocythemia. Blood 2002;100:1596-1601.
25. Anastasi J, Vardiman W. Chronic myelogenous leukemia and chronic myeloproliferative diseases. In: Knowles DM (Eds). Neoplastic Hematopathology. 2nd edn. Philadelphia. PA Lippincott Williams and Wilkins, 2001:1745-19.

26. Bock O, Schule J, Mengel M, Busche G, Serinsoz E, Kreipe H. Thrombopoietin receptor (Mpl) expression by megakaryocytes in myeloproliferatives disorders. J Pathol 2004;203:609-15.
27. Cesar JM, de Miguel D, Garcia Avello A, Burgaleta C. Platelet dysfunction in primary thrombocythemia using the platelet function analyzer, PFA-100. Am J Clin Pathol 2005;123:772-77.
28. Meschengieser S, Blanco A, Woods A, et al. Intraplatelet levelof vWF: Ag and fibrinogen in Myeloproliferative disorders. Thromb Res 1987;48:311-19.
29. Falanga A, Marchetti M, Barbui T, Smit CW. Pathogenesis of thrombosis in essential thrombocythemia and polycthemia vera: The role of neutrophils. Semin Hematol 2005;42:239-47.
30. Falanga A, Marchetti M, Vignoli A, Balducci D, Barbui T. Leukocyte-platelet interaction in patients with essential thrombocythemia and polycythemia vera. Exp Hematol 2005;33:523-30.
31. James C, Ugo V, Le Couedic JP, et al. A unique clonal JA mutation leading to constitutive signalling causes polycythaemia vera. Nature 2005;434:1144-48.
32. Kralovics R, Passamonti F, Buser AS, et al. A gain-of function mutation of JAK2 in myeloproliferative disorders. N Engl J Med 2005;352:1779-90.
33. Campbell PJ, Scott LM, Buck G, et al. Definition of subtypes of essential thrombocythaemia and relation to polycythaemia vera based on JAK2 V617F mutation status: A prospective study. Lancet 2005;366:1945-53.
34. Vannucchi AM, Antonioli E, Guglielmelli P, et al. Characteristic and clinical correlates of MPL 515W>L/K mutation in essential thrombocythemia. Blood 2008:112:844-47.
35. Scott LM, Scott MA, Campbell PJ, Green AR. Progenitors homozygous for the V617F mutation occur in most patients with polycythemia vera, but not essential thrombocythemia. Blood 2006;108:2435-37.
36. Dupont S, Masse A, James C, et al. The JAK2 617V>F mutation triggers erythropoietin hypersensitivity and terminal erythroid amplification in primary cells from patients with polycythemia vera. Blood 2007;110:1013-21.
37. Beer PA, Campbell PJ, Scott LM, et al. MPL mutations in myeloproliferative disorders: Analysis of the PT-1 cohort. Blood 2008;112:141-49.
38. Pikman Y, Lee BH, Mercher T, et al. MPLW515L is a novel somatic activating mutation in myelofibrosis with myeloid metaplasia. PLoS Med 2006;3:e270.
39. Sirhan S, Lasho TL, Hanson CA, Mesa RA, Pardanani A, Tefferi A. The presence of JAK2V617F in primary myelofibrosis or its allele burden in polycythemia vera predict chemosensitivity to hydroxyurea. Am J Hematol 2008;83:363-65.
40. Ruggeri M, Finazzi G, Tosetto, Riva S, Rodeghiero F, Barbui T. No treatment for low-risk essential thrombocythemia: Results from a prospective study. Br J Haematol 1998;103:772-77.
41. Landolfi R, Marchioli R, Kutti J, Gisslinger H, Tognoni G, Patrono C, et al. Efficacy and safety of low-dose aspirin in polycythemia vera. N Engl J Med 2004;350: 14-24.
42. Elliott MA, Tefferi A. Thrombosis and haemorrhage in polycythemia vera and essential thrombocythaemia. Br J Haematol 2005;128:275-90.
43. Finazzi G, Ruggeri M, Rodeghiero F, Barbui T. Efficacy and safety of long-term use of Hydroxyurea in young patients with essential thrombocythemia and a high-risk of thrombosis. Blood 2003;101:3749.
44. Finazzi G, Caruso V, Marchioli R, Capnist G, Chisesi T, Finelli C, et al. Acute leukemia in polycythemia vera. An analysis of 1638 patients enrolled in prospective observational study. Blood 2005;105:2664-70.

45. Lofverberg E, Noderson I, Walhlin A. Cytogenic abnormalities and leukemic transformation in hydroxyurea-treated with philadelphia chromosome negative chronic myeloproliferative disease. Cancer genet Cytogenet 1990;49:57-67.
46. Sterkers Y, Preudhomme C, Lai J-L, Demory J-L, Caulier MT, Wattel E, et al. Acute myeloid leukemia and myelodyslastic syndromes following essential thrombocythemia treated with hydroxyurea: High proportion of cases with 17p deletion. Blood 1998;91:616-22.
47. Finazzi G, Ruggeri M, Rodeghiero F, Barbui T. Second malignancies in patients with essential thrombocythemia treated with busulphan and hydroxyurea: Long-term follow-up of a randomized clinical trial. Br J Haematol 2000;110:577-83.
48. Finazzi G, Harison C. Essential Thrombocythemia. Semin Hematol 2005;42: 230-38.
49. Fruchtman SM. Treatment paradigms in the management of myeloproliferative disorders. Semin hematol 2004;41:18-22.
50. Storen EC, Tefferi A. Long-term use of anagrelide in young patients with essential thrombocythemia. Blood 2001;97:863-66.
51. Lengfelder E, Griesshammer M, Hehlmann R. Interferon-alpha in the treatment of essential thrombocythemia. Leuk Lymphoma 22:135-142,1996{suppl 1}.
52. Griesshammer M, Bergmann L, Pearson T. Fertility, pregnancy and the manage-mant of myeloproliferative disorders. Baillieres Clin Haematol 1998;11:859-74.
53. Griesshammer M, Grunewald M, Michiels JJ. Acquired thrombophilia in pregnancy: Essential thrombocythemia. Semin Thromb Hemost 2003;29:205-12.
54. Vantroyen B, Vanstraelen D. Management of essential thrombocythemia during pregnancy with aspirin, interferon alpha-2a and no treatment. A comparative analysis of the literature. Acta Haematol 2002;107:158-69.
55. Verstovek S, Kantarjian H, Pardanani A, et al. A phase I/II study of ICNB018424, an oral, selective JAK inhibitor, in patients with primary myelofibrosis and postPV/ET myelofibrosis [abstract]. J Clin Oncol. 2008:26 (May 20 suppl). Abstract #7004.
56. Guerini V, Barbui V, Spinelli O, et al. The histone deacetylase inhibitor ITF2357 selectively targets cells bearing mutated JAK2 (V617F). Leukemia 2008;22:740-47.
57. Kiladjian JJ, Cassinat B, Chevret S, et al. Pegylated interferon alpha-2a induces complete hematological and molecular responses with low toxicity in polycythemia vera. Blood 2008 July 23. Epub ahead of print.

Chapter 20
Current Management of Idiopathic Thrombocytopenic Purpura

Tulika Seth

Idiopathic thrombocytopenic purpura (ITP), is a benign condition which causes great anxiety and stress in both its acute and chronic forms. Clinical management decisions have traditionally been guided by individual training and experience. The supporting literature had been in the form of observational reports and case series. Practice guidelines and several important studies in clinical hematology practice have highlighted the important questions in the field. Recent laboratory investigations have produced valuable new information on the pathophysiology. Many guidelines for management have been devised for pediatric and adult patients.[1-4] However, though acute ITP can be successfully and promptly managed, chronic ITP can still be a difficult disease entity causing much distress to the patients as they traverse the multitude of treatment regimens.

It is important to exclude secondary causes if ITP prior to initiating treatment as these disorders warrant special attention and require specific therapeutic interventions.

We shall review some of the current practice guidelines in this report.

Diagnosis

A thorough history and physical examination is required, many patients may present with dengue, drug related complications and other infections. A detailed hematological evaluation is required after with a complete blood count, and peripheral smear. Care is to be taken to exclude pseudo-thrombocytopenia due to EDTA-dependent platelet agglutination. Exclude HIV and Hepatitis B and C by performing the required baseline tests. An autoimmune screen to exclude other underlying autoimmune diseases may be performed, if symptomatic.[3,5]

Bone marrow examination is a required procedure, particularly in the Indian context where most patients will be treated with steroids, due to cost considerations and follow-up of patients cannot be assured due to patient noncompliance. However, if the case appears as a typical ITP and intravenous gammaglobulin is to be given, then the bone marrow evaluation may be deferred. Patients older than 60 years have a higher risk of myelodysplatic syndrome or lymphoproliferative disorders and warrant a bone marrow examination. Prior to performing a splenectomy patients should have a bone marrow examination to exclude other differentials.

Special cases may need evaluation of a direct Coomb's test to exclude coexisting immune hemolytic anemias in Evans syndrome; Immunoglobulin levels are needed if there is a history of recurrent infections, severe allergy, reactions to IVIG or prior blood transfusions (common variable immunodeficiency or IgA deficiency).

Helicobacter pylori infection work up may be needed in chronic refractory patients as suggested by the literature.[1,3,5]

Management

As ITP has varied presentations and there are some differences in adult and pediatric patients there is no uniform treatment. Guidelines are available for both Adult and pediatric ITP.[1-7] Special care is needed during acute emergency management. Then there is chronic patient management and refractory cases or pregnant women need different treatment strategies

- Acute
  - Emergency
  - Nonemergency
- Chronic
  - Stable
  - Nonstable
  - Special cases

Acute

Pediatric acute ITP may not need treatment, as it is a benign self-limiting disorder, usually with mild clinical symptoms and has a low-risk for serious bleeding (approximately 3% with intracranial hemorrhage). Hence many cases can be observed and therapy started only in children with overt signs of bleeding and platelet counts that are in the range that may cause significant hemorrhage. Based on these guidelines, intervention is reserved for the few children who have overt hemorrhage and platelet counts below 20×10^9/L or those who have organ- or life-threatening bleeding irrespective of the circulating platelet count.[1,2,4]

Though many centers set at $< 20 \times 10^9$/L as a limit to start therapy, this cut off depends on availability of supportive care, accessibility of patients to the hospital and their awareness level. Many centers may set a higher cut off for treatment depending on their resources. Children with acute ITP and mild clinical disease may be managed expectantly with supportive advice and a 24 hours contact point, irrespective of the platelet counts. The full blood counts should be repeated within 10 days of diagnosis, to evaluate for any evidence of any a serious marrow disorder. Subsequent counts are not required to be monitored until resolution of clinical symptoms and for documenting remission or there are other clinical indicators suggesting their need.[1,2]

Emergency Treatment

Patients with profound mucocutaneous, e.g. hematuria, extensive skin bleeds or suspected internal bleeding need immediate hospitalization. Patients who present with platelet counts of less than 20,000/µL with a history of significant bleeding, or if any concern regarding compliance to treatment need to be admitted. Emergency treatment is similar for both adults and children.

Emergent treatment includes any of the treatment regimens:
- IV Immunoglobulin 1 g/kg for 1-2 days
- IV Anti-D 75 µg/kg - single dose
- IV Methylprednisolone 30 mg/kg (Max. 1 gm/day) for 3 days
- Addition of IV Vincristine to the above regimens
- Addition of fVIIa if uncontrolled bleeding.

Supportive care in the form of platelet transfusion for serious hemorrhage and hemostatic agents, e.g. tranexamic acid or €-aminocaproic acid are needed (unless there is hematuria, when they are contraindicated). Hormonal preparations are useful for controlling menorrhagia which can be so severe as to cause anemia and even require blood transfusions.[1,2]

The use of immunotherapy with anti-D or IVIg avoids the need for a marrow since immunotherapy, in contrast to glucocorticoids, has no masking effect on the diagnosis of acute lymphoblastic leukemia, or may result in tumor lysis from lymphomas. However, both anti-D and IVIg share the problem of drug reactions including fever, chills, urticaria, and particularly headache. In a patient with a platelet count below 10,000/ml and a severe headache, a CT scan is required to rule out an intracerebral hemorrhage. Less common complications from immunotherapy include severe acute hemolytic anemia with possible renal failure with both anti-D and IVIg.

IVIg can raise the platelet count rapidly, but should be reserved for emergency treatment of serious bleeding symptoms or in children undergoing procedures likely to induce blood loss. It is effective given as a single dose of 0.8-1 g/kg. Lower doses have fewer side effects in younger children and may still be effective. Platelet transfusions should only be given for intracranial hemorrhage or other life-threatening bleeding, and the requirement is in much larger doses than for marrow failure. Platelets should not be given alone, but under cover of immunomodulatory treatment such as high dose intravenous steroids or IVIg. Although the platelet count may not increase substantially, bleeding often can be controlled by this measure. 80-90% of initially responsive patient will require additional therapy within 6 months, only < 5% will be primary refractory to first line therapy.[1,2]

Acute ITP

Although observation may be the best option for most patients with ITP, there are several primary therapies available for patients with significant bleeding.

Nonemergent Treatment

- Corticosteroids — prednisolone
- High dose dexamethasone
- IV immunoglobulin
- Anti- D
- Splenectomy
- Corticosteroid

If a child has mucous membrane bleeding and more extensive cutaneous symptoms, high dose prednisolone 4 mg/kg/day is effective. It can be given as a very short course (maximum 4 days). There are no direct comparisons of low dose (1-2 mg/kg/day) with high dose therapy. If lower doses of 1-2 mg/kg/day are used the treatment should be given for no longer than 14 days, irrespective of response.

In adults 2/3rd of patients will respond to prednisolone at 1-2 mg/kg/day for 4-6 weeks, with a slow taper over several weeks. Corticosteroids have a direct effect on vascular integrity and they reverse thinning of endothelium. Hence, purpuric bleeding stops 3-4 days before actual platelet count rise. Corticosteroids should be rapidly tapered and stopped in patients who fail to respond after 4 weeks.[1]

IV Immunoglobulin (IVIg)

Effective in elevating the platelet count in 75-85% of patients, of which 50% will achieve normal platelet counts. Responses may be transient and after 3–4 weeks following IVIg treatment the platelet counts may fall. Immunoglobulin (IVIg) in acute ITP has many applications, it may be used in emergency, preparation for splenectomy in Rh negative, DCT positive patients in particular, may help to defer splenectomy in children, and can be used in pregnancy.

Anti-D Ig

Is given as a single IV infusion of 50-75 µg/kg, similar response as IVIg in efficacy and rapidity with an initial response rate of 71%. This product is less expensive than IVIg. However, this product can only be given to Rh (D) positive patients who do not have a positive antiglobulin test, or active hemolysis, anemia, cirrhosis of liver, or renal insufficiency. Studies suggest it has limited efficacy in postsplenectomized patients. The utility of anti-D has been shown in ITP emergency management as an alternative to IVIg and to prepare for splenectomy.

Splenectomy

- Splenectomy is rarely indicated in childhood ITP,[5,6] may be required selected cases of acute ITP in adult patients.

Chronic ITP

Children and adults with chronic ITP usually do not need active therapy but should be followed up regularly. They need to be counseled regarding their platelet counts, which may continue to abnormal for a long period. They need reassurance that therapy is only required for bleeding episodes and that there is little risk because of mild or moderate thrombocytopenia. Stable chronic ITP does not require treatment but only observation.

Only 15-20% become chronic, very few refractory, chronic refractory ITP are patients who fail to respond to first line treatment or require unacceptably high doses of corticosteroids to maintain a safe platelet count. Most adult patients have good response to therapy (without necessarily normal platelet count) have a normal life span when compared to general population.[1,2]

Splenectomy is an excellent option for chronic symptomatic adult patients. To date considered the Gold Standard for treatment of ITP, CR-66% (Median follow-up 29 months) and an excellent safety profile as mortality rates are 1% for laparotomy, 0.2% for laparoscopy. Due consideration needs to be taken in individual cases regarding risk of post-splenectomy sepsis, which may be an issue for rural or poor patients. Splenectomy is rarely indicated in childhood ITP. It is occasionally justified for life-threatening bleeding and a platelet count below $10 \times 10^9/L$ (children ages 3 to 12) or 10 to $30 \times 10^9/L$ (children ages 8 to 12 years) and for children with chronic unremitting and severe ITP whose disease has been present for more than 12-24 months with significant impairment of quality of life or sequelae of therapy (Grade C recommendation). Generally Indian patients are averse to splenectomy, even though it is an effective and cost efficient modality of treatment. In our experience this is usually the last line of treatment for both adults and children in India, because of patient choice.[1,2]

Splenectomy Sparing Options for Chronic ITP

These may be a necessity in patients unwilling, or not suitable candidates for splenectomy.

Options for Chronic ITP

- High dose steroids
- Intermittent infusion of anti-D (Rh + patients)
- Anti-CD20 antibody — Rituximab
- Danazol
- Dapsone
- Immunosuppressive agents including azathioprine and cyclophosphamide, mycophenolate mofetil
- Combination therapy
- Thrombopoietic growth factors

High Dose Steroids

Dexamethasone for adults is given as a dose of 40 mg/d for 4 days, initial response rate 85%, with 6 months response rate of 50%. However, needs good supportive care to manage steroid side effects. Repeated doses 40 mg/d for 4 days every 15 days for 4 cycles—showed similar results, the median duration of response is usually 8 months (4-24 months), also has been used in children at a lower dose.

Other schedules which are effective are 40 mg of dexamethasone daily for 4 d, repeated every 28 d for six cycles, methylprednisolone was given at 30 mg/kg/d for 3 d, 20 mg/kg/d for 4 d then 5, 2 and 1 mg/kg/d each for 1 week.[1,2,5]

Intermittent Infusions of Anti-D

This is recommended when platelet < 30,000/µl, it carries a 43% response rate. It may defer splenectomy but may not prevent the need for splenectomy, this is safe in children.[1,5-7]

Rituximab

Is given in adults at a dose of 375 mg/m^2 once a week for 4 weeks with an overall response rate of 55% and durable responses which last for 6 months to 1 year (Median duration- 74 weeks). The rise in platelets is seen in some patients after 1-2 infusions and, peaks by 6-10 weeks. This is not influenced by splenectomy, hence is an option postsplenectomy. Due to concerns in pediatric patients, it is to be used with caution in only selected children. Side effects include serum sickness, reactivation of Hepatitis B in carriers and progressive multifocal leukoencephalopathy.[1,2]

Intravenous Gammaglobulin (IVIg)

This is given usually in a dose of 1 g/kg per day for one or two consecutive days, often in combination with corticosteroids, may be repeated every 2–3 weeks.[1,2] Cost is the major barrier to repeated use in Indian patients.

Vincristine

Most effective when used in combination with other agents, has been used for 2-4 weeks and indefinately. 10% response rate for refractory ITP, vincristine 1-1.5 mg/m^2, max 2 mg, or vinblastine 4-6 mg/m^2, max 10 mg, IV have been safely used.[1,2]

Azathioprine

It is associated with 20-40% response rates, and takes a median time of 4 months for response. Dose of 1-3 mg/kg/day (given at bedtime) to maintain ANC 1500/µl. Implicated with side effects of, e.g. elevation of serum transaminases, diarrhea, nausea and depression.[1,2]

Danazol

Has response rates of 20-40% at a dose of 10-15 mg/kg/day for 4-6 months. It is usually used to defer splenectomy, and as a steroid sparing agent. May be associated with increase in cholesterol, masculization, menstrual changes, cholestatic hepatic injury and rarely associated with neoplasia.[1,2]

Dapsone

Has been used at a dose of 75-100 mg orally, in adults. It has response rate of 50%, the median duration of treatment required to achieve a response of 21 days, associated with little toxicity, however, G-6-PD should be ruled out before initiation.[1,2]

Cyclophosphamide

Has been used in combination with prednisolone and vincristine in refractory ITP, usual dose is 1-1.5 gm/m^2 every 3 weeks. The common side effects are alopecia, hemorrhagic cystitis, infertility and a risk of development of leukemia.

Others

Cyclosporine and mycophenolate mofetil and combination therapies have also been used in a few studies.

Thrombopoietic Growth Factors

Romiplostim (TPO peptide), Eltrombopag, (TPO nonpeptide) AKR-501 and TPO against antibodies. Minibodies are being used and have shown efficacy in trials, Indian experience is lacking.[1,2]

All of these treatments should be reserved for patients with chronic, symptomatic disease. Patients who have a concomitant autoimmune disease (e.g. SLE) or congenital or acquired immunodeficiency require treatment of the underlying problem. Chronic, refractory ITP in children or adults remains a challenge, this group has the greatest risk of serious bleeding, particularly among the elderly. Evidence for treatment for ITP needs more prospective, randomized clinical trials.[1,2,4]

Surgical guidelines for ITP patients: In general, patients with platelet counts exceeding 30,000/µl require no treatment unless they are undergoing any procedure likely to induce blood loss including surgery, dental extraction or delivery.

Recommendation for "Safe" Platelet Counts in Adults (BCSH)[3]

- Minor surgery > 50,000/µl
- Major surgery > 80,000/µl
- Dentistry > 10,000/µl
- Extractions > 30,000/µl
- Regional dental block > 30,000/µl.

REFERENCES

1. Arnold DM, Kelton JG. Current options for the treatment of idiopathic thrombocytopenic purpura. Semin Hematol 2007;44(4 Suppl 5):S12-23.
2. McMillan R. Immune-mediated thrombocytopenias: Focus on chronic immune thrombocytopenic purpura. Semin Hematol 2007;44(4 Suppl 5):S1-2.
3. Guidelines for the investigation and management of idiopathic thrombocytopenic purpura in adults, children and pregnancy. British journal of Hematology 2003,120,574-96.
4. Beardsley DS. ITP in the 21st century. Hematology Am Soc Hematol Educ Program 2006:402-07.
5. Kalpatthi R, Bussel JB. Diagnosis, pathophysiology and management of children with refractory immune thrombocytopenic purpura. Curr Opin Pediatr 2008;20: 8-16.
6. Buchanan GR, Adix L. Current challenges in the management of children with idiopathic thrombocytopenic purpura. Pediatr Blood Cancer 2006;47:681-84.
7. Tarantino MD, Bolton-Maggs PHB. Update on the management of immune thrombocytopenic purpura in children. Curr Opin Hematol 2007;14:526-34.

Chapter 21

Minimal Residual Disease (MRD) Detection in Acute Leukemia

Seema Tyagi, Sanjeev Kumar Gupta

SUMMARY

Minimal residual disease (MRD) detection provides important information on treatment response and has a strong correlation with the risk of relapse and thus, gradually becoming a crucial constituent of many modern treatment protocols. Early detection and monitoring of MRD has a proven role in clinical management of acute lymphoblastic leukemia (ALL) as well as in acute myeloid leukemia (AML). The advantages and limitations of various MRD detection techniques and their application in different types of acute leukemia will be highlighted in this review.

What is Minimal Residual Disease (MRD)?

Minimal residual disease (MRD) refers to the persistence of resistant malignant cells in the bone marrow and/or peripheral blood which are detectable by highly sensitive assays when the patient appears to be in complete remission. Postinduction therapy, one million or more leukemic cells may persist, even when the residual cells are undetectable, i.e. the patient appears to be in complete molecular remission.[1]

Bradstock et al (1981) provided the first account of MRD detection when they reported that the anti-TdT (terminal deoxynucleotidyl transferase) antibody in combination with an anti-T-cell antibody could identify MRD in the bone marrow of patients with T-ALL (T-acute lymphoblastic leukemia) in morphologic remission.[2] In the subsequent years, the development of multicolor flow cytometry (FCM) and DNA and mRNA based molecular techniques have provided sensitive, precise, and reliable tools for MRD detection resulting in their widespread use in hematological malignancies.[3]

The Rationale for Testing the Minimal Residual Disease in Acute Leukemia

Monitoring response to treatment by periodic evaluation of bone marrow aspirates is an integral part of the acute leukemia management. The status of residual leukemic and the normal marrow components, based on cellular morphology, provide an indication of the sensitivity of leukemic cells to chemotherapy and of the degree of hematopoietic regeneration activity occurring during various treatment intervals. However, the resemblance of leukemic cells to normal hematopoietic progenitors makes it difficult to separately identify them even for an experienced hematopathologist, unless leukemic cells have striking morphological traits, such as Auer rods. In the absence of such findings, a patient with less than 5% blasts is considered in remission but may still harbor ~ 10^{10} leukemic cells and may remain undertreated. These small numbers of leukemic cells may also be missed by comparatively lesser sensitive techniques like conventional cytogenetics and fluorescent *in situ* hybridization (FISH). Similarly, the morphological similarities between leukemic cells and normal hematopoietic cells (e.g. hematogones) may lead to overestimation of the leukemia burden resulting in over-treatment thus necessitating the need to develop sensitive and objective methods to measure minimal residual disease.[4]

Clinical Importance of MRD Detection

MRD detection finds various clinical applications these days, the most important of which is prognosis. The early detection of the expansion of resistant leukemic cells is associated with a higher risk of relapse. Thus, accurate and precise measurement of MRD can help in early prediction of relapse and in selection of patients for treatment intensification based on the poor response to therapy. Conversely it may help identify the good responders who may be the candidates for de-intensification of treatment avoiding the toxic effects of unnecessary chemotherapy. MRD detection has also proved useful in predicting the optimal timing of hematopoietic stem cell transplantation (HSCT) and better understanding of the mechanisms of drug resistance.[1,3,5]

Basic Principle of MRD Assays

The common principle underlying all MRD assays is that molecular and cellular changes induced by the leukemogenic process are used to distinguish leukemic cells from normal.[6] These leukemia associated features are identified using various techniques at diagnosis or relapse and then used to monitor MRD.[4]

What is the Optimal MRD Technique?

Optimal MRD technique should be patient specific (or at least leukemia specific), with satisfactory sensitivity (at least 10^{-4}, i.e. one malignant cell among 10,000 normal cells), applicable for the vast majority of patients, have stable target during the course of disease, feasible (easy standardization and less turn around time) as well as show intralaboratory and interlaboratory reproducibility.[5]

What are the Sensitive MRD Detection Techniques Available?

The three approaches which appear to be suitable for MRD detection in acute leukemia are:
1. Multiparameter flow cytometric (FCM) immunophenotyping.
2. Real-time quantitative polymerase chain reaction (RQ-PCR)-based detection of fusion gene transcripts or breakpoints or aberrant/overexpressed genes, e.g. WT-1.
3. RQ-PCR-based detection of clonal immunoglobulin (Ig) and T-cell receptor (TCR) gene rearrangements.

While flow cytometry relies on protein expression, fusion genes are generally detected at messenger RNA levels, and Ig/TCR junctions are RQ-PCR targets at the DNA level.

Table 21.1 summarizes the applicability and sensitivity of the most widely used assays in childhood leukemia.

Table 21.1: Methods for monitoring MRD in childhood leukemia[4]

Method	ALL		AML	
	% of cases with marker	Sensitivity	% of cases with marker	Sensitivity
Flow cytometric detection of abnormal phenotypes	98%	10^{-4}	93%	10^{-3}-10^{-4}
PCR amplification of genes encoding Ig and TCR proteins	90%	10^{-4}-10^{-5}	< 10%	
RT-PCR amplification fusion transcripts	< 50%	10^{-3}-10^{-5}	< 20%	10^{-3}-10^{-5}

1. Quantification with Multiparameter Flow Cytometric (FCM) Immunophenotyping

One of the distinguishing features of leukemic cells is the expression of immunophenotypic cell markers in abnormal patterns. Multiparametric flow cytometry traces these leukemia-associated aberrant immunophenotype (LAIP) as the result of *cross-lineage* antigen expression, e.g. CD7 in AML, *maturational asynchrony*, i.e. simultaneous presence of early and late antigens, e.g. CD21 on CD19/34 positive precursor B-cells, *under/overexpression* (e.g.underexpression of CD38 in ALL and overexpression of CD11a, CD44 in ALL) or *absence* of antigen, ectopic antigens (TdT positive cells in CSF), *unique* antigens, e.g. NG2 in ALL identified by antibody 7.1 and various combinations of above-mentioned features. These LAIP are absent or present at low frequency in normal bone marrow. The antibody panels which allow for identification of these LAIPs are chosen keeping in mind the differential antigen expression intensity, which has to be known from normal expression, to choose the appropriate fluorochromes and avoid possible steric hindrance and quenching for antigens in close vicinity on the cell membrane. Extensive list of antibody panels proposed to identify these LAIPs has been recently reviewed by Bene et al.[1]

The sensitivity of flow cytometric approach depends on two main factors: The degree of dissimilarity between the immunophenotypes of leukemic cells and those of normal cells, and the number of cells available for study. In nearly all patients with acute lymphoblastic leukemia (ALL), leukemic lymphoblasts express immunophenotypes that are sufficiently distinct to allow the detection of one leukemic cells among 10 000 normal cell (sensitivity 10^{-4}).[7,8]

FCM in T-ALL

The normal equivalents of T lineage ALL cells are immature T cells which are confined to the thymus. Thus, MRD studies in patients with T-ALL is based on searching for immature T cells in the bone marrow or in the peripheral blood as only leukemic T lymphoblasts circulate. The most useful immunophenotypes for this task are coexpression of T cell markers such as CD3 and CD5 with TdT or CD34.[9]

FCM in B-ALL

The normal equivalents of B lineage ALL cells are B cell progenitors which normally reside in the bone marrow, and may also be found in the peripheral blood. Therefore, MRD studies in B-ALL differentiate leukemic cells from their normal counterparts based on the immunophenotypic differences. For example, myeloid associated markers CD13, CD15, CD33 and CD65, and the mature B cell-associated marker CD21 can be expressed by CD19+CD34+ B lineage ALL cells, unlike normal B cell progenitors which do not or very weakly express these markers. Expression of CD19, CD10, TdT and CD34 in B lineage ALL can be significantly different (higher or lower) than that of their normal counterparts and CD38 and CD45 (or CD45RA) are often underexpressed in leukemic cells. In efforts to prevent false-negative MRD findings due to immunophenotypic shifts, extensive antibody panels are advised.[9] The marker combination used in childhood ALL by one of the study groups and its applicability in different cases is shown in Table 21.2. LAIPs can be identified in up to 98% of childhood ALL (Table 21.1).

Coustan-Smith et al[10] (2006) reported a simplified assay based on a three-color combination (CD19/CD10/CD34), which when applied on day 19 of induction was highly significant for predicting relapse in childhood B-lineage ALL. This was based on the observation that normal immature CD19 cells become undetectable after 2 weeks of chemotherapy in B-ALL patients. Thus, any such cells detected in B-ALL on day 19 of induction would likely be residual leukemic cells. The results were comparable with those using more extensive antibody panels and so this assay may be especially valuable in resource limited settings.

Krampera et al[11] studied the utility of flow cytometric detection of MRD in adult ALL patients and found that 61/64 (95.3%) of cases had at least one LAIP and 35/64 (57.3%) had two or more LAIP as compared to

Table 21.2: Marker combinations used to study MRD in childhood ALL[9]

Leukemia cell lineage	Marker combination	Applicability, %[a]
T lineage ALL (n = 39)	TdT/CD5/CD3(CD19/CD33/HLA-Dr)	92
	CD34/CD5/CD3(CD19/CD3/HLA-Dr)	21
B lineage ALL (n = 169)	CD19/CD34/CD10/CD38	52
	CD19/CD34/CD10/CD58	49
	CD19/CD34/CD10/CD45	47
	CD19/CD34/CD10/TdT	43
	CD19/CD34/CD10/CD66c	31
	CD19/CD34/TdT/IgM	17
	CD19/CD34/CD10/CD22	11
	CD19/CD34/CD10/CD13	10
	CD19/CD34/CD10/CD15	10
	CD19/CD34/CD10/CD21	6
	CD19/CD34/CD10/CD33	6
	CD19/CD34/CD10/NG-2	5
	CD19/CD34/CD10/CD65	4

n = Number of cases studied.
[a] Percentage of patients within each type of leukemia in whom MRD could be studied with the listed antibody combination. Percentages were calculated by including only cases in which intensity of antigen expression was sufficiently different from that of normal bone marrow cells (sensitivity of detection 1 in 10^4).

physiologic B-cell precursors in adult bone marrow with a sensitivity of 10^{-4}. They showed that marker combinations for childhood ALL are also applicable to adult cases.

FCM in AML

Detection of MRD in acute myeloid leukemia (AML) requires the identification of leukemia-associated aberrant immunophenotype (LAIP) that can distinguish leukemic myeloblasts from normal myeloid precursors. These include expression of markers normally not expressed on myeloid cells, e.g. CD2, 7, 19, coexpression of markers normally expressed at different stages of maturation, e.g. CD15/33/34 positive cells, as well as overexpression and under expression of myeloid markers, e.g. HLA-DR negativity. These changes are summarized in Table 21.3.

Distinctive markers can be identified in most patients with acute myeloid leukemia (AML) however MRD detection by flow cytometry in AML presents some specific difficulties. Due to their immunophenotypic heterogeneity, AML cells usually spread across many areas of each dot plot instead of forming the tight cluster typical of ALL cells. Therefore, with any given marker combination, only a fraction of cells may appear to be phenotypically abnormal. In addition, AML cells often have light scattering properties similar to that of normal cells with high autofluorescence.[9] Thus, in approximately 40% of patients the routine sensitivity that can be achieved is not higher than one in 1000, owing to a partial overlap between the phenotype of leukemic cells and those of normal hematopoietic cells.[12]

Table 21.3: Leukemia-associated aberrant immunophenotypes (LAIP) in myeloblasts[13]

LAIP class	Examples
Cross-lineage expression of lymphoid antigens	CD33+ CD2+ CD34+; CD34+ CD13+ CD19+
Overexpression	HLA– DR++ CD33++ CD34++; CD64++ CD4++CD45++
Lack of expression of antigen	HLA– DR– CD33+ CD34+
Asynchronous expression of antigens	CD15+ CD33+ CD34+; CD65+ CD33+ CD34+

+ indicates expression; ++ overexpression; – no expression.

Although no real consensus exists, it is commonly accepted that a cluster of between 10 and 100 MRD cells should be identified in a given sample to ensure that MRD cells have been seen. Thus, to achieve a sensitivity of between 1×10^{-4} to 1×10^{-5}, approximately 10^5 to 10^6 leukocytes must be screened, stressing the value of assessing MRD in samples with normalized cell counts.[1]

Advantages of FCM

It is widely applicable to > 95% cases of precursor B-ALL and T-ALL and > 90% AML cases, rapid (turnaround time 1-2 days) and relatively cheap. It is directly quantitative compared to PCR which estimates the leukemic cell number based on the transcripts which may vary from cell to cell. Another important advantage here is the discriminating ability of flow between viable and apoptotic cells. In addition, FCM also analyses the normal hematopoietic component simultaneously.

Limitations of FCM

Sensitivity of FCM is limited (10^{-3}-10^{-4}), however is sufficient for identifying high-risk ALL patients. The latest ≥ 6 color flow cytometers promise better sensitivity and specificity of MRD detection. Modulation of antigen expression occurs during the treatment, may change the leukemia-specific immunophenotype into a normal lymphoid phenotype.[14] Immunophenotype of leukemia cells may also be different at diagnosis and relapse. Therefore, following of at least two leukemia specific immunophenotypes per patient has been recommended to prevent false-negative results.[5]

The major difficulty in detecting MRD for patients with common B-ALL (CD10+) is to differentiate blast cells from hematogones, which can be quite abundant in young children and in regenerating bone marrow after transplantation or cessation of chemotherapy. The combination CD34/CD19/CD10/CD38 is quite pertinent to differentiate these cell types, based on the difference in fluorescence intensity displayed by hematogones and blasts.[1]

There is a growing need for intralaboratory as well as interlaboratory standardization especially with the advent of highly sensitive flow cytometers and increasing technical complexity. Recently, people have reported on the reproducibility of MRD detection in FCM in multi-center studies.[15,16]

In addition to the skills necessary for reliable leukemia immunophenotyping, productive MRD studies by flow cytometry require great care to avoid sample contamination at all stages of processing as well as a detailed knowledge of the immunophenotypic patterns found in normal and regenerating bone marrow cells, particularly of immature myeloid and lymphoid cells.[7] Hence, flow cytometry based MRD monitoring requires expertise beyond that needed for leukemia immunophenotyping. Without such specific expertise, the likelihood of errors in MRD estimates is very high; laboratories that are unprepared to perform the assay correctly should resist the pressure to deliver MRD results until the methodology has been validated.[4]

2. RQ-PCR-based Quantification of Leukemia-associated Fusion Genes or Overexpressed Genes

Another leukemia-associated feature that can be used to distinguish leukemic from normal cells is represented by chromosomal abnormalities. Chromosomal translocations in leukemia result in fusion genes which are very good and stable disease-specific markers as they are directly linked to leukemogenesis. The most frequent fusion transcripts detected by reverse-transcriptase RT-PCR in ALL are: t(1;19)(q23;p13) with the E2A-PBX1 fusion gene, t(4;11)(q21;q23) with the MLL-AF4 fusion gene, the two main types of t(9;22)(q34;q11) with BCR-ABL fusion genes, t(12;21)(p13;q22) with the TEL-AML1 fusion gene, and the intrachromosomal microdeletion on 1p32 with the SIL-TAL1 fusion gene. Similarly, t (8;21)(RUNX1-RUNX1T1), inv 16 (CBFB-MYH11) and t(15;17) (PML-RARA) in AML can be used as target for amplification.

With the addition of targeted imatinib mesylate therapy for BCR-ABL+ ALL, BCR-ABL transcripts have become the first-choice marker for MRD monitoring by RT/RQ-PCR.[17,18] In contrast, advantage of MRD monitoring is not yet clear in ALL cases with TEL-AML1 fusion gene with good prognosis.

Advantages

This approach is relatively easy, rapid (2-3 days), highly sensitive (10^{-4} – 10^{-6}) and leukemia-specific. An advantage of monitoring MRD by targeting fusion transcripts is the strong association between the molecular abnormality and the leukemic clone, irrespective of the presence of intraclonal differentiation and cellular changes caused by therapy.

Limitations

Applicable to only a minority of patients as these leukemia specific markers can only be identified in around 40-45% of B-ALL, 15-35% of T-ALL and around 20% of AML.

Cross contamination of RT-PCR products between patient samples is a major pitfall resulting in up to 20% of false-positive results.[19] This cross-contamination is difficult to recognize, as leukemia-specific fusion gene transcripts are not patient-specific markers. Another disadvantage of targeting fusion transcripts is that the number of transcripts per leukemic cell may vary among patients with the same genetic abnormality and among different cells within the leukemic clone, and might be affected by therapy.[20] Therefore, precise quantitation of MRD with this technique can be difficult.

RQ-PCR-based Quantification of Aberrant/Overexpressed Genes

The new molecular MRD markers in AML include quantification of somatic mutations using mutation specific, e.g. (NPM1)[21] and aberrantly expressed genes, e.g. ecotropic virus integration-1 (EVI1).[22] In the absence of disease-specific molecular markers, the over expression of tumor suppressor gene, e.g. WT-1, have been used. WT-1 is reported to be overexpressed in approximately 70% of AML patients and is therefore considered to be a specific feature of AML.[23] There is evidence that all patients with higher levels of WT-1 in peripheral blood postinduction therapy subsequently relapsed, with a median of 12 months after diagnosis.[24] The presence of FLT3-ITD at diagnosis in AML is reported to be associated with a 8.5-fold higher frequency of MRD cells after the first course of chemotherapy compared to those with wildtype FLT3.[25] Although these mutations are relatively common in normal karyotype AML, their potential as MRD markers is unclear due to the need to design patient specific assays and mutant alleles instability.

3. RQ-PCR-based Quantification of Junctional Regions of Ig and TCR Gene Rearrangements

RQ-PCR-based detection and quantification of junctional regions of clonal Ig and TCR gene rearrangements is the most widely used strategy of MRD monitoring in ALL. The immunoglobulin and T-cell receptor gene rearrangements during normal B and T-lymphocyte development, respectively, generate unique fusions of variable, diversity and joining (VDJ) segments, interspersed by random nucleotide (N) insertion and/or deletion.

These B and T-clonal recombinations generate patient-specific DNA length and sequences which represent ideal molecular markers for detection and quantification of leukemic cells among normal lymphocytes in remission samples.[1] Although this MRD strategy is the most laborious, expensive and time consuming, it has a good reproducibility not only within the same laboratory but also between different laboratories. The junctional regions of clonal Ig and TCR gene rearrangements are fingerprint-like sequences for each lymphoid malignancy and can be identified in the vast majority of ALL patients.[5]

Advantages

This method has a good sensitivity (10^{-4} -10^{-5}), depending on the type of gene rearrangement and the size of junctional region. It is applicable for most ALL patients (90-95%). Applicable for virtually all patients, if IGH, IGK-Kde, TCRG, and TCRD gene rearrangements are used as targets. It is patient specific and rapid during follow-up if junctional region is identified and if RQ-PCR is used. The target identification has been standardized within the European BIOMED-1 and BIOMED-2 networks. RQ-PCR for MRD detection has been standardized by the European Study Group for MRD detection in ALL (ESG-MRD-ALL).[5]

Limitations

It is time consuming at diagnosis because of identification of the junctional regions and sensitivity testing. It is relatively expensive. Another limitation is its limited applicability in AML (< 10%).

The reliability of the method can be affected by the presence of multiple rearrangements in the same leukemic cell population. Thus, a minor clone at diagnosis may become predominant during the course of the disease and remain undetected because only a major clone present at diagnosis is being monitored.[26] Therefore, it is widely accepted that preferably at least two Ig/TCR targets should be followed per patient because of a chance of clonal evolution. Two sensitive targets (10^{-4}) are available in nearly 80% of patients.[5]

Some Ig/TCR gene rearrangement junctions (particularly of TCRG), although unique for a particular patient, are so similar to rearrangements in the normal Ig/TCR repertoire that nonspecific amplification might occur from non-leukemic lymphocytes at low or even moderate levels resulting in false positivity. Therefore, the sensitivity of this MRD approach cannot easily be further improved.

Comparison of MRD Techniques

The three major MRD techniques provide information expressed as seemingly identical MRD levels. The three methodologies differ in their sensitivity and applicability. Therefore, MRD data obtained with different techniques are hardly interchangeable. Small single-center studies have shown that results of MRD detection by flow cytometry and quantitative PCR of Ig/TCR gene rearrangements are largely comparable especially with higher MRD levels of >10^3 where both techniques seem to give comparable results (< 3-fold difference). However, in samples with MRD levels < 10^3, many discrepancies between the two techniques have been found; this hampers the recognition of low-risk patients.[27,28] Consequently, usage of different MRD techniques for different patients within the same treatment protocol should be avoided. Kerst et al[29] studied minimal residual disease (MRD) in 45 childhood acute lymphoblastic leukemia patients by flow cytometry and real-time PCR and showed that both MRD assays yield generally concordant results. The combined use of MRD techniques should enable MRD monitoring in virtually all patients and prevent false-negative results due to clonal evolution or phenotypic shifts.

The Rationale and Prognostic Significance of MRD in ALL

A high cure rate has been achieved in acute lymphoblastic leukemia (ALL) with the advent of modern chemotherapy supplemented with the hematopoietic stem cell transplantation (HSCT) in high-risk patients. Still, a substantial number of ALL patients relapse and the risk of relapse does not always correlate with conventional prognostic factors such as age, blast count at diagnosis, immunophenotype at diagnosis, presence of chromosome aberrations, response to steroid, etc.

Several studies have demonstrated that monitoring of minimal residual disease (MRD) in childhood[8,30] and adult[31] acute lymphoblastic leukemia (ALL) significantly correlates with *clinical outcome*. MRD detection is particularly useful for evaluation of *early treatment response* and consequently for improved front-line *therapy stratification*. Treatment intensification or HSCT may be considered in children with high MRD levels at the end of induction treatment. In comparison treatment de-intensification may be considered in children with undetectable MRD at the end of induction especially ultrafast responders with MRD clearance within first 2 weeks of the induction.

MRD information is also significant for children with high-risk primary ALL and relapsed ALL planned for allogeneic hematopoietic stem cell *transplantation*. Maximal reduction of MRD pre-transplant is desirable for successful allo-HSCT. Patients with high pretransplant MRD levels are at very high-risk for ALL relapse.[32]

Clinically Significant Levels and Timing of MRD

Different MRD study groups have taken different cut off levels for prognostication and also different time points for estimating MRD. Several prospective studies in childhood ALL demonstrated that the most relevant information comes from detection of MRD in bone marrow at the early phases of treatment, particularly at the end of induction treatment.[5]

The 0.01% threshold is commonly used to define MRD positivity, simply because this represents the typical limit of detection for routine flow cytometric and molecular assays. Nevertheless, it is possible to achieve a routine sensitivity of 0.001% by PCR in clinical samples. The current 0.01% threshold has proven to be clinically informative.

Coustan-Smith et al found that patients who had MRD of 0.01% or higher in bone marrow at any time point during treatment had a significantly higher risk of relapse.[8] Investigators of the Children's Oncology Group (COG) monitored MRD in peripheral blood specimens collected on day 8 and in bone marrow specimens collected on day 29 (end of remission induction therapy) in 2143 children with B-lineage

ALL. The presence of MRD (0.01% or higher) at either interval predicted a poorer outcome. The MRD results obtained in the day 29 bone marrow were the strongest prognostic indicator, superior to other commonly used prognostic parameters in childhood ALL.[30]

Cave et al[33] found a cut-off level of 0.1% at the end of remission induction and thereafter to be particularly informative. Investigators of the I-BFM study group reported that patients with 0.1% or higher MRD on days 33 and 78 had a particularly high relapse rate;[34] those of the Austrian BFM group also reported that the cut-off level of 0.1% on day 33 was particularly informative.[35] For the Dana-Farber Cancer Institute ALL Consortium, a MRD threshold of 0.1% best predicted relapse hazard.[36] The I-BFM group uses MRD levels on days 33 and 78 as a guide for treatment intensification,[34] and other groups worldwide are planning to introduce MRD in their risk-assignment schema.

Prognostic Significance of MRD in AML

MRD studies in adult AML patients using either reverse transcription RT-PCR amplification of fusion transcripts[37] or flow cytometry[38] have demonstrated the potential clinical usefulness of monitoring MRD in AML.

Similarly, Children's Oncology Group investigators detected MRD in the bone marrow of 41 of 252 children with AML, all of whom had achieved remission.[39] These patients had a 4.8 times higher relapse hazard in a multivariate model, with MRD being the strongest prognostic factor. MRD study by flow cytometry in 46 children with *de novo* AML enrolled in the St. Jude Children's Research Hospital AML97 study showed that the mean 2-year survival estimates for patients with MRD positivity (0.1% or higher) after induction therapy was 33% as compared to 72% for those with lower levels or no detectable MRD. Among patients tested after the first cycle of remission induction therapy, those in morphological remission but with detectable MRD were 3.8 times more likely to die than those who were MRD negative.[4]

Can MRD be Determined in Peripheral Blood?

In patients with B-lineage ALL, MRD is usually present at 1 log higher levels in bone marrow than in peripheral blood.[40] However, the presence of MRD in peripheral blood in such cases denotes more aggressive leukemia with an extremely high-risk for recurrence. In T-ALL, MRD levels in peripheral blood are similar to those in bone marrow.[41] In these patients, sequential MRD testing can be performed in blood, which will spare patients the discomfort of bone marrow aspirations. In AML also, significant concordance has been shown between peripheral blood and bone marrow MRD levels (coeffient of correlation (r) = 0.86 and 0.82 at end of induction and consolidation respectively) by Maurillo et al.[42]

Interlaboratory Standardization

In an era of multi-center clinical trials and wide accessibility of MRD studies by Q-PCR the need for standardization of MRD studies is essential. However, standardization of RNA based studies has proved to be complex because mRNA is labile and cDNA synthesis adds to the difficulties in establishing interlaboratory quality assurance. Such difficulties are minimal with the highly stable genomic DNA, as the latter can be made available easily and the quantity included in MRD assays can be measured with much greater accuracy than RNA. Hence, considerable progress has been made in standardization of Ig and TCR rearrangement studies. Methods to standardize the lab results to enable interlaboratory comparisons like International Standardised Ratio (ISR) used for calculating the standard BCR-ABL1 ratio may be extended to other MRD assays also in future.[43]

Future of MRD Studies in Acute Leukemia

MRD detection is one of the successful examples where complicated basic research was transferred into high-technology laboratory diagnostics. MRD diagnostics is very likely to be included in all acute leukemia treatment protocols as MRD data provides the most optimal evidence of the *in vivo* response to treatment, thus providing the clinician a better knowledge and control of the clinical course in individual patients. Introduction of newer targeted therapies will create additional applications of MRD monitoring and may result in newer techniques for MRD detection like microarrays and immunobeads. An EQA program is necessary to minimize interlaboratory variations and ensure uniformity of protocols being followed in all diagnostic MRD laboratories.

REFERENCES

1. Bene MC, Kaeda JS. How and why minimal residual disease studies are necessary in leukemia: A review from WP 10 and WP 12 of the European leukemia net. Haematologica 2009;94:1135-50.
2. Bradstock KF, Janossy G, Tidman N, Papageorgiou ES, Prentice HG, Willoughby M. et al. Immunological monitoring of residual disease in treated thymic acute lymphoblastic leukaemia Leuk Res 1981,5:301-9.
3. Campana D. Minimal residual disease in acute lymphoblastic leukemia Semin Hematol 2009;46:100-06.
4. Campana D. Status of minimal residual disease testing in childhood haematological malignancies. Br J Haematol, 2008;143:481-89.
5. Szczepanski T. Why and how to quantify minimal residual disease in acute lymphoblastic leukemia? Leukemia 2007;21:622-26.
6. Szczepanski T, Orfao A, Van der Velden VH, San Miguel JF and Van Dongen, JJ. Minimal residual disease in leukaemia patients. Lancet Oncology 2001;2: 409-17.
7. Campana D, Coustan-Smith E. Detection of minimal residual disease in acute leukemia by flow cytometry. Cytometry, 1999;38;139-52.

8. Coustan-Smith E, Sancho J, Behm FG, Hancock ML, Razzouk BI, Ribeiro RC, et al. Prognostic importance of measuring early clearance of leukemic cells by flow cytometry in childhood acute lymphoblastic leukemia. Blood, 2002;100: 52-58.
9. Campana D, Coustan-Smith E. Minimal Residual Disease Studies by Flow Cytometry in Acute Leukemia. Acta Haematol 2004;112:8-15.
10. Coustan-Smith E, Ribeiro RC, Stow P, Zhou Y, Pui CH, Rivera GK, et al. A simplified flow cytometric assay identifies children with acute lymphoblastic leukaemia who have a superior clinical outcome. Blood 2006; 108:97-102.
11. Krampera M, Perbellini O, Vincenzi C, Zampieri F, Pasini A, Scupoli MT, et al. Methodological approach to minimal residual disease detection by flow cytometry in adult B-lineage acute lymphoblastic leukemia. Haematologica 2006; 91:1109-12.
12. Coustan-Smith E, Ribeiro RC, Rubnitz JE, Razzouk BI, Pui CH, Pounds S, et al. Clinical significance of residual disease during treatment in childhood acute myeloid leukemia. Br J Haematol 2003;123,243-52.
13. Kern W, Haferlach C, Haferlach T, Schnittger S. Monitoring of minimal residual disease in acute myeloid leukemia. Cancer 2008;112:4-16.
14. Gaipa G, Basso G, Maglia O, Leoni V, Faini A, Cazzaniga G, et al. Drug-induced immunophenotypic modulation in childhood ALL: Implications for minimal residual disease detection. Leukemia 2005;19:49-56.
15. Dworzak MN, Gaipa G, Ratei R, Veltroni M, Schumich A, Maglia O, et al. Standardization of flow cytometric minimal residual disease evaluation in acute lymphoblastic leukaemia: Multicentric assessment is feasible. Cytometry B Clin Cytom 2008;74:331-40.
16. Irving J, Jesson J, Virgo P, Case M, Minto L, Eyre L, et al. Establishment and validation of a standard protocol for the detection of minimal residual disease in B lineage childhood acute lymphoblastic leukemia by flow cytometry in a multi-center setting. Haematologica 2009;94:870-74.
17. Scheuring UJ, Pfeifer H, Wassmann B, Bruck P, Gehrke B, Petershofen EK, et al. Serial minimal residual disease (MRD) analysis as a predictor of response duration in Philadelphia positive acute lymphoblastic leukemia (Ph+ALL) during imatinib treatment. Leukemia 2003;17:1700-06.
18. Wassmann B, Pfeifer H, Stadler M, Bomhauser M, Bug G, Scheuring UJ, et al. Early molecular response to post-transplantation imatinib determines outcome in MRD+ Philadelphia-positive acute lymphoblastic leukemia (Ph+ ALL). Blood 2005;106:458-63.
19. Gleissner B, Rieder H, Thiel E, Fonatsch C, Janssen LA, Heinze B, et al. Prospective BCR-ABL analysis by polymerase chain reaction (RT-PCR) in adult acute B-lineage lymphoblastic leukemia: Reliability of RT-nested-PCR and comparison to cytogenetic data. Leukemia 2001;15:1834-40.
20. Gabert J, Beillard E, van der Velden V, Bi W, Grimwade D, Pallisgaard N, et al. Standardization and quality control studies of 'real-time' quantitative reverse transcriptase polymerase chain reaction of fusion gene transcripts for residual disease detection in leukemia—a Europe Against Cancer program. Leukemia 2003; 17:2318-57.
21. Mecucci C, Tschulik C, Martelli MF, et al. Nucleophosmin gene mutations are predictors of favourable prognosis in acute meylogenous leukaemia with normal karyotype. Blood 2005;106:3733-39.
22. Lugthart S, van Drunen E, van Norden Y, van Hoven A, Erpelinck CA, Valk PJ, et al. High EVI-1 levels predict adverse outcome in acute myeloid leukaemia: Prevalence of EVI-1 overexpression and chromosome 3q26 abnormalities underestimated. Blood 2008;111:4329-37.

23. Ostergaard M, Olesen LH, Hasle H, Kjeldsen E, Hokland P. WTI gene expression: An excellent tool for monitoring minimal residual disease in 70% of acute myeloid leukaemia patients—results from a single-centre study. Br J Haematol 2004:125:590-600.
24. Cilloni D, Messa F, Arruga F, Defilippi I, Gottardi E, Fava M, et al. Early prediction of treatment outcome in acute myeloid leukaemia by measurement of WTI transcript levels in peripheral blood samples collected after chemotherapy. Haematologica 2008;93:921-24.
25. Hess CJ, FelierN, Denkers F, Kelder A, Merle PA, Heinrich MC, et al. Correlation of minimal residual disease cell frequency with molecular genotype in patients with acute myeloid leukaemia. Haematologica 2009;94:46-53.
26. Szczepan ski T, Willemse MJ, Brinkhof B, van Wering ER, van der Burg M, van Dongen JJM. Comparative analysis of Ig and TCR gene rearrangements at diagnosis and at relapse of childhood precursor- B-ALL provides improved strategies for selection of stable PCR targets for monitoring of minimal residual disease. Blood 2002; 99:2315-23.
27. Malec M, Bjorklund E, Soderhall S, Mazur J, Sjogren AM, Pisa P, et al. Flow cytometry and allele-specific oligonucleotide PCR are equally effective in detection of minimal residual disease in ALL. Leukemia 2001; 15:716-27.
28. Neale GAM, CoustanSmith E, Pan Q, Chen X, Gruhn B, Stow P, et al. Tandem application of flow cytometry and polymerase chain reaction for comprehensive detection of minimal residual disease in childhood acute lymphoblastic leukemia. Leukemia 1999;13:1221-26.
29. Kerst G, Kreyenberg H, Roth C, Well C, Dietz K, Coustan-Smith E, et al. Concurrent detection of minimal residual disease (MRD) in childhood acute lymphoblastic leukaemia by flow cytometry and real-time PCR. Br J Haematol, 2005;128,774-82.
30. Borowitz MJ, Devidas M, Hunger SP, Bowman WP, Carroll AJ, Carroll WL, et al. Clinical significance of minimal residual disease in childhood acute lymphoblastic leukemia and its relationship to other prognostic factors. A Children's Oncology Group study. Blood 2008;111:5477-85.
31. Bruggemann M, Raff T, Flohr T, Go'kbuget N, Nakao M, Droese J, et al. Clinical significance of minimal residual disease quantification in adult patients with standard-risk acute lymphoblastic leukaemia. Blood 2006; 107:1116-23.
32. Knechtli CJ, Goulden NJ, Hancock JP, Grandage VL, Harris EL, Garland RJ, et al. Minimal residual disease status before allogeneic bone marrow transplantation is an important determinant of successful outcome for children and adolescents with acute lymphoblastic leukaemia. Blood 1998;92:4072-79.
33. Cave H, van der Werff ten Bosch J, Suciu S, Guidal C, Waterkeyn C, Otten J, et al. Clinical significance of minimal residual disease in childhood acute lymphoblastic leukaemia. European Organization for Research and Treatment of Cancer-Childhood Leukemia Cooperative Group. N Engl J Med 1998;339:591-98.
34. Flohr T, Schrauder A, Cazzaniga G, Panzer-Grumayer R, van der Velden V, Fischer S, et al. Minimal residual disease-directed risk stratification using real-time quantitative PCR analysis of immunoglobulin and T-cell receptor gene rearrangements in the international multicenter trial AIEOP-BFM ALL 2000 for childhood acute lymphoblastic leukaemia. Leukemia 2008;22:771-82.
35. Dworzak MN, Froschl G, Printz D, Mann G, Potschger U, Muhlegge N, et al. Prognostic significance and modalities of flow cytometric minimal residual disease detection in childhood acute lymphoblastic leukaemia. Blood 2002;99:1952-58.
36. Zhou J, Goldwasser MA, Li A, Dahlberg SE, Neuberg D, Wang H, et al. Quantitative analysis of minimal residual disease predicts relapse in children with B-lineage acute lymphoblastic leukemia in DFCI ALL Consortium Protocol 95-01. Blood 2007;110:1607-11.

37. LoCoco F, Ammatuna E. Front line clinical trials and minimal residual disease monitoring in acute promyelocytic leukemia. Current Topics in Microbiology and Immunology 2007;313,145-56.
38. Buccisano F, Maurillo L, Ganei V, Del PG, Del Principe MI, Cox MC, et al. The kinetics of reduction of minimal residual disease impacts on duration of response and survival of patients with acute myeloid leukemia. Leukemia 2006;20, 1783-89.
39. Sievers EL, Lange BJ, Alonzo TA, Gerbing RB, Bernstein ID, Smith FO, et al. Immunophenotypic evidence of leukemia after induction therapy predicts relapse: Results from a prospective Children's Cancer Group study of 252 acute myeloid leukemia patients. Blood 2003;101,3398-3406.
40. Coustan-Smith E, Sancho J, Hancock ML, Razzouk BI, Ribeiro RC, Rivera GK, et al. Use of peripheral blood instead of bone marrow to monitor residual disease in children with acute lymphoblastic leukemia. Blood 2002;100:2399-402.
41. van der Velden V, Jacobs DC, Wijkhuijs AI, Comans-Biner WM, Willemse MI, HablenK, et al. Minimal residual disease levels in bone marrow and peripheral blood are comparable in children with T cell acute lymphoblastic leukemia (ALL), but not in precursor-B-ALL. Leukemia 2002;16:1432-36.
42. Maurillo L, Buccisano F, Spagnoli A, Poeta GD, Panetta P, Neri B, et al. Monitoring of minimal residual disease in adult acute myeloid leukemia using peripheral blood as an alternative source to bone marrow. Haematologica 2007;92:605-11.
43. Branford S, Fletcher L, Cross NCP, Muller MC, Hochhaus A, Kim DW, et al. Desirable performance characteristics for BCR-ABL measurement on an international reporting scale to allow consistent interpretation of individual patient response and comparison of response rates between clinical trials. Blood 2008;112:3330-38.

Index

A

Abdominal
    ultrasound 190
    apoptosis in bone marrow 67
    cytogenetics 228
    localization of immature precursor 70
    platelet aggregation 228
Absolute neutrophil count 50
Acquired erythrocytosis 192
Activation of endothelial cells 79, 181
Acute
    bleeding 12
        episodes 11, 15
    episode of thrombosis 87
    ITP 240
    lymphoblastic leukemia 37, 142, 149, 159, 211
    myeloblastic leukemia 34
    myeloid leukemia 49, 95, 142, 149, 211, 212
    promyelocytic leukemia 35
    respiratory distress syndrome 82
Afibrinogenemia 3, 4, 5
Alemtuzumab 163
Alkylating agents 213
Allogeneic
    BMT 43
    hematopoietic stem cell
        transplantation in hematologic disorders 141
    SCT 142
    transplantation in
        ALL 150
        chronic lymphocytic leukemia 152
        chronic myeloid leukemia 152
        myelodysplastic syndrome 153
        NHL 154
    stem cell transplantation 74
Amaurosis fugax 82
Aminoglycosides 53
Amsacrine 213
Anagrelide 232
Androgens 200
Anemia 67, 228
Antenatal screening 175
Antiangiogenesis 161
Anticardiolipin test 85
Antimetabolites 213
Antimicrotubule agents 213
Antiphospholipid syndrome 77, 90
Anti-thymocyte globulin 70, 197
Aplastic anemia 50, 153, 194
Apoptosis inducers 161, 162
Approach to polycythemia 187
Arachidonic acid 111
Arterial
    oxygen saturation 190
    thrombosis 81
Artery thombosis 82
Ascites 82
Aspergillus 32
Aspirin resistance 110, 116
Autoimmune disease 50
Autologous stem cell transplantation 19, 29
Avastin 162
Azacitidine 70
Azathioprine 213, 243

B

Bacterial contamination 136
Bevacizumab 162
Bimolane 213
Bleeding
    episodes 9
    in dengue fever 179
Blood and
    bone marrow features 100
    marrow transplantation 50
Blood
    component support 145
    smear 100
Bone marrow 100
    blasts 69
    evaluation 95
    failure 95
    studies 190
    transplantation 141, 201
Borrelia 79
Breast cancer therapy 216
Budd-Chiari syndrome 82
Busulfan 213

C

C. albicans 32
C. tropicalis 32

Carboplatin 213
Carcinomas of breast 211
Cardiac valves 82
Carmustine 213
Catastrophic antiphospholipid syndrome 83
Causes of thrombocythemia 229
Center for International Blood and Marrow
    Transplant Research 40, 148
Central
    and State Screening Program 172
    Government Program 171, 172
    nervous system 2
    venous access devices 50
Cerebrovascular disease 115
Cervix 211
Cesarean section 2
Cetuximab 162
Chest X-ray 190
Chlorambucil 107, 213
Chlorpromazine 79
Chorionic villous sampling 175
Chronic
    ITP 242
    lymphocytic leukemia 38, 100, 142, 152
    lymphoproliferative disorders 99
    myeloid leukemia 38, 142, 150, 160, 226
    myeloproliferative neoplasms 211
Ciclosporin 197, 198
Ciprofloxacin 31
Cisplatin 213
Classification of
    antiphospholipid syndrome 86
    catastrophic antiphospholipid
        syndrome 83
    chronic lymphoproliferative
        disorders 99
Clauss method 3
Clinical
    features of APS 80
    use of aspirin 112
Clonal hematopoiesis 228
Colony stimulating factors 56, 146
Column agglutination technology 137
Complete blood count 100, 190
Complications of autologous stem cell
    transplantation 32
Congenital
    afibrinogenemia 3
    erythrocytosis 188
    neutropenia 50
Conventional care regimens 74
Cord blood 148
    stem cell transplantation 148
    transplants 148
Coronary
    artery diseases 61
    heart disease 115
Corticosteroids 200

Creutzfeld Jakob disease 137
Current
    management of idiopathic
        thrombocytopenic purpura 238
    pathogenesis and therapy in essential
        thrombocythemia 226
Cutaneous necrosis 82
Cyclophosphamide 213
Cytogenetic molecular risk in acute myeloid
    leukemia 35
Cytogenetics 191
Cytokine storm in dengue fever 182
Cytopenia 67

D

Dacarbazine 213
Dactinomycin 213
Danazol 244
Dapsone 244
Daunorubicin 213
Decitabine 70, 73
Deep
    vein thrombosis 61
    venous thrombosis 81
Deferoxamine 70
Dengue hemorrhagic fever 179
Dexamethasone 20
Diagnosis of APS 85
Diarrhea 32
Digital gangrene 83
Dihydroxybusulfan 213
Discriminant factors 174
Docetaxel 213
Donor
    hemovigilance 137
    lymphocyte infusions 43
    requirement 143
Doxorubicin 213
Dysfibrinogenemia 3, 4, 5

E

Emergency treatment 240
Empirical use of glycopeptides 54
Endocrine glands 83
Endothelial cell activation in dengue virus
    infection 182
Engraftment syndrome 33
Enzyme-linked immunosorbent assay 11
Epidemiological studies and TAFI 61
Epigenetic alterations 67
Epratuzumab 163
Erlotinib 162
Erythropoietin 70
Esophageal perforation 82
Essential thrombocythemia 226
Etoposide 213

European
　bone marrow transplant registry 43
　group for blood and marrow
　　transplantation 40
Evaluation of erythrocytosis 187
Evidence-based management of fever in
　neutropenic patient 49
Evolution of hemovigilance 130
Ewing sarcoma 211

F

Factor
　V deficiency 7
　VII deficiency 10
　X deficiency 12
　XI deficiency 13
　XIII deficiency 14
Factors related to pregnancy loss 79
Failure of engraftment 146
Fanconi anemia 94
Fludarabine 213
Follicular lymphoma 99
Food and drug administration 74
Free health insurance 169
French hemovigilance system 132
Future therapies 234

G

Galiximab 163
Gangrene of digits 82
Gastrointestinal stromal tumor 161
GB syndrome 81
Gefitinib 161
General population screening strategies 170
Genetic alterations 68
Graft
　rejection 146
　versus host disease 146
Granulocyte colony stimulating factor 30, 49

H

Hairy cell leukemia 99, 106, 108
Headache 89
Health care related vigilance systems 131
Helicobacter pylori 239
HELLP syndrome 84
Hematologic neoplasms 211
Hematopoietic
　growth factors 70, 72, 146
　stem cell transplantation 215
Hematuria 82
Hemoglobinopathy screening tests 173
Hemopoietic growth factors 196
Hemorrhagic cystitis 33
　disease 32
Hemovigilance 129
　systems 131

High dose
　chemotherapy 30, 31
　cyclophosphamide 200
　steroids 243
High oxygen affinity hemoglobin 189
HLA-identical sibling donor transplantation
　201
Hodgkin's
　disease 142
　lymphoma 39,
Home message 16, 25, 90, 139
Hospital transfusion committees 139
Hydroxyurea 232
Hypofibrinogenemia 3
Hypomethylating agent 70, 73

I

Idiopathic thrombocytopenic purpura 238
Imatinib mesylate 161
Immune
　complications 137
　destruction of platelets 181
　mediated 68
Immunomodulatory drugs 70, 73
Immunophenotype 102
Immunoradiometric assay 11
Immunosuppressive
　agents 201
　drugs 70, 200
　therapy 72, 197
Immunotherapy 161
Increased acute phase reactants 228
Indications for allogeneic
　stem cell transplantation 142
　transplants 148
Induction and stem cell mobilization 20
Inherited abnormalities of fibrinogen 2
Inhibition of protein C activation system 79
Inhibitors of TAFI 63
Initial antibacterial therapy 51
Intergroup francais DU myelome 19
International
　Prognostic Scoring System 38, 68
　Workshop on Chronic Lymphocytic
　　Leukemia 100
Intravenous gammaglobulin 243
IPSS scoring 69
Iron
　chelation 70
　deficiency 228
Ischemic colitis 82
Itraconazole 31

K

Klebsiella pneumoniae 135

L

Leg ulcers 82
Lenalidomide 70
Leptospira 79
Leukodepletion of cellular blood
    components 137
Limitations of IPSS 68
Livedo reticularis 83
Lomustine 213
Low-molecular weight heparin 5
Lumiliximab 163
Lung 211
Lupus anticoagulant
    hypothrombinemia syndrome 82
    test 84
Lymphocyte doubling time 104
Lymphomas 153
Lymphoplasmacytic lymphoma 99

M

Maintenance therapy 44
Malignant disorders 142
Management of
    aplastic anemia in
        older patients 207
    pregnancy 205
    catastrophic APS 88
    pregnancy morbidity 88
    thrombosis 87
Mandatory antenatal screening 169
Mantle cell lymphoma 99, 100
Marginal zone lymphoma 100
Marrow examination 105
Matched unrelated donor bone marrow
    transplantation 203
Mechlorethamine 213
Melphalan 30, 213
Menorrhagia 4
Methotrexate 213
Micrornas expression 104
Migraine 81
Minimal residual disease 165, 246
Mismatched donor transplantation 204
Mitomycin C 213
Mitoxantrone 213
Molecular
    basis for inherited abnormality of
        fibrinogen 3
    biology 5, 7, 8, 13
    defects 6
    genetics 103
    studies 230
Morphology of therapy related myeloid
    neoplasms 218
Mucositis 32
Multicentric studies 168
Multidisciplinary approach 133
Multinational association for supportive
    care in cancer 51
Multiple
    myeloma 42, 142, 211
    sclerosis 211
Mycobacterium tuberculosis 32
Myeloablative conditioning 43, 143
Myelodysplastic syndrome 38, 67, 142, 152,
    212, 231
Myeloproferative disorders 226
Myocardial infarction 82, 115
Myocarditis 82

N

National
    Cancer Institute-Sponsored Working
        Group 100
    Comprehensive Cancer Network 70
    Institute of
        Health 133
        Health Study 72
        Immunohematology 179
    Screening Program 169
Natural history of aplastic anemia 195
Nausea 32
Nephritic syndrome 82
Nervous system 81
Neuroblastoma 211
Neutropenia 67
Neutropenic episode 49
Newborn screening program 169
Nitrogen mustard 213
Nonemergent treatment 241
Non-Hodgkin lymphoma 39, 142, 211
Nonmalignant
    diseases 142
    disorders 211
Nonmyeloablative conditioning 144
Nucleotide excision repair 218

O

Options for chronic ITP 242
Oral
    acyclovir 31
    fluconazole 31
Osteosarcoma 211
Outcome of hemovigilance 135
Ovary 211

P

Paclitaxel 213
Pancreatitis 82
Pathobiology of myelodysplastic syndrome 67
Peripheral
    activation of platelets 180

artery disease 115
blood stem cell transplantation 147
Phenytoin 79
Phytohemagglutinin 95
Platelet
    activation 79
    dysfunction 179
    physiology 111
    transfusion 70
Pneumocystis carinii 32
Polycythemia vera 187, 189
Population screening 170
Post-transfusion purpura 134
Prednisone 20
Pregnancy 5, 7, 8, 9, 13, 14, 16
    morbidity 84, 86
Premarital
    test 169
    thalassemia screening 169
Preparatory regimen 31
Prevalence of aspirin resistance 118
Prevention of infection 196
Primary
    myelofibrosis 226
    thromboprophylaxis 87
Primitive neuroectodermal tumor 211
Procainamide 79
Procarbazine 213
Production of proinflammatory and procoagulant state 79
Prognosis assessments in MDS 68
Progression-free survival 41
Prolymphocytic leukemia 99, 106
Properties of TAFI 60
Prostate 211
Proteinuria 82
Prothrombin
    complex concentrates 12
    deficiency 5
Psoriasis 211
Psychosis 81
Pulmonary
    and cardiac disease 32
    arterial thrombosis 82
    complications 32
    embolism 81
    hemorrhage 82
    hypertension 82
Purine analogues 108

Q

Quinidine 79
Quinolones 31

R

Rapid alert system 135
Rare coagulation disorders 1

Rational for erythropoietin 72
Razoxane 213
Red cell transfusion 70
Reduced-intensity conditioning 144
Regional analgesia 2
Relevance of secondary leukemia 212
Renal
    and liver function tests 190
    artery 82
    artery thrombosis 82
    vein 82
Retinal vein 82
Retinitis 82
Rhabdomyosarcoma 211
Rheumatoid arthritis 211
Rituxan 163
Rituximab 162, 163, 243
Role of
    autologous stem cell transplantation in hematological malignancies 29
    International Society of Blood Transfusion in hemovigilance 138
    prophylactic antibacterial agents 54

S

Screening test 95, 173
Second transplants 23
Secondary
    leukemia 211
    thromboprophylaxis 87
Seizure disorders 211
Semustine 213
Serum
    ferritin 190
    markers 104
Severe
    aplastic anemia 153
    congenital neutropenia 211
Skin 82
Small
    lymphocytic lymphoma 100
    molecules 161
Solid
    phase red cell adherence 137
    tumors 211
Source and dose of stem cells 202
Splenectomy sparing options for chronic ITP 242
Splenic
    lymphoma with villous lymphocytes 99
    marginal zone lymphoma 100
Spontaneous bleeding 4, 14
    episodes 8
Standardized mortality ratio 207
Staphylococcus aureus 52
State Blood Transfusion Councils 139

Stem cell
    infusion 31
    mobilization 30
    source 142
    transplantation 141
Stroke 61
Sulphamethoxazole 55
Surgery 4, 8

T

Target population 168
Technical aspects of allogeneic
    transplantation 144
Teniposide 213
Testicular 83
    tumors 211
Thalassemia
    control 168
    screening and control program 167
Thalidomide 70
Therapy-related
    leukemia 216
    myeloid neoplasms 212
Thiotepa 213
Thrombin time 3
Thrombin-activable fibrinolysis inhibitor 60
Thrombocytopenia 67, 89
Thrombopoietic growth factors 244
Thromboprophylaxis in patients with
    recurrent thrombosis 88
Topoisomerase II inhibitors 213
Total
    body irradiation 31
    nucleated cells 144
Toxicity related to conditioning 146
Transfusion
    associated circulatory overload 134
    errors 136
    related acute lung injury 134
    transmitted infections 134
Transfusional support 195
Transplant related mortality 40

Transplantation for follicular lymphoma 41
Trastuzumab 162
Treatment
    modality in MDS 70
    of infection 196
    response score 72
Treponema 79
Trimethoprim 55
Tumor relapse 147

U

Umbilical cord blood transplantation 204
Unrelated donor umbilical cord blood
    transplantation 205
Use in clinical practice 106

V

Vaginal delivery 2
Valvulopathy 89
Vancomycin resistant enterococci 54
Varicella zoster 32
Vascular thrombosis 80, 86
Veno-occlusive disease 32, 33, 146
Venous
    access 145
    thrombosis 81
Vinblastine 213
Vincristine 20, 213, 243
Vindesine 213
Viral disease transmission 137
Viridians streptococci 53
Vomiting 32
von Willebrand factor 181, 229

W

Wegener granulomatosis 211
Wilm's tumor 69, 211
World Health Organization 68
    Classification of Hematopoietic
        Neoplasias 100
    Prognostic Scoring System 68